VITAMINS: NUTRIENTS AND THERAPEUTIC AGENTS

Edited by A. HANCK and D. HORNIG

W0228396

International Journal for Vitamin and Nutrition Research
Internationale Zeitschrift für Vitamin- und Ernährungsforschung
Journal international de Vitaminologie et de Nutrition

Supplement No. 27

VITAMINS

NUTRIENTS AND THERAPEUTIC AGENTS

Edited by A. Hanck and D. Hornig
Basle, Switzerland

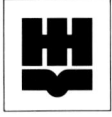

Hans Huber Publishers Bern Stuttgart Toronto

CIP-Kurztitelaufnahme der Deutschen Bibliothek

Hanck, A. and Hornig, D.
VITAMINS: NUTRIENTS AND
THERAPEUTIC AGENTS
A. Hanck and D. Hornig
Bern, Stuttgart, Toronto: Huber, 1985

ISBN 3-456-81419-4

©1985 Hans Huber Publishers, Bern
Printed in Switzerland
by Druckerei Heinz Arm, Bern

Contents

DAZA, C.H.: Vitamin Deficiencies in Latin America and the Carribbean   9

MORA, J.O.: Nutritional Status of the Colombian Population   19

SCHAEFER, A.E.: Principles and Applications of Nutrition Survey Findings   33

BAKER, H. and FRANK, O.: Sub-Clinical Vitamin Deficits in Various Age Groups.   47

PIETRZIK, K.: Concept of Borderline Vitamin Deficiencies   61

MEJÍA, L.A.: Vitamin A Deficiency as a Factor in Nutritional Anemia .   75

CHAVEZ, A., MATA, A. and SANDOVAL, J.: Possibilities of Enriching Sugar with Micronutrients in Mexico.   85

LAYRISSE, M.: Iron Deficiency in Latin America, Causes and Prevention   105

WILSON, D., NETTO, O.B., SIMAO DA COSTA, A., STEINER, A., DE FATIMA NUNES MARUCCI, M. and BARBOSA, M.C.: Effect of Vitamin A on Visual Accuracy   117

TOLBERT, B.M.: Metabolism and Function of Ascorbic Acid and its Metabolites.   121

HORNIG, D.H. and GLATTHAAR, B.E.: Vitamin C and Smoking: Increased Requirement of Smokers   139

BUZINA, R. and SUBOTIČANEC, K.: Vitamin C and Physical Working Capacity   157

STEKEL, A., OLIVARES, M., PIZARRO, F., AMAR, M., CHADUD, P., CAYAZZO, M., LLAGUNO, S., VEGA, V. and HERTRAMPF, E.: The Role of Ascorbic Acid in the Bioavailability of Iron from Infant Foods . . .   167

HALLBERG, L.: The Role of Vitamin C in Improving the Critical Iron Balance Situation in Women.   177

HANCK, A. and WEISER, H.: Analgesic and Anti-Inflammatory Properties of Vitamins.   189

HAUSER, G.A.: Vitamin Requirements in Human Pregnancy   207

GUNN, A.D.G.: Vitamin B_6 and the Premenstrual Syndrome (PMS) . . .   213

BIESALSKI, K.: Aspects of Vitamin A Metabolism in Sensory Epithelia (Inner Ear, Olfactory Bulbus, Pineal Gland) 225

BASU, T.K.: Drug-Vitamin Interaction........................... 247

SEIB, P.A.: Oxidation, Monosubstitution and Industrial Synthesis of Ascorbic Acid – A Review................................... 259

BAUERNFEIND, J.C.: Antioxidant Function of L-Ascorbic Acid in Food Technology... 307

KLAEUI, H.: Ascorbic Acid as a Flour and Bread Improver 335

MILATOVIČ, L.: The Use of L-Ascorbic Acid in Improving the Quality of Pasta... 345

SCHMIDT, K. and MOSER, U.: Vitamin C – A Modulator of Host Defense Mechanism... 363

WEISBURGER, J.H.: Causes of Gastric and Esophageal Cancer. Possible Approach to Prevention by Vitamin C 381

WILSON, D.: Vitamin C Deficiency in São Paulo State, Brazil......... 403

Author Index... 411

Key Word Index 413

Foreword

In the past decade leading experts on vitamins have met repeatedly in order to exchange new ideas concerning the action of vitamins under physiological conditions as well as in the prevention and therapy of diseases. As a consequence, new research projects were started all over the world to obtain a better understanding of these ideas. It was felt that the new findings from this research should be presented continuously, and that other vitamins should also be included in this evaluation.

From November 24 to 26, 1983, prominent researchers met again at Cartagena, Colombia. The topics treated at the Cartagena meeting have had a conspicuous impact on our knowledge of borderline vitamin deficiency, of vitamin requirements in man, of the role of vitamins in prevention of cardiovascular diseases and cancer and of the possible use of vitamins as therapeutic agents in various diseases. Health authorities must be made aware that borderline vitamin deficiency should not be neglected, since it may impair functions as diverse as, for example, a person's work capacity or his immune system.

New ways of formulating recommended dietary allowances should be found, because modern life has created new conditions. We have to take into account life-style factors such as smoking or drinking habits, or the medication of chronic diseases, since these may enhance the vitamin requirements. In comparison with non-smokers for example, smokers need about 40% more vitamin C to maintain their body stores.

The present volume contains 26 contributions, each of them dealing with a special topic whose interest is nonetheless general. In making the reported findings available to a broader public, the editors hope that this volume will help to improve public health and to extend the therapeutic arsenal through the addition of safe and effective treatments.

GEORG BRUBACHER

Vitamin Deficiencies in Latin America and the Carribean

C.H. Daza

Pan American Health Organization, Washington, DC, USA

Key Words: Vitamin deficiencies · Assessment of nutritional status of population groups · Public health significance of vitamin deficiencies · Prevention and control · Food fortification · Nutrition education

Abstract: Hunger, undernutrition and some specific nutritional deficiencies affect particularly the poor people of Latin America and the Caribbean. Malnutrition as a result of faulty diets and excess food intake is also of increasing concern among affluent groups for its close association with hypertensive cardiovascular diseases, diabetes and some degenerative processes. Protein-energy malnutrition interacts with diarrheal and acute respiratory infections, determining high morbidity and mortality rates in children under five years of age. Survivors of this vicious circle of malnutrition-infection-malnutrition cannot fully develop their genetic potential and usually become stunted due to impaired physical growth or they may be intellectually handicapped due to lack of adequate psychomotor development during the early stages of life. Vitamin deficiencies, particularly of vitamin A, riboflavin and folate, affect the most vulnerable population and are intimately associated with the broader and more serious problem of protein-energy malnutrition. Iron and iodine deficiencies are also prevalent in some groups and areas of the region. Several countries have put into action preventive and control measures by means of food fortification and vitamin supplementation. Food and nutrition education activities in the community are an integral part of the primary health care strategy. The Pan American Health Organization and its two specialized nutrition centers – INCAP in Guatemala and CFNI in Jamaica – along with other international and bilateral agencies support national governments in developing strategies for the control of malnutrition and the achievement of "Health for All by the Year 2000".

Introduction

Hunger, undernutrition and some specific nutritional deficiencies are of great social and economic significance in Latin America and the Caribbean, seriously affecting the health and well-being of the population, particularly of those in the low-income groups. On the other hand, malnutrition as a result of faulty diets and excess food intake is an emerging problem closely related to overweight and its association with hypertensive cardiovascular pathology, late-onset diabetes and some degenerative diseases.

The prevalence of protein-energy malnutrition (PEM) is accompanied by high morbidity and mortality rates in children as a result of its interaction with diarrheal and acute respiratory diseases which is a common epidemiological trait in developing countries.

The persistence of the vicious circle of malnutrition-infection-malnutrition also determines retardation of a child's physical growth which is often accompanied by substandard mental development and low psychosocial performance.

Moreover, the nutritional status has a definite effect on an individual's capacity to do physical work in terms of both the duration and productivity of this work. And in Latin America and the Caribbean, where mechanization is still limited, the achievement of maximum individual output is of obvious economic consequences. Needless to say, the fulfilment of optimal development of each individual's genetic potential is mandatory to effectively contribute to his own well-being and to that of the society to which he belongs [1].

In this context, vitamin deficiencies should be seen as an important although not isolated part of the broader and more serious problem of hunger and protein-energy malnutrition affecting a substantial number of mothers and children in rural areas and deprived communities of fast-growing metropoles.

From the public health point of view, vitamin deficiencies in Latin America and the Caribbean do not appear to be a problem of great magnitude and, whenever present, they can be related to inadequate intake, recurring infections and/or malabsorption diseases. However, since vitamin A, riboflavin and folate deficiencies have been consistently reported in various national studies, it seems appropriate to reassess the current situation in order to establish a clearer and more reliable picture of vitamin deficiencies in the Americas.

Nutritional Problems

During the last twenty years several food and nutrition surveys have been carried out by the countries of the Americas with the support of the Pan American Health Organization (PAHO), the Institute of Nutrition of Central America and Panama (INCAP), the Caribbean Food and Nutrition Institute (CFNI), the United States National Institutes of Health and the Center for Disease Control (US/NIH/CDC), the Food and Agriculture Organization (FAO), and various national groups of nutrition specialists [2–16].

Based on the above studies and other available information, a review of the most prevalent nutritional problems in this region was made a few years ago, concluding that although the countries of Latin America and the Caribbean differ markedly in many respects – ecology, cultural background, social and economic status, and political systems – on the whole their people have a diet notably deficient in energy, protein, vitamin A, riboflavin, iron, folates, and iodine [17].

It is pertinent to say that the majority of surveys were carried out in the 1960s with the support of the Interdepartmental Committee on Nutrition for National Defense (ICNND), later named Office for International Research (OIR), which developed a well standardized methodology for the collection and analysis of data regarding food intake, anthropometry, clinical examination and biochemical determinations [18]. The subjects under study were usually military conscriptees and a limited number of civilians including mothers and children.

It is evident from the results of nutrition surveys carried out in Latin America and the Caribbean that vitamin A deficiency is a severe and widespread problem as determined by food intake and retinol serum levels. In other studies xerophthalmia was detected in 9.7 % of preschool children suffering from protein-energy malnutrition [19].

More specifically, over 67 % of the families surveyed in Central America and Panama [3] were shown to have a vitamin A intake of less than one half of the daily recommended allowance [20]; in El Salvador, the deficit reached 88 percent of the families (Table I).

Tab. I: Distribution of families by adequacy of vitamin A intake [3]

Country	Number of families surveyed	Level of adequacy of vitamin A in diet		
		less than 50 %	50–99 %	100 % or more
Costa Rica	414	70	18	12
El Salvador	278	88	10	2
Guatemala	200	67	16	17
Honduras	323	83	11	6
Nicaragua	331	68	21	11
Panama	352	74	18	8

Regarding serum levels of retinol, Table II shows that the prevalence of vitamin A deficiency in children under 15 years of age ranged from 14.9 % in Nicaragua to 36.5 % in El Salvador. Children up to 4 years of age were the most frequently affected group in all countries.

Tab. II: Prevalence of vitamin A deficiency in children under 15 years [3]

Country	Prevalence by age group, %			
	0–4 years	5–9 years	10–14 years	0–14 years
Costa Rica	32.5	25.6	11.7	23.3
El Salvador	43.5	43.5	22.4	36.5
Guatemala	26.2	16.2	11.1	17.8
Honduras	39.5	29.5	21.9	30.3
Nicaragua	19.8	18.5	6.4	14.9
Panama	18.4	12.1	9.7	13.4

Iron deficiency anemia is also highly prevalent in mothers and children. In some countries folate deficiency was found to be associated with anemia ranging in the general population from 13.0% in Honduras to 36.0% in Nicaragua; in pregnant women from 4.3% in Brazil to 39.0% in Argentina; and in children from 13% in Grenada to 34.0% in Barbados [4, 5, 11, 21].

In general, the nutrition surveys have not detected clinical signs of overt ascorbic acid, riboflavin, thiamine, or niacin deficiencies, probably due to the fact that the intake of these nutrients was only marginally below the recommended allowances. In Guyana for instance, less than 80% of the recommended intake for these nutrients was found in about 25, 65, 15 and 43% of both rural and urban populations, respectively [2].

The ICNND surveys included biochemical determinations of serum vitamin C, red cell riboflavin and urinary excretion of thiamine, riboflavin and N-methylnicotinamide. In general, the findings were within "acceptable" values with few individuals in the "low" and "deficient" range, correlating rather closely with the results of the food intake assessment and the clinical examination regarding these nutrients.

The fact is that protein-energy malnutrition in children under five years of age is the most serious nutritional problem in this region, with a prevalence of approximately 20% according to weight for age deficit (grades II and III of the Gomez classification). On the other hand, maternal malnutrition during pregnancy and lactation creates enough of a social and economic burden to make it a leading public health problem too and a serious obstacle to national development in many countries, because it affects not only the mother but also the fetus and the newborn, determining great prevalence of low-birth weight which is frequently accompanied by high morbidity and mortality rates [22].

In summing up the situation, it is evident that although single vitamin deficiencies in general do not appear to represent a serious public health problem in Latin America and the Caribbean both in terms of significance and magnitude, the effects of the association of vitamin A, riboflavin and folate deficiencies with malnutrition, particularly protein-energy malnutrition, is a matter that merits future research.

It is indeed necessary to update the information on the vitamin status in the countries of this region through well-designed epidemiological surveys giving emphasis to the study of high risk groups of the population, i.e., mothers and children of low-income groups.

Priority Programs

In planning action programs one of the constraints in analysing current nutritional situations is, as previously discussed, that the past nutrition surveys fail to provide reliable data to establish the actual magnitude of the problem and a clear understanding of its functional significance in terms of individual performance, levels of health and the most important conditioning factors. Since nutrition surveys usually present their data as a national average, this can lead to a serious error of interpretation, especially regarding the food intake of the more needy segments of the population which differs greatly from national figures.

For planning and action purposes it is essential to determine what is happening in the various situations and socioeconomic settings within each country. This information should be readily available to the policy and decision makers to understand the nature, magnitude and significance of the nutrition problems allowing them to identify the large disparities that exist between population groups in different geo-economic contexts, to establish the importance of certain basic foods in satisfying the nutritional requirements, and to make the most appropriate decisions in each circumstance.

In addition, it is essential to develop simple and reliable indicators for the continuous surveillance of the nutrition and health status of the population, the monitoring of ongoing programs and the evaluation of specific interventions [22].

It is recognized that the factors determining the availability, consumption and biological utilization of food, and therefore the nutritional status of the people, are to be found in different development sectors. The adequacy of food availability and its consumption is directly influenced by factors such as national food production and distribution, the level and trend of wages for low income groups, the rate of unemployment and underemployment, and the cost of a minimum but adequate diet.

The habits, traditions and beliefs which help to shape the actual consumption of an adequate diet are also important determinants in assessing the feasibility of any food and nutrition program. Regarding the absorption and utilization of nutrients at the cellular level, the following factors are of particular importance: environmental sanitation, including the availability of drinking water and the disposal of excreta and solid wastes, morbidity from infectious and parasitic diseases, immune status of the population, and other determinants of the quality of life such as education and housing.

Since food and nutrition are key components of the well-being profile that each Government in the Americas has decided to set as a goal for its people, high priority has been assigned to the prevention and control of malnutrition. "Health for All by the Year 2000" must be achieved through strategies based on coordinated health care and extended services by means of primary health care and effective community participation [23].

The regional strategies adopted by the Governments of the Americas call for actions aimed at increasing the availability and improving the consumption of basic foods combined with specific activities for preventing and correcting malnutrition with special emphasis on the most vulnerable population groups. Moreover, the plan of action which is being implemented by the Pan American Health Organization and its member countries [24] includes as an important objective the reduction of malnutrition and the promotion of optimum nutritional status in the population by means of intersectoral integrated approaches.

Specific emphasis is given to improving the surveillance and monitoring of the nutritional status of vulnerable population groups as an integral activity of primary health care, the institution of early preventive and control measures for those at high risk, the prevention and control of specific nutritional deficiencies, the development of intersectoral policies and approaches for the improvement of overall food and nutrition status, through food production, availability, distribution and safety. It also includes the development of operational research, appropriate technologies for the monitoring of food and nutrition trends, education for nutrition improvement; the establishment of effective information exchange mechanisms, and the training in nutrition of health and allied personnel at all levels.

Coordination with other sectors, specially agriculture, education, food industry and national development planning units is essential for the implementation of this plan, as is the active involvement of individuals, families and communities. Therefore, effective intersectoral programs with community participation should be developed to achieve the maximum impact of these activities.

Regarding the prevention and control of specific nutritional deficiencies the Pan American Health Organization has collaborated in developing national programs including a technical group meeting which was convened in Washington, DC to develop guidelines for food fortification in Latin America and the Caribbean [25]. However, the implementation of this feasible measure has been handicapped in some countries by the lack of enforcement of appropriate legislation, e. g. in the case of salt iodination for endemic goiter control and sugar fortification with retinol palmitate for the prevention of vitamin A deficiency.

Regarding the latter intervention the Institute of Nutrition of Central America and Panama carried out a thorough evaluation in Guatemala in 1975–1977, and it is clear that the program contributed to fulfil the population requirements for this essential nutrient [26].

Conclusions

According to the available information, vitamin deficiencies in general do not appear to represent a serious health problem in Latin America and the Caribbean. Nevertheless it is not a problem to be neglected. Vitamin A has been identified as one of the most frequent deficiencies from the dietetic and biochemical point of view. Clinical manifestations of hypovitaminosis A – various grades of xerophthalmia – have been reported in a few countries. Riboflavin and folate deficiencies particularly affect mothers during pregnancy and lactation, placing a potential health risk to the newborn and the growing child.

Since the information on vitamin deficiencies in this region is the result of national surveys carried out about 15 years ago, it seems appropriate to update the information through well-designed epidemiological studies focusing on the high-risk groups of the population. Nutritional surveillance systems should include, when feasible, selected biochemical determinations of those vitamins which seem to be deficient in selected countries.

In the meantime, some interventions such as the fortification of sugar with vitamin A should be promoted in the Central American countries with an ongoing assessment of the situation. Other programs such as the fortification of wheat flour with thiamine, riboflavin, niacin, iron and calcium should be reviewed in the light of the actual deficiencies and the feasibility of this intervention.

Supplementation of vitamins and other nutrients for mothers and children attending local health services should be implemented whenever deficiencies are identified.

Nutrition education should be an integral component of primary health care aiming at supporting healthy diets and the consumption of nutritious and locally produced foods. Academic training in nutrition and health sciences should address the problem of vitamin deficiencies as part of the overall problem of hunger and malnutrition in the countries of Latin America and the Caribbean.

References

1   Pan American Health Organization. Technical discussions on national food and nutrition policies: final report and condensed background working document. Bull PAHO *10,* 347–362, 1976.
2   Government of Guyana/PAHO/CFNI/FAO. The National Food and Nutrition Survey of Guyana. PAHO Sci No 323. PAHO, Washington, DC, 1976.
3   INCAP/CDC-Nutrition Program. Nutritional evaluation of the population of Central America and Panama: regional summary. DHEW Publication No HSM-72-8120. US Dep Hlth Educ Welfare, Washington, DC, 1972.
4   INCAP/DIR/NIH/Ministerios de Salud. Evaluación nutricional de la población de Centro América y Panamá: Costa Rica, El Salvador, Guatemala, Honduras, Nicaragua y Panamá (seis volúmenes). INCAP, Guatemala City, 1969.
5   Government of Barbados/PAHO/CFNI/FAO. The national food and nutrition survey of Barbados. PAHO Sci Publ No 237. PAHO, Washington, DC 1972.
6   Interdepartmental Committee on Nutrition for National Defense. Paraguay: Nutrition Survey, May–August 1965. US Government Printing Office, Washington, DC, 1967.
7   Interdepartmental Committee on Nutrition for National Defense. Bolivia: Nutrition Survey. US Government Printing Office, Washington, DC, 1964.
8   Interdepartmental Committee on Nutrition for National Defense. Northeast Brasil: Nutrition Survey, March–May 1963. US Government Printing Office, Washington, DC, 1965.
9   Interdepartmental Committee on Nutrition for National Defense. Venezuela: Nutrition Survey, May–June 1963. US Government Printing Office, Washington, DC, 1964.
10 Interdepartmental Committee on Nutrition for National Defense. Uruguay: Nutrition Survey, March–April 1962. US Government Printing Office, Washington, DC, 1963.
11 Interdepartmental Committee on Nutrition for National Defense. The West Indies, Trinidad and Tobago, St. Lucia, St. Kitts, Nevis and Anguilla: Nutrition Survey, August–September 1961. US Government Printing Office, Washington, DC, 1962.
12 Interdepartmental Committee on Nutrition for National Defense. Colombia: Nutrition Survey, May–August 1960. US Government Printing Office, Washington, DC, 1961.
13 Interdepartmental Committee on Nutrition for National Defense. Chile: Nutrition Survey, March–June 1960. US Government Printing Office, Washington, DC, 1961.
14 Interdepartmental Committee on Nutrition for National Defense. Ecuador: Nutrition Survey, July–September 1959. US Government Printing Office, Washington, DC, 1960.
15 Interdepartmental Committee on Nutrition for National Defense. Peru: National Survey of the Armed Forces, February–May 1959. US Government Printing Office, Washington, DC, 1960.
16 Sebrell, H W *et al:* Nutritional Status of middle and low income groups in the Dominican Republic. Archivos Latinoamericanos de Nutrición, Vol XXII, suppl July 1972.
17 Lechtig, A, Arroyave, G: The nutrition problem in Latin America: definition, causes, and remedial actions. Bull PAHO *11,* 319–331, 1971.
18 Interdepartmental Committee on Nutrition for National Defense. Manual for nutrition surveys; 2nd Ed. Nat Inst Hlth, Bethesda, Md, 1963.

19 Pan American Health Organization. Hypovitaminosis A in the Americas. Report of a PAHO technical group meeting. PAHO Sci Publ No 198. PAHO, Washington, DC, 1970.

20 Instituto de Nutrición de Centro América y Panamá. Recomendaciones dietéticas diarias para Centro América y Panamá. INCAP, Guatemala City, 1973.

21 Pan American Health Organization. Analysis of PAHO collaborative studies of nutritional anemias in Latin America and the Caribbean. RD 8/14, June 1969.

22 Daza, C H, Lechtig, A: Programs to improve the nutrition of pregnant and lactating women. Bull PAHO *14,* 22–34, 1980.

23 Pan American Health Organization. Health for all by the year 2000: strategies. PAHO Off Doc No 173. PAHO, Washington, DC, 1980.

24 Pan American Health Organization. Health for all by the year 2000: plan of action for the Implementation of regional strategies. PAHO Off Doc No 179. PAHO, Washington, DC, 1982.

25 Pan American Health Organization. Guidelines for food fortification in Latin America and the Caribbean. Report of a PAHO Technical Group Meeting. PAHO Sci Publ No 240. PAHO, Washington, DC, 1972.

26 Arroyave, G *et al:* Evaluation of sugar fortification with vitamin A at the national level. PAHO Sci Publ No 384. PAHO, Washington, DC, 1979.

C.H. Daza, MD, MSc, MPH, Regional Advisor in Nutrition, Pan American Health Organization, 525, Twenty-third Street, NW, Washington, DC 20037, USA

Nutritional Status of the Colombian Population

Results of the 1977–80 National Health Survey

J.O. Mora

Department of Community Medicine, Colombian School of Medicine, Bogotá, Colombia

Key Words: Nutritional status · Colombian population · Anthropometry · Iron deficiency anemia · Vitamin deficiencies

Abstract: The overall results of the Colombian National Health Survey (CNHS) in regard to the evaluation of the nutritional status of the Colombian population are reported in brief. The CNHS was carried out in a probabilistic sample representative of the non-institutional population of the country and included anthropometric measurements and laboratory examinations for the assessment of the nutritional status. Using the WHO anthropometric classification of nutritional status, about 20% of the children under five years have a deficient weight-for-age (general malnutrition), close to 25% show growth retardation (chronic malnutrition), and 6% have an inadequate weight-for-height (acute malnutrition). The period of high risk for malnutrition extends over the first two years of life. In the adult population, about 20% are underweight, while the prevalence of frank overweight reaches 5% of the males and 16% of the females. Specific nutrient deficiencies are not frequent in Colombia, except for iron deficiency anemia. Hypovitaminosis A is a public health problem in the population under 15 years of age while folate and vitamin B$_{12}$ deficiencies are uncommon. Information on specific deficiencies of other vitamins and minerals is scanty.

Introduction

Infant and preschool malnutrition is the most important public health problem of developing countries, where the reported prevalence rates are usually above 50% among children under five years [1]. Specific mineral and vitamin deficiencies have also been reported as frequent. Most of the data, however, appear to have been drawn from small scale surveys of selected population groups, usually from low income communities to which special nutrition and health programs are addressed. Prevalence studies using large, statistically selected samples of the entire population are uncommon in developing countries. Therefore, very often the available figures cannot be applied to the population as a whole; they represent usually not well defined portions of the population. Nevertheless, international reports and comparisons among countries and regions are based on these figures [2, 3].

From 1977 to 1980 the Colombian Ministry of Health undertook a National Health Survey (NHS) in cooperation with the Colombian Association of Medical Schools. The survey, conducted in a representative sample of the total population, included enough clinical, anthropometric and laboratory data to provide a valid assessment of the nutritional status of the Colombian population.

Study Sample and Methods

The CNHS was conducted between July 1977 and December 1980 in a probability sample of the non-institutional populations; people staying in institutions (e. g. military personnel, hospitalized patients, etc.), as well as those living in the underpopulated oriental plains and jungle areas of the country, were excluded. The sample as a whole was representative of 98.7 % of the population, at five major regions and at the national level, and included 9 869 randomly selected households with 52 762 persons from which information was collected through home interviews. Data on family composition, dwelling conditions, recent morbidity, health care demand, satisfaction and costs, mortality, incapacitation, family income, fertility, features of last pregnancy and delivery, as well as on the socioeconomic, educational, occupational and current work situation were gathered.

Tab. I: Sample size and reference population by age and sex

Age group, years	Males		Females		Both sexes	
	sample	population, × 1 000	sample	population, × 1 000	sample	population, × 1 000
0– 4	912	1 666	850	1 499	1 762	3 165
5– 9	624	1 539	579	1 374	1 203	2 912
10–14	515	1 542	504	1 509	1 019	3 052
15–24	736	2 482	818	2 554	1 554	5 036
25–34	589	1 450	763	1 473	1 352	2 924
35–44	422	1 093	598	1 100	1 020	2 192
45–54	463	835	595	904	1 058	1 739
55–64	359	546	380	573	739	1 120
65 and older	249	393	305	479	554	872
Total	4 869	11 545	5 392	11 466	10 261	23 011

A random subsample of 10 621 individuals of the 52 762 composing the basic sample was drawn for clinical and laboratory examinations. The age and sex distribution of this subsample is shown in Table I. Clinical examinations included weight and height (or length) measurements of the total subsample, and head circumference of children under five years of age. Laboratory examinations comprised blood and urine tests commonly used in the nutritional assessment of population groups, as follows:

Analyses in blood (fasting specimens). Hemoglobin (cyanomethemoglobin method, duplicate); hematocrit (micro-method, duplicate); total protein (micro-biuret method); albumin, globulin and fractions alfa 1, alfa 2, beta and gamma (electrophoresis in cellulose acetate); total serum iron and total iron binding capacity (spectrophotometric method by atomic absorption); vitamin A and carotenes (Carr-Price method); vitamin B_{12} (microbiologic assay with *Lactobacillus leichmanni);* folic acid (microbiologic assay with *Lactobacillus casei).* Serum levels of folates and vitamin B_{12} were assessed only in subjects under 15 years.

Analyses in urine (fasting specimens). Iodine (photometric method); creatinine (Folin-Wu method); urea nitrogen (diacetyl-monoxime method).

Anthropometric measurements were taken by trained and standardized examiners (auxiliary nurses) following standard techniques [4]; weight was taken with beam scales having 12 kg and 125 kg capacity in individuals below and above two years of age, respectively, and the results were registered to the nearest 5 g and 250 g. Recumbent length was measured in children under two years using standard measuring boards. Height of those above this age was measured with non-elastic measuring tapes placed on a regular vertical wall, the subject standing up against the wall; a triangular mobile head piece with a wedge on one side was put perpendicular to the wall at the top of the head. Length or height were recorded to the nearest millimeter.

Standard quality control procedures were used in data collection, and the field supervisors constantly surveyed the quality of measurement techniques. Further steps in data quality control were introduced throughout data processing by which potential inconsistencies and errors were detected and corrected; in the few cases in which this was not possible, the data were deleted. Expected ranges were set up for each measurement at any given age to identify data deserving closer verification.

Selected anthropometric data and the results of the laboratory assessment of some specific nutritional deficiencies are reported here. Age, weight and length or height data were used to obtain weight-for-age, lenght or height-for-age, and weight-for-height indicators by contrasting the observed values against those proposed as international physical growth reference values by the WHO [5]. The nutritional status of children under 5 years was estimated by the WHO classification [6]. For each indicator, the third percentile of the reference population was taken as a point below which general malnutrition, chronic malnutrition or stunting, and acute malnutrition or wasting were qualified; a so-called "alarm zone" of high risk cases was set up between the third and the tenth percentiles. The two-by-two Waterlow classification combining height-for-age and weight-for-height was also used [7].

Weight and height data of the adult population were used to estimate a weight-for-height indicator, on the basis of which the nutritional status of adults was classified. Such indicator was calculated as the percent ratio between the observed weight and that desirable for the height, according to Jelliffe [4].

The prevalence of anemia (Table II) was estimated as the proportion of the population with hematocrit values below certain cut-off points adapted from those established for the Central American population [8].

Transferrin saturation was calculated as the percent ratio between serum iron and total iron binding capacity. Deficient levels were regarded as indication of iron deficient erythropoiesis. Cut-off points used for deficient values were 10 % for individuals below 5 years, 12 % for those between 5 and 12 years and 16 % for those older than 12 years of age [9, 10].

Serum levels of protein, albumin, vitamin A, folates and vitamin B_{12} were categorized as low or deficient (Table III), according to Sauberlich [11].

Tab. II: Prevalence of anemia

Age group, years	Cut-off point of hematocrit, %
0.5–4	32
5–12	34
13–17	
Males	38
Females	37
18–44	
Males	40
Females (pregnant)	34
Females (non pregnant)	37
45 and above	
Males	38
Females	36

Tab. III: Serum level categories, according to SAUBERLICH [11]

Test	Category	
	low	deficient
Protein, g/dl	6.0– 6.4	less than 6.0
Albumin, g/dl	3.0– 3.4	less than 3.0
Vitamin A, µg/dl	10– 19	less than 10
Folate, ng/ml	3– 5	less than 3
Vitamin B_{12}, pg/ml	100–150	less than 100

Results

Adopting the WHO classification, the prevalence of general malnutrition in children under 5 years was found to 19.4 %, of which 16.9 % was mild and 2.5 % moderate to severe. About 611 000 children under five were malnourished, 533 000 of them mildly and 78 000 moderately to severely (Table IV). The total prevalence of malnutrition increased with age up to the second year and tended to remain stable afterwards; a similar pattern was seen for the different degrees of severity. About 19.7 % of the children, a proportion similar to that of malnutrition, were at high risk of malnutrition (their weight was at the lower 10 % level of the distribution of the reference population).

The prevalence of retarded height (chronic malnutrition or stunting) reached 25.9 % (788 000 children), a figure somewhat greater than that for general malnutrition; 18.7 % (570 000) showed mild growth retardation, whereas 7.2 % (218 000) had a moderate to severe degree (Table V). Similarly to

Tab. IV: Nutritional status of children under five years of age according to the modified WHO weight-for-age classification

Age group, months	Well-nourished, %	At risk, %	Malnourished, %		
			mildy	moderately to severely	total
0– 5	86.8	10.2	2.6	0.4	3.0
6–11	72.3	12.8	13.2	1.7	14.9
12–23	55.5	17.6	21.1	5.9	26.9
24–35	55.0	24.9	18.1	1.9	20.1
36–47	54.9	23.1	20.2	1.8	22.0
48–60	55.5	23.5	18.9	2.1	21.0
Total	60.9	19.7	16.9	2.5	19.4
Population, × 1000	1919	622	533	78	612

weight-for-age indicators, low values stabilized after two years. About 16 % of the under five population would be at risk of height retardation.

Tab. V: Nutritional status of children under five years of age according to the modified WHO height-for-age classification

Age group, months	Adequate height/age, %	At risk, %	Low height/age (stunting), %		
			mild	moderate	total
0– 5	87.8	8.7	2.9	0.6	3.5
6–11	77.6	10.4	9.2	2.8	12.0
12–23	44.8	21.9	25.0	8.3	33.3
24–35	55.2	20.1	17.5	7.2	24.7
36–47	50.0	14.4	24.2	11.4	35.6
48–60	52.3	14.1	24.7	8.9	33.6
Total	58.3	15.8	18.7	7.2	25.9
Population, × 1000	1776	481	571	218	789

Weight-for-height deficits (acute malnutrition or wasting) were less frequent than weight-for-age or height-for-age retardation. The overall prevalence was 6.0 % with only 0.8 % moderate to severe cases, and it was heavily concentrated in the first two years of life, being relatively uncommon afterwards (Table VI); moderate to severe forms were seen only from 6 to 23 months. Overall, 182 000 children under five would have wasting, and some 323 000 (10.7 %) would be at risk. The Waterlow two-by-two classification of nutritional status combines weight-for-height and height-for-age indicators, providing estimations of the relative frequency of wasting and stunting. Around 24 % of the under five population exhibited stunting only, with adequate weight for their retarded height (736 000 children); 4.3 % were just wasted (130 000) and only 1.7 % (51 000) showed combined deficits of weight-

Tab. VI: Nutritional status of children under five years, according to the modified WHO-weight-for-height classification

Age group, months	Adequate weight/ height, %	At risk, %	Low weight-for-height (wasting), %		
			mildly	moderately to severely	total
0– 5	85.9	8.3	5.8	–	5.8
6–11	78.0	12.0	6.9	3.1	10.0
12–23	76.3	11.7	10.1	1.9	12.0
24–35	84.5	11.4	4.1	–	4.1
36–47	91.0	7.9	1.1	–	–
48–60	83.9	12.2	4.0	–	3.9
Total	83.3	10.7	5.2	0.8	6.0
Population, × 1000	2 526	323	159	23	183

Tab. VII: Nutritional status of children under five years, according to the water-low height/age-weight/height classification

Age group, months	Well-nourished, %	Wasted, %	Stunted, %	Wasted and stunted, %
0– 5	90.9	5.6	3.3	0.2
6–11	78.5	9.5	11.5	0.5
12–23	58.3	8.4	29.7	3.6
24–35	72.7	2.6	23.2	1.5
36–47	64.0	–	34.9	0.7
48–60	64.8	1.3	31.2	2.6
Total	69.7	4.3	24.2	1.7
Population, × 1000	2 113	131	737	52

for-height and height-for-age, most of them in the age group 12–23 months (Table VII).

The results of analyses published elsewhere [12] show that global and chronic malnutrition were associated with demographic variables (urban or rural residence, family size and number of children below five years), socio-economic conditions (family and per-capita income, mother or father level of formal education), household sanitary conditions (water supply, excreta and garbage disposal), and the presence of intestinal parasites (ascaris, trichuris trichura, and hookworm infestation). All these associations were in the expected direction, e. g. the prevalence of malnutrition was higher in the rural population, it increased with decreases in either family and per capita income, in the level of education of mother or father, or in the quality of household sanitary conditions, and it went up in the presence of parasitic infections.

As seen in Table VIII, about 13.9% of the adult male population and 13.5% of the females had low weight-for-height, below 80% of standard weight-for-height, indicative of undernutrition. On the other hand, obesity was observed in close to 5% of the males and 16% of the females. Under-nutrition was more frequent in the rural population, whereas the prevalence of obesity (weight-for-height above 120%) was about three times greater among women living in towns and cities than among rural women; obesity in males was somewhat more frequent in towns and cities too. Overall, more than 800 000 adults of each sex were classified as undernourished, and more than one million as obese.

Tab. VIII: Undernutrition and obesity among the adult population, by urbanization level

Urbanization level	Males, %		Females, %	
	undernutrition	obesity	undernutrition	obesity
Rural areas	16.0	2.5	14.6	14.6
Towns (2 500 – 100 000 inhabitants)	11.7	7.3	14.3	18.4
Cities (above 100 000 inhabitants)	12.6	6.0	12.0	16.2
Total	13.9	4.8	13.5	16.1
Population, × 1 000	819	285	878	1 050

Serum protein levels were low in 6.5% of the population and deficient in 4.6%; low levels were more frequent among children under 5 and adults above 45 years (Table IX). Low levels of albumin reached 12.3% of the

Tab. IX: Prevalence of low and deficient levels of serum total protein and albumin, by age group

Age group, years	Total protein, %		Albumin, %	
	low	deficient	low	deficient
0– 4	9.8	5.7	11.6	3.8
5–14	6.5	3.4	12.7	2.7
15–44	5.6	4.1	11.0	3.9
45 and above	6.7	6.4	15.7	5.9
Total	6.5	4.6	12.3	4.1
Population, × 1000	1 367	967	2 586	862

population, without great differences by age group; deficient serum albumin levels were found in 4.1 % of the population, their frequency being lowest in the 5- to 14-year age group.

Nutritional anemias represented the second major nutritional problem of the country. Even though a substantial improvement was apparent, the anemic population amounted to more than three million; the highest prevalence figures were found among pregnant and non-pregnant women, followed by those over 45 years and by the adolescents (Table X). Close to 24 % of the pregnant women were anemic. The overall prevalence of anemia reached about 13 %.

Tab. X: Prevalence of anemia by age group, as estimated from hematocrit values

Age group, years	Prevalence, %	Population, × 1000
0.5– 4	10.6	317
5–12	11.2	620
13–17		
Males	18.9	305
Females	14.8	248
18–44		
Males	9.7	387
Females (pregnant)	23.6	109
Females (non pregnant)	17.1	678
45 and above		
Males	10.5	187
Females	14.7	286
Total	12.9	3 138

Iron deficiency anemia was frequent, particularly among pregnant women (30.3 %); 17.4 % of the non-pregnant women, 16.0 % of the children under five, and 14 % of the adults older than 45 years were also iron deficient (Table XI). The overall prevalence was about 15 % and well above three million persons of all ages were affected. Deficient levels of folates were found in 7.2 % of children under 15 years (close to 600 000 individuals), while serum vitamin B_{12} levels were deficient only in 2.7 % of the child population (Table XII).

Tab. XI: Prevalence of iron deficieny anemia, by age group

Age group, years	Prevalence, %	Affected population, × 1000
0.5– 4	16.0	239
5–12	12.8	597
13–17		
Males	22.0	345
Females	19.1	307
18–44		
Males	10.0	382
Females (pregnant)	30.3	132
Females (non pregnant)	17.4	667
45 and above		
Males	12.1	211
Females	15.6	292
Total	15.1	3 173

Serum vitamin A levels below 10 µg/dl (deficient) were not found at all; 12.4 % of the total population had low serum levels (between 10 and 19 µg/dl). The prevalence of low levels reached public health importance (point

Tab. XII: Prevalence of deficient levels of serum folates (less than 3 ng/ml) and vitamin B_{12} (less than 100 µg/ml) among the population under 15 years

Age group, years	Folates, %	Vitamin B_{12}, %
0– 4	7.0	2.3
5–14	7.3	2.9
Total	7.2	2.7
Population, × 1000	590	208

prevalence above 15 %) among children under 15 years of age, with prevalence figures between 22.4 and 24.1 % (Table XIII). Low levels were less frequent in the adult population (6.7–7.2 %).

Tab. XIII: Prevalence of low serum vitamin A levels (10–19 µg/dl), by age group, Colombia, 1977–1980

Age group, years	Prevalence, %	Affected population, × 1 000
0– 4	24.1	330
5–14	22.4	1 256
15–44		
Males	4.7	220
Females (pregnant)	15.3	74
Females (non pregnant)	7.9	368
45 and above	7.2	254
Total	12.4	2 503

Comments

Infant and preschool protein-calorie malnutrition remains an important public health problem in Colombia. Two of every five children under five years of age suffer from general malnutrition and retardation in linear growth or are at high risk of being affected. The period of highest risk for malnutrition and physical growth retardation encompasses the first two years of life; new cases of malnutrition are uncommon thereafter.

The first two years of life and, particularly, the crucial period between 6 and 18 months, are characterized by two major adverse events in the life of many children in developing countries:

a) weaning, when breast feeding is either progressively or abruptly replaced by artificial feeding carrying the dual risk of dietary inadequacies and food contamination; b) the decline of natural immunity accompanied by an increased exposure to infection, particularly to gastrointestinal infections leading to diarrhea, vomiting, dehydration and physical growth retardation or death.

It is usually the combination of these interrelated series of events that leads to malnutrition and growth failure among Colombian children. The relative importance of dietary inadequacies (attributable to family food shortage and/or faulty feeding practices) and infection (chiefly diarrheal diseases) in the etiology of infant and preschool protein-calorie malnutrition may vary among regions and communities. In some cases, dietary deficiencies predominate, frequently as protein-calorie deficits, especially in extremely poor communities or families; in others, diarrheal diseases play a major causal role, even in the absence of primary food restrictions.

It has been known for a long time that infection may adversely affect physical growth and aggravate mild to moderate malnutrition; however, the demonstration that, under real life conditions, diarrheal diseases by themselves greatly contribute to the causation of infant malnutrition in Colombian communities without food scarcity is relatively recent [13, 14]. Studies have consistently shown that many poor families in Colombia, as in other countries [15], manage to provide adequate or only marginally deficient diets to young children while they are healthy, but that diarrheal diseases substantially reduce intake and increase nutrition requirements of the child thus conducing to infant malnutrition.

It is interesting to point out that the prevalence of wasting, commonly regarded as an indication of acute dietary deficiency, is remarkably lower in Colombia and in other Latin American countries [16], than in regions of the world where food scarcity is frequent, whereas the prevalence of stunting, often associated with inadequate sanitary and other environmental conditions, does not greatly differ between countries and regions [17]. Similarly to other transitional societies, Colombia is experiencing a gradual shift from the health problems typical of underdevelopment (infectious diseases, undernutrition, high fertility rates, etc.) to those affecting affluent societies (chronic diseases, overnutrition, accidents, low fertility rates, etc.). As a matter of fact, a moderate but steady decline in the incidence of infection has been observed in Colombia, together with an increasing importance of cardiovascular and other chronic diseases, and accidents as causes of death; similarly, a significant, though not dramatic, reduction in the prevalence of infant and preschool malnutrition over the past 15 years has been documented [12], whereas overnutrition and obesity are already present in a relatively high proportion of the adult population, particularly in the large cities, with clear preference for the females.

Iron deficiency anemia remains a serious health problem in the country, affecting mostly women (especially during pregnancy), as well as the adolescent population [18]. Although hookworm infestation may play an important role in some regions where it is endemic, iron deficiency is for the most part due to low bioavailability of iron in the Colombian diet, which is heavily based on vegetable foods (cereals and starchy roots). Unfortunately, no systematic effort has been undertaken toward the prevention and control of iron deficiency anemia in Colombia.

Specific nutrient deficiencies of vitamins and minerals have not been looked for in Colombia. Except for iron deficiency anemia, they do not appear to represent a serious problem. It has been shown in this report that the frequency of folate and vitamin B_{12} deficiencies is relatively low among children; unfortunately, they have not been assessed in pregnant women, the most susceptible group to be affected. The prevalence of vitamin A deficiency among the population under 15 years reaches public health significance and should deserve special attention.

There is no indication so far that vitamin C deficiency may be a serious problem in Colombia; however, in view of the important role of vitamin C in substantially increasing non-heme iron absorption, more information is certainly needed on the bioavailability of ascorbic acid in the local diets, as well as on the actual consumption by the population and the eventual role of vitamin C fortification of foods as a means of increasing iron absorption and preventing iron deficiency anemia. It is known that non-hem iron represents about 82 % of the total iron supply for the Colombian population [19].

Very little is known regarding the status of other vitamins (thiamine, riboflavin, niacin, etc.) and of trace minerals in the Colombian population, except for iodine deficiency and endemic goiter, which are currently under control, and the need for fluorine fortification as a means of reducing the high prevalence of dental caries [20].

References

1   OPS/OMS: Condiciones de salud del niño en las Américas. Organización Panamericana de la Salud. PAHO Sci Publ No 381. PAHO, Washington, DC, 1979.
2   BENGOA, J M: Recent trends in the public health aspects of protein-calorie malnutrition. WHO Chronicle 24, 552-561, 1970.
3   BENGOA, J M: The problem of malnutrition. WHO Chronicle 28, 3-7, 1974.
4   JELLIFFE, D B: The assessment of the nutritional status of the community (with special reference to field surveys in developing nations of the world). WHO Monogr Ser No 53. WHO, Geneva, 1966.
5   World Health Organization. Measurement of nutritional impact. WHO, Geneva, 1979.
6   World Health Organization. A growth chart for international use in maternal and child health care. Guidelines for primary health care personnel. WHO, Geneva, 1978.
7   WATERLOW, J C, RUTISHAUSER, I H E: Malnutrition in man. Symposia of the Swedish Nutrition Foundation XII. In: CRAVIOTO et al (ed.). "Early malnutrition and mental development", pp. 13-26. Almquist and Wiksell, Uppsala, 1974.
8   VITERI, F E et al: Normal haematological values in the Central American population. Br J Haematol 23, 189-197, 1972.
9   KOERPER, M A, DALLMAN, P R: Serum iron concentration and transferrin saturation in the diagnosis of iron deficiency in children: Normal developmental changes. J Pediat 91, 870-874, 1977.

10   INACG. Iron deficiency in women. A report of the International Nutritional Anemia Consultative Group (INACG). Nutrition Foundation, Washington, DC, 1981.

11   SAUBERLICH, H E et al: Laboratory tests for the assessment of nutritional status. CRC Press, Cleveland, 1974.

12   MORA, J O: Situación nutricional de la población Colombiana en 1977–80. Vol I. Resultados antropométricos y de laboratorio. Comparación con 1965–66. Estudio Nacional de Salud. Ministerio de Salud, Instituto Nacional de Salud, Asociación Colombiana de Facultades de Medicina, Bogotá, 1982.

13   MORA, J O et al: La enfermedad diarreica en la etiología de la desnutrición infantil en Colombia. Instituto Colombiano de Bienestar Familiar, Bogotá, 1983.

14   KOOPMAN, J S et al: Food, sanitation, and the socioeconomic determinants of child growth in Colombia. Am J Pub Hlth 71, 31–37, 1981.

15   MATA, L: The children of Santa Maria Cauque. A prospective field study of health and growth. MIT Press, Cambridge, 1978.

16   ANDERSON, M A: Comparison of anthropometric measures of nutritional status in preschool children in five developing countries. Am J Clin Nutr 32, 2339–2345, 1979.

17   KELLER, W, FILMORE, C M: The prevalence of protein-energy malnutrition. Wld Hlth Stat Quart 36(2), 129–167, 1983.

18   MORA, J O, RODRIGUEZ, E: Situacion nutricional de la poblacion colombiana en 1977–80. Vol II: Anemias nutricionales. Ministerio de Salud, Instituto Nacional de Salud, Asociación Colombiana de Facultades de Medicina. Estudio Nacional de Salud, Bogotá, 1984.

19   BOHORQUEZ, C et al: Hoja de balance de alimentos. Colombia, 1976. Instituto Colombiano de Bienestar Familiar, Bogotá, 1978.

20   MONCADA, O, ERAZO, B: Morbilidad oral. Colombia, 1977–80. Estudio Nacional de Salud. Ministerio de Salud, Instituto Nacional de Salud, Asociación Colombiana de Facultades de Medicina, Bogotá, 1984.

J.O. Mora, MD, Chairman, Department of Community Medicine, Colombian School of Medicine, Calle 134 No. 12-81, Bogotá, Colombia

Principles and Applications of Nutrition Survey Findings

A.E. Schaefer

Emeritus Director, Swanson Center for Nutrition, Inc., Omaha, Nebraska, USA

Key Words: Nutrition survey applications

Abstract: Objectives of a nutrition survey must be defined as precisely as possible. The primary goals should be to assess nutrition health status, identify major problems, prevalence, location, causes and resources (manpower, economics, agriculture, education and health services) for potential practical solutions. The nutritional health status of a population group is not static, thus there is need for continued surveillance of the effects of changes in food supply and of economic and social changes on the health of the population. The methods employed may be limited to one assessment method such as anthropometric measurements or combinations of physical examinations, biochemical, dietary and food availability studies. The survey sample should be defined to enable inferences from the sample to population groups. Simplicity of a survey reference, methodologies to be employed, cost, personnel and time are directly related to sample size. Priorities of methodologies should be established and guidelines for interpreting the data be considered. For continued monitoring to document change, it is essential to develop a simple data retrieval system.

Applications of survey findings will be described utilizing four different areas – the US Government's response to the 1968–70 nutrition survey findings, progress in Bangladesh since the 1962–64 survey, Jordan's follow-up program, and INCAP's follow-up and research in Central America and Panama. Bangladesh in 1962–63 identified a high prevalence of vitamin A deficiency blindness in children. This was instrumental in the fortification with vitamins A and D of all US dry skim milk powder and the launching of the UNICEF vitamin A capsule program in Bangladesh, Indonesia and other countries. Establishing the Institute of Nutrition and Food Science at the University of Dacca (Bangladesh) was a direct follow-up activity. Recently their staff discovered the dramatic effect of vitamin C in the prevention and treatment of neurolathyrism, and tetanus toxicity. The nutrition surveys in the Near East stimulated numerous follow-up activities including research on the human requirement for zinc, chromium, selenium, and vitamin E, as well as self-help applied programs to combat malnutrition.

Introduction

The first edition of the "Manual for Nutrition Surveys" published in 1957 [1] by the Interdepartmental Committee on Nutrition for National Defense (ICNND) served as a guide for collecting and interpreting data for an assessment of the nutritional status of population groups. The 1963 second edition [2] incorporated experience gained from 18 country surveys. The ICNND surveys totalling over 35 country surveys during the period of 1956–67 had the primary objective of assisting developing countries to assess their nutritional status, define existing problems of malnutrition, and to identify means for solving critical nutrition problems by maximum utilization of the country's own resources. The interpretative guidelines were developed for use with the field methods employed and were intended as guidelines to be updated as research findings dictated.

In 1971 the Pan American Health Organization (PAHO) convened a technical workshop in Buenos Aires, Argentina, to develop guidelines for the establishment of a data system for the assessment of nutrition and health status [3]. The basic purpose was to utilize relevant health data already being collected in relation to other data to be collected to assess the nutritional health and food status and to evaluate the effectiveness of intervention programs. The majority of the Latin American countries had already conducted a nutrition survey in various population groups. The Director General of PAHO urged that valid survey tests, analyses and observations by low cost procedures are made adaptable to national nutrition surveys and monitoring of change. He likewise urged the development of techniques to determine human and economic loss due to malnutrition.

The fundamental consideration in planning a nutrition survey is to define its objectives as precisely as possible. Regardless of the scope, its primary goals should be to assess the nutrition health status and to identify: the major nutrition problems and prevalence, location, cause and available resources for potential practical solutions. Since the nutritional health status of a population group is not static, there is need for continued surveillance of the effects on health of the changing food supply, economic and social conditions. Where resources are limited, a nutrition survey needs to be restricted to the nutritionally critical areas in which large gains in health and efficiency can be obtained. This is essential to gain political support.

Sampling Considerations

A survey is carried out to enable inferences from the sample to the population. Generally, stratifications are made of the whole population based on prior information suggestive of sub-populations more nearly homogeneous in nutritional status than the total. Simplicity of a survey reference, methodologies to be employed and cost in terms of money and personnel are directly related to sample size and type of sampling. The logistics of presenting the subjects for study is the greatest cost item.

Screening-surveys. In some cases when a full-scale nutrition survey is not possible, it is desirable to screen small communities in a given area or region in order to select locations for action programs on a reasonable priority basis. In this case, children under five years of age can be used as an indicator of community nutrition problems. Measures of height and weight in combination with an abbreviated food consumption questionnaire and the determination of hemoglobin values could serve for an approximate evaluation of the nutritional status and for the identification of community problems. For this purpose the following sample sizes are suggested: communities with 800 inhabitants: all preschool children; communities with 900–1200 inhabitants: 65 % of preschool children; communities with 1200–1500 inhabitants: 50 % of preschool children; communities with 1500–2000 inhabitants: 40 % of preschool children; communities with 2000–3000 inhabitants: 30 % of preschool children; communities with 3000–5000 inhabitants: 20 % of preschool children; communities with 5000 inhabitants: 15 % or less to ensure sample of about 150 preschool children.

The sample sizes given by this scheme will allow approximate estimates of the proportion of children within lower bound groupings of weight for age; height for age; weight for height; and hemoglobin deficits. The dietary inquiry should allow identification of gross calorie, protein or vitamin deficiencies as established from food group consumption patterns.

The sample of preschool children to be studied should be randomly chosen from a complete roster of preschool children in the community. For large communities, when it is not possible to establish a roster for all children in the community, such roster could be established for randomly selected sectors for a composite sample of approximately 150 children.

Probability sampling. The application of probability sampling techniques is essential to validate statistical inferences from the samples studied to the total population under consideration.

Expert statistical advice should be obtained in the early planning stages of the survey. Likewise, and as soon as field procedures are defined, it is advisable to establish a viable system for the processing of the information.

Nutrition Assessment Procedures and Priorities (Classed 1–3)

Sample. (1) Random cluster stratification of vulnerable population groups, i.e., 0 to 5-year-old children and pregnant women.
(2) Other groups (urban poor, rural poor).
(3) Random probability survey. Examples are described for Ecuador and the West Indies in the literature [2].

Anthropometric measurement. (1) Height and weight for age.
(2) Arm circumference, skinfold thickness, head circumference.

Physical examination. (1) Short form key indicator lesions [2].
(2) Pediatric – maternal questionnaire.

Biochemical analysis (dependent upon sample size; could be 1 in 5 or 1 in 10 of those measured anthropometrically). (1) Hemoglobin and hematocrit.
(2) Serum iron, rbc folate on a subsample.

(2) Vitamin A and serum albumin on 1 to 5-year-olds and pregnant women.

(3) Other vitamins (vitamin C, riboflavin etc.) (2) Urinary iodine for adolescent girls.

Parasitological analysis. (1) Fecal analysis on subsample if risk suspected.

Dietary studies. (1) 24 hour recall on subsample of an anthropometric sample. (1) Food frequency pattern. (2) Home food weighing. (3) Food composite chemical analysis.

Agriculture. Food production, processing, storage, marketing and pricing (urban *vs.* rural).

Guidelines for Interpreting Nutrition Information

The primary purpose of guides for evaluating nutrition data – dietary, biochemical, anthropometric and physical – is to permit, within the limits of knowledge and methods, realistic, uniform interpretation of such data. Dietary data represent the situation at a given limited time. In no case should dietary nutrient intake be used by itself to define a nutritional deficiency state. Likewise, it must be appreciated that current food nutrient composition tables contain only (mean) nutrient values for relatively few nutrients, especially trace minerals, folic acid, vitamin B_{12}, types of fiber, etc. (Tables I and II).

Tab. I: Guidelines for evaluation of nutrient intake (protein and calcium)

Age, years	Body weight, kg	kcal/day	kcal/ kg/day	Protein safe levels[1]						Calcium[2], mg
				g/kg body weight	total intake/person/day, g (different protein scores)					
					100[3]	80[3]	70[3]	60[3]		
Children										
½–1	9.0	1 000	112	1.53	14	17	20	23		550
2–3	13.4	1 360	101	1.19	16	20	23	27		450
4–6	20.0	1 830	91	1.01	20	26	29	34		450
7–9	28.1	2 190	78	0.88	25	31	35	41		450
10–12	37.4	2 470	66	0.84	30	37	42	49		650
Males										
13–15	51.3	2 900	57	0.72	37	46	53	62		650
16–18	62.9	3 070	49	0.60	38	47	54	63		550
Adult	65.0	3 000	46	0.57	37	46	53	62		450
Females										
13–15	49.9	2 490	50	0.63	31	39	45	52		650
16–18	54.4	2 310	43	0.55	30	37	43	50		550
Adult	55.0	2 200	40	0.52	29	36	41	48		450
Pregnant		+ 350			+ 9	+ 11	+ 13	+ 15		1 100
Lactating		+ 550			+ 17	+ 21	+ 24	+ 28		1 100

[1] Adapted after meeting of the Expert Committee on Energy Requirements [17].

[2] Adapted from INCAP [8].

[3] Scores are estimates of protein quality relative to egg, milk protein taken as 100. Corrected protein requirements for 80–70–60 score may overestimate safe level needs for both adult males and females.

Biochemical analyses of nutrient tissue levels or functional tests provide objective data identifying the degree of tissue saturation or depletion and are indicative of nutritional status of longer

Tab. II: Guidelines for evaluation of nutrient intake (iron and vitamins)

Age, years	Iron, mg animal fodd, % [15]			Vitamin A, µg retinol [8]	Vitamin D, µg [15]	Vitamin C, mg [15]	Vitamin B_{12}, µg [15]	Folate, µg [15]	Thiamin, mg [16]	Riboflavin, mg [16]	Niacin equivalent, mg [16]
	10	10–25	25								
½–1	10	7	5	300	10	20	0.3	60			
2–3				300	10	20	0.9	100			
4–6		7		300	10	20	1.5	100			
7–9		7		400	2.5	20	1.5	100			
10–12	10	7	5	600	2.5		2.0	100			
Males											
13–15	18	12	9	750	2.5	30	2.0	200	0.4/	0.6/	6.6/
16–18	18	12	9	750	2.5	30	2.0	200	1 000 cal	1 000 cal	1 000 cal
Adult	9	6	5	750	2.5	30	2.0	200			
Females											
13–15	24	16	12	750	2.5	30	2.0	200			
16–18	24	16	12	750	2.5	30	2.0	200			
Adult	28[1]	19[1]	14[1]	750	2.5	30	2.0	200			
Pregnant	30	20	15		10	50	3.0	400			
Lactating	24	16	12		10	50	2.5	300			

[1] Iron requirement for a menstruating female.

duration. Biochemical assessment for the specific nutrient analysed permits an estimation of the prevalence of subjects that are in a «risk» category with an estimate as to how severe or how mild the condition may be. Furthermore, it indicates, in general terms, the percentage of the population that have tissue levels along the scale from "deficient" or "extreme risk" to "acceptable" or "adequate". These same guidelines can be applied to an individual (Tables III and IV).

In general, the guidelines for interpretation have regarded "adequate" or "acceptable" levels as that level above which objective evidence of health *improvement* does not occur. Likewise, those levels designated as "severe" risk or "deficient" are those levels which may be expected to be associated with definite, although not necessarily severe, physical-physiological impairment due to insufficiency of a nutrient in a measurable proportion of individuals. In this later state histological and physiological alterations are clearly evident in a majority of the subjects. The guidelines are *not* intended to be diagnostic for an individual but should be followed up with additional studies such as saturation and therapeutic tests.

Physical examinations are directed at identifying "indicator lesions" of nutritional deficiencies which may come and go unpredictably in "mild deficiency states". Few, if any, of the physical signs of suboptimal nutrition are specifically diagnostic. Other factors or vectors in the environment may result in similar lesions and the concomitant presence of several deficiency states may obscure the appearance of clear cut physical signs.

Anthropometric data, i.e., weight for height, height and weight for age, and skinfold thickness, are extremely useful in characterizing the general health status of individuals or population groups. One must keep in mind that growth retardation or weight loss may be, and often is, due to a combination of factors such as infectious disease and inborn errors, as well as undernutrition. Anthropometric data obviously do not identify the cause of malnutrition.

Of equal importance to collecting the data is the statistical analysis of the data and the development of recommendations for action. When intervention programs are proposed they should include a mechanism for monitoring and evaluating progress.

Tab. III: Guides for interpretation of hematology data, 0–750 m altitude

Age, years	Hemoglobin, g %			Hematocrit, %			Serum iron, µg/100 ml [2]	
	extreme risk [12]	low risk [12]	anemia [13]	extreme risk [12]	low risk [12]	anemia [13]	extreme risk	low risk
1–4	11.3	11.8	11	32.6	34.3	33	< 30	< 50
5–8	10.9	11.5	12	33.0	34.6	36		
9–12	11.8	12.3		35.3	36.6		< 30	< 50
13–16								
Male	12.4	12.9	13	36.9	38.2	39	< 30	< 60
Female	12.7	13.0	12	38.0	39.0	36	< 30	< 60
17–20								
Male	13.4	13.8		40.8	41.9		< 30	< 60
Female	12.9	13.4		38.5	39.6		< 30	< 60
21–49								
Male	13.3	14.0		40.2	42.1		< 30	< 60
Female	11.8	12.4		35.2	36.9		< 30	< 60
50								
Male	12.2	13.0	13	35.0	37.7	39	< 30	< 50
Female	12.1	12.7	12	36.5	38.2	36	< 30	< 50
Pregnant, 1st half	9.5[1]	11.0[1]	11			33	< 30	< 60
Pregnant, 2nd half	9.0[1]	10.4[1]	11			33	< 45	< 60

[1] According to the ICNND [2].

Tab. IV: Guides for interpretation of blood data [2, 8, 14]

	Extreme risk	Low risk	Probably normal
Serum albumin (electrophotometric method), g/100 ml [2]	< 2.80	2.80–3.49	3.50+
Serum albumin during 1st half of pregnancy [2]	< 3.00	3.0–3.99	4.00+
Serum albumin during 2nd half of pregnancy [2]	< 3.00	3.0–3.49	3.50+
Plasma ascorbic acid, mg/100 ml [2]	< 0.10	0.10–0.19	0.20+
Plasma vitamin A, µg/100 ml [2]	< 10	10–19	20+
Serum folacin, ng/ml [8, 14]	< 3.0	3.0–5.9	6.0+
Serum vitamin B_{12}, pg/ml [8, 14]	< 100	100–149	150+
Red blood cell folacin, ng/ml [8, 14]	< 140	140–159	160+
Red blood cell riboflavin, µg/100 ml RBC [2]	< 10	10.0–14.9	15.0+
Transferrin saturation index, % [8]	< 15	15.0–19.9	20.0+

Application of Findings

United States – problems and action programs. We had the opportunity in the US in 1967 to remind our Government that we knew more about the nutrition problems in over 30 developing countries than we did about the US. In rapid order we launched a survey in ten US states [4], concentrating on families living in the lower quartile of income areas. An examination of over 43 000 family members on whom physical, anthropometric, biochemical and dietary data were obtained revealed the following:

a) Obesity (i.e., over 20% of ideal weight) in 30% over age 35.

b) Growth retardation in 15% of the preschool age children from poor families, with a higher prevalence in the migrants (Hispanic), Native Americans and poor blacks.

c) Anemia of the "low risk" category in 10–15% of the children, teenagers, pregnant women, and elderly.

d) Biochemical evidence of marginal to low risk status for vitamin A (in migrants and very poor) and of riboflavin, and folic acid in the elderly and poor.

Many of the poor were not enrolled in the food distribution program. Likewise they had limited, if any, access to a health delivery system. Children were not participating in the school lunch program, and nutrition education in our schools and through health clinics was virtually nonexistent. This was especially true for the urban population. The 1968–70 nutrition survey helped stimulate congressional action which resulted in a rapid expansion of the family food assistance and child nutrition programs [5]. A few examples are given in Table V.

Tab. V: Food assistance program

Year	Food distribution and stamps, $ billions	Amount spent on child nutrition, $ billions
1969	1.0	0.2
1971	2.9	1.0
1973	3.0	1.2
1976	6.0	2.3
1980	8.0	3.2

Year	School lunch program, millions participating	
	total	free and reduced lunches
1969	22	2.2
1971	24	5.0
1976	27	11.0

Since the government bureaucrats were not enthusiastic about the need to update nutrition education, legislation was defeated each year until the agriculture bill for 1977 provided special funding to each state to launch a

Nutrition Education and Training Program. Each state received an allocation of $ 0.50 per school child per year, providing an overall budget of $ 27 million. This was reduced in 1978 to 15 million and in 1979 to 5 million. In spite of the lack of adequate funding, new innovative nutrition education materials were developed and implemented in many schools. Nutrition education must be dynamic and updated continuously so as to stay abreast of the changing food supply, as well as changing life styles.

It is essential to evaluate government nutrition programs so as to document economic and health gains. Our Swanson Center for Nutrition staff had the opportunity to evaluate the supplementary feeding program for women, infants and children (WIC) in the native American tribes in Nebraska and in a random population sample under a USDA grant. In our Nebraska study, the prevalence of hemoglobin levels in the children of less than 11 g/100 ml of blood was reduced from 15.8 to 9.8 % within six months of initiating the WIC program which consisted of furnishing milk and enriched cereals to the eligible families.

Jordan – problems and action programs. The ICNND nutrition survey in the Kingdom of Jordan in 1962 [6] identified serious calorie-protein malnutrition, vitamin A deficiency, and anemia in children. Low levels of intake and biochemical evidence of vitamin A and riboflavin deficiency were found among all segments of the population.

Follow-up programs based upon the survey findings were implemented by the government over a five-year period and included:

a) Establishment of an interdepartmental committee on nutrition for Jordan – 1962.

b) Publication of a nutrition reference book and training aids by the committee and the Ministry of Health – 1963.

c) Initiation of a year-long detailed nutrition study of nearly 3 000 infants from November 1962 to October 1963 [7].

d) Presentation findings of the pediatric study at a nutrition conference held for the Jordanian medical profession in 1965.

e) Collaboration with US ICNND investigators in studying severe calorie-protein malnutrition and vitamin E, chromium and selenium, 1964–66.

f) Mandated for the enrichment of vegetable oils with vitamins A and D in 1966.

Central America and Panama. Activities by INCAP and ICNND survey teams during and after the surveys of 1965–67 [8] were as follows:

a) Etiology of anemias with new guidelines for interpretation.

b) Evaluation of effect of anemia on work performance.

c) Evaluation of salt iodination in Guatemala and extension to other countries.

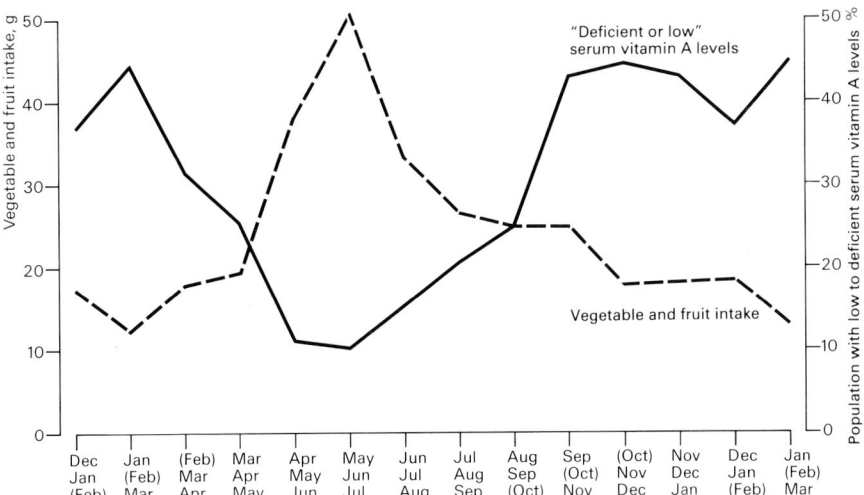

Fig. 1: East Pakistan Nutrition Survey: seasonal correlation of intake of leafy green vegetables and ripe fruit with serum vitamin A levels; quarterly averages. ——————— = Percentage of population with "deficient" or "low" serum vitamin A levels. – – – – = Intake of leafy green vegetables and ripe fruit.

d) Evaluation of dietary and biochemical assessment methodologies.

e) Established of a master serum bank followed by immunological studies.

f) Evaluation of bone maturation by wrist bone x-ray to determine physiological *vs.* chronological age.

g) Evaluation of enrichment of sugar with vitamin A.

Bangladesh. From 1962 to 1964 Bangladesh (then called East Pakistan), with assistance from the ICNND, FAO and UNICEF, conducted a comprehensive nutrition survey of 2 340 households over a two-year period which involved a cyclic stratified population sample during each season [9].

The study revealed a high prevalence of vitamin A deficiency, resulting in an estimated 40 000 blind children per year. The number of blind children diagnosed in the hospitals correlated with the reduced intake of carotene rich foods (yellow and green fruits and vegetables) in autumn and winter from an average of 50 g/person/day to 20 g. With the reduced intake of carotene rich foods the percent of individuals having plasma vitamin A levels of less than 20 μg/100 ml increased from 15 to 40 % (Figs. 1 and 2).

The other major problems identified were growth stunting in children, severe anemia in pregnant and lactating women and children, and goiter.

The survey findings served as the basis for the government's five-year plan for agriculture and health programs. Without doubt, the most significant ac-

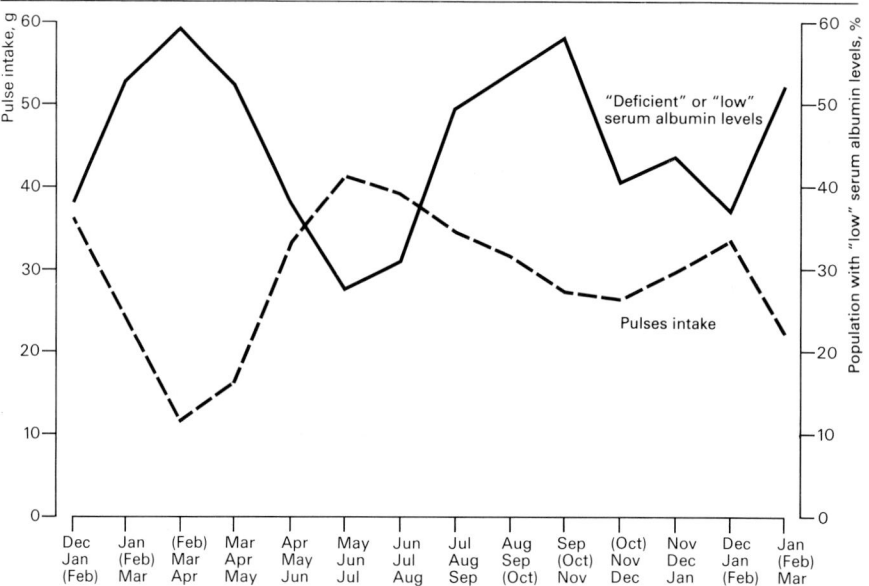

Fig. 2: East Pakistan Nutrition Survey: seasonal correlation of pulse intake with serum albumin levels; quarterly averages. ——————— = Percentage of "deficient" or "low" serum albumin levels. – – – – = Intake of pulses.

complishment was the establishment of a functional Institute of Nutrition and Food Science at the University of Dacca. This institute, headed since its inception in 1964 by Dr. Kamal Ahmad, has succeeded in the face of adversity – drought and famine, civil war, and floods. The staff was instrumental in monitoring nutritional health and in building a tremendous new edifice, staffed completely by MDs and PhDs trained in England, Australia, USA and Canada. Of great importance has been their ability to work with and receive support from UNICEF, FAO, WHO, foundations and bilateral aid.

In 1975–76 they re-surveyed the country [10]. Their findings revealed that as a result of the civil war, floods and droughts, the nutritional status of children and mothers was even worse than in 1962–64. For example, 16 % of children 0–5 years of age were both wasted and stunted suffering from acute and chronic undernutrition. An estimated 80 000 suffered from night blindness with still thousands going blind each year in spite of a large UNICEF supported campaign of administering vitamin A capsules once per year to preschool children. Goiter was found in 12–31 % of the pregnant lactating women. 82 % of the children and mothers were anemic. Vitamin A intake was very marginal which probably contributed to the high incidence of iron deficiency anemia. In 1975 over 100 000 cases of neurolathyrism were reported in just the province of Bihar.

Bangladesh is a good example of what can be accomplished in an economically depressed country. Over the years a cadre of technicians has been trained to work at the village level to test and evaluate applied programs directed at:

1) Nutrition education at the family level.
2) Nutrition education in schools and use of schools to launch a vegetable gardening program.
3) Initiation of home extension programs in rural villages.
4) Assistance in a de-worming project.
5) Assistance in installation of tube wells for pure water.
6) Assistance in home fish culture.
7) Assistance in organizing health clinics.
8) Support of basic and applied research involving:
   a) iodization of salt;
   b) identification of a local small fish as a superior source of vitamin A;
   c) development of a local infant food supplement;
   d) discovery of a herbal extract which is very effective in the cure of tuberculosis and also effective in treatment of various infectious diseases and parasitic manifestations.

The recent discovery by the Institute staff of the role of vitamin C in the treatment and prevention of neurolathyrism is worthy of special attention [11]. This recent discovery clearly identifies a new physiological role for ascorbic acid. The consumption of the legume *L. sativa* (Khesari) takes place especially in times of drought. However, in some areas of Bangladesh and India this prolifically growing legume is consumed by the poor in quantities greater than the usual staple cereals. Consumption of Khesari for approximately two months leads to neurolathyrism characterized by paralysis of lower limbs, tremor and ataxic gait. Until recently it has been impossible to produce experimental lathyrism in common laboratory animals. Dr AHMAD suggested that if there existed a nutritional relationship to neurolathyrism it would have to be based upon the difference in nutrient requirements between man and most experimental animals. Obviously vitamin C fulfilled this assumption. This led to the discovery that adult guinea pigs and monkeys fed a cooked Khesari diet supplemented with all the vitamins except vitamin C became paralyzed in 3–7 weeks while those receiving vitamin C remained normal (Table VI). Moving from animals to man it was demonstrated that when vitamin C was added to the diet, neurolathyrism was prevented. For man AHMAD believes that a serum vitamin C level of above 0.4 mg/100 ml is essential. New cases of neurolathyrism (within two months of first symptoms) recover within two weeks of intravenous administration of 500–1 000 mg ascorbic acid/day. This observation that vitamin C administered to human patient in doses of 500–1 000 mg/day cured paralysis fully or partially, was confirmed by researchers in India.

Tab. VI: Vitamin C and neurolathyrism

Animals	Treatment	Vitamin C	No. of Animals	Observation
Guinea pigs	fed *L. sativa*	none	35	9 died, all paralyzed
Guinea pigs	fed *L. sativa*	5 mg/day	20	normal
Guinea pigs	injected extract of *L. sativa*	none	30	25 paralyzed in 30 to 150 min
Guinea pigs	*L. sativa*	5 mg	20	normal
Adult monkeys	fed *L. sativa*	none	6	5 of 6 neurological symptoms in 3 months
	fed *L. sativa*	20 mg/day	6	normal

Dr AHMAD extended these observations to the toxicity of monosodium glutamate (MSG). When vitamin C deficient guinea pigs or monkeys are administered MSG they develop the same type of neural symptoms as animals fed *L. sativa*. Ascorbic acid protects them. Other substances such as D-glucuronic acid, reduced glutathione, or D-gluconic acid lactone do not show any protective effect. He did observe that high levels of D-gulono lactone and iso-ascorbic acid were effective in preventing neurological symptoms, however, these compounds were less active than ascorbic acid. (Drs KAMAL AHMAD and KHURSHEED JAHAN gave me permission to include their findings in this paper).

Conclusions

Obviously not all countries are prepared to monitor nutritional status employing population survey procedures. However, every country is capable of predicting times and areas where malnutrition problems may arise from the following "indicators" – rainfall, drought, unemployment, crop yields, cost of an average diet, infant mortality and morbidity. Irrespective of the state of health delivery every clinic regardless of size should have personnel trained to recognize overt physical lesions which are indicative of malnutrition such as night blindness, edema in children or young adults, wasting and growth stunting, severe anemia. There is need to establish guidelines to ensure uniform collecting and reporting of these data. In the developed countries, too, health personnel must be alert to seek out the nutritionally vulnerable groups, i. e., the poor, the elderly, the dieter. Nutritional deficiencies once eradicated, such as goiter, pellagra, and rickets will only appear under certain circumstances.

One simple surveillance method can prove invaluable: the systematic assessment of height and weight of 7-year-olds on a well defined random population sample at routine intervals (1–4 years).

References

1   Interdepartmental Committee on Nutrition for National Defense. Manual for nutrition surveys, pp 1–138. US Government Printing Office, Washington, 1957.
2   Interdepartmental Committee on Nutrition for National Defense. Manual for nutrition surveys, 2nd ed.; pp 1–310. US Government Printing Office, Washington, 1963.
3   Pan American Health Organization. General guidelines for establishment of a data system for the assessment of nutrition and health status, p 59. PAHO, Washinton, DC, 1973.
4   US Department of Health, Education, and Welfare. Ten-state nutrition survey, 1968–70; HSM No. 72–8134. US Department of HEW, Washington, 1972.
5   White House Conference on Food, Nutrition and Health, pp 1–341. US Government Printing Office, Washington, 1969.
6   Interdepartmental Committee on Nutrition for National Defense. Nutrition Survey, the Hashemite Kingdom of Jordan in April-June 1962, pp 1–327. US Government Printing Office, Washington, 1962.
7   Pharaon, H M et al: A year-long study of the nutriture of infants and preschool children in Jordan. Trop Pediat African Child Hlth 2, 3–39, 1965.
8   Institute of Nutrition of Central America and Panama. Nutritional evaluation of the population of Central America and Panama, regional summary 1965–67, pp 1–165. INCAP, Guatemala, 1971.
9   Ministry of Health, Government of Pakistan and Nutrition Section Office of Institute of Research, NIH. Nutrition survey of East Pakistan, March 1962-January 1964, pp 1–426. US Department of HEW, Washington, 1966.
10 Ahmad, K U et al: Nutrition survey of rural Bangladesh 1975–76, pp 1–235. Institute of Nutrition and Food Science, Dacca, 1977.
11 Ahmad, K U, Jahan, K: Facts and fancies on neurolathyrism and mode of action of ascorbic acid in its prevention and cure. Nutr News (Bangladesh) 2, 1–2, 1983.
12 Viteri, F E et al: Normal hematological values in Central American populations. Br J Haemat 23, 189 (1972).
13 WHO: Nutritional anemias. Tech Rep Scr Wld Hlth Org No 405, (1968).
14 O'Neal, R M et al: Guidelines for classification and interpretation of group blood and urine data collected as part of the National Nutrition Survey. Pediat Res 4, 103–106 (1970).
15 FAO/WHO: Requirements of ascorbic acid, vitamin D, vitamin B_{12}, folate and iron (adjustments made for age groups). FAO Rep No 47 (1970).
16 FAO/WHO: Requirements of vitamin A, thiamine, riboflavin and niacin. FAO Rep No 41 (1961).
17 WHO/FAO: Report of the ad hoc Committee on Energy and protein requirements, Rome No 522 (1973).

Arnold E. Schaefer, PhD, Professor of Nutrition, Department of Food Science and Technology, 132 Filley Hall, East Campus, University of Nebraska, Lincoln, Nebraska 68583, USA

Sub-Clinical Vitamin Deficits in Various Age Groups

H. Baker and O. Frank

New Jersey Medical School, Newark, New Jersey, USA

Key Words: Vitamins · Maternal · Fetal · Children · Adults · Elderly · Vitamin supplementation

Abstract: Thiamin, biotin, vitamin B_{12}, folate, pantothenate, riboflavin, nicotinates, vitamin B_6, vitamins A, E, C, and β-carotene were estimated in the blood of mothers and in the cord blood of their neonates at parturition. Circulating vitamin levels were analysed in 68 neonates born to mothers with no laboratory evidence of hypovitaminemia. The higher incidence of hypovitaminemia in gravidas not taking vitamins concerned folate, thiamin, vitamins A, C, B_{12}, B_6, and nicotinate in descending order. A similar relationship held for neonates from these mothers.

The above vitamins were also analysed in 642 10- to 13-year-old New York City School children belonging to Chinese, Puerto Rican, Black, and Caucasian families. All groups studied showed distinct vitamin patterns. Clinical impressions of the nutrition status did not correlate with the calculated inadequate protein intake in some children. Thiamin, biotin, and ascorbate were all markedly below the mean values for the total study population when protein intake was inadequate. It is suggested that the combination of the extreme thiamin, biotin, and ascorbate deviations from the mean for the total population may form part of the pattern common to inadequate protein nutriture in children.

The above vitamin profile of 473 elderly persons was compared with that of 204 healthy volunteers (controls aged 20–50). Hypovitaminemia was not obvious for biotin, pantothenate, riboflavin, vitamins A, E, and carotenes in either the institutional or non-institutional elderly. In the 473 elderly studied, vitamin B_6, nicotinate, and vitamin B_{12}, in that order, were the most commonly deficient vitamins; folate, thiamin and ascorbate deficits comprised a lesser percentage. Of the elderly subjects, 39 % showed vitamin deficits despite oral vitamin supplementation. Ingested folylpolyglutamates proved to be a poor source of folates for the elderly subjects, whereas synthetic folylmonoglutamate served as a good source. Intramuscular rather than oral vitamin supplementation is an effective method for maintaining adequate blood levels of vitamins in the elderly.

Introduction

In this report we present a survey of our experience involving imbalances of circulating vitamins seen in various age groups, e.g. neonates, teenagers, and the elderly. The easier quantitation permitted by sensitive and specific protozoan techniques [1] has helped to clarify the significance of vitamins not merely in classic nutritional deficiencies but for metabolic disturbances generally.

As with other constituents of blood or serum, deviation of vitamin titers from "normal" can mean different things: lowered intake or absorption, increased utilization, increased demand, increased excretion or vitamin dependencies, e.g. in the case of inborn errors of vitamin B_6 or biotin metabolism [2, 3]. Nutritional deficiency states lacking overt signs can be recognized. Subclinical malnutrition – as the phrase implies – is not obvious, but real; it foretells imminent biochemical and clinical lesions. It remains to be determined how malnutrition in the form of subclinical deficiencies contributes to ill health and senescence.

Neonates

Gestation is more than imposition of fetal growth upon the mother: the stress for the mother is exacerbated when the maternal diet is inadequate since nutritional demands of the mother and fetus heighten as pregnancy progresses. All this can be inferred from the intense metabolic and developmental changes in the fetus during gestation. Maternal undernutrition can be disastrous to fetus and neonate. The damage caused by maternal malnutrition emphasizes the need for quantitating metabolites critical for gestation. Serious undernutrition during pregnancy increases the risks of intrauterine growth retardation, prematurity, and abortion – all seem to reflect cellular malfunction. For example, during pregnancy, megaloblastic anemia is commonly due to disturbances in vitamin B_{12} and/or folate metabolism. These disorders adversely affect the fetus who is especially vulnerable to such injury [4]. Maternal vitamin B_6 and biotin deprivation may result in neurologic disorders, irritability, convulsions, behavioral disorders, abnormalities in development, and severe mental retardation in newborn infants. Large doses of vitamin B_6 and biotin [2, 3] may reverse some of these effects. As most vitamins and enzymes cross the placenta into the fetal circulation [5, 6], maternal malnutrition can evidently deplete fetal coenzymes and thereby impair metabolism and embryogenesis.

Documentation of the vitamin status in pregnancy could permit assessment of the extent to which a maternal vitamin imbalance not only affects the outcome of pregnancy for the mother but fetal and newborn development as well. To begin with, a vitamin profile of both mother and neonate should be established. A start has already been made [6, 7].

Table I presents vitamin levels in neonates born to mothers, who disclaimed ingesting supplemental vitamins and who showed no evidence of hypovitaminemia. Based on the findings given in Table I, an extremely high incidence of folate and thiamin hypovitaminemia was noted in 71 and 53 % respectively, of pregnant subjects not ingesting supplemental vitamins. A similar relationship held for the neonates of these mothers, i.e., a high incidence of maternal hypovitaminemia gave rise to a high incidence of neonatal vitamin values that fell below the mean for this population. Mothers taking vitamins were not exempt from varying degrees of thiamin, folate, vitamins C, A, B_6, B_{12}, and nicotinate hypovitaminemia, but the incidence was lower than in mothers not ingesting vitamins. Vitamin values in neonates of mothers ingesting vitamins were almost always above the mean for the neonate population in contrast to neonates from mothers not ingesting vitamins [7]. Untreated hypovitaminemic mothers gave birth to infants with significantly depressed blood levels of vitamins B_{12}, B_6, and folate when compared with neonates of untreated normovitaminemic mothers [7].

Tab. I: Circulating vitamin levels in neonates born to 68 mothers without evidence of hypovitaminemia (95 % confidence limits)

Vitamin	Range with median
pg/ml	
Vitamin B_{12}	180–650–1 400
Biotin	525–810–1 436
ng/ml	
Folate	11– 33– 62
Thiamin	50– 84– 200
Vitamin B_6	24– 51– 84
Riboflavin	265–392– 660
Pantothenate	451–995–1 700
Vitamin A	180–250– 430
β-Carotene	110–220– 440
µg/ml	
Vitamin C	7– 13– 19
Vitamin E	1– 3– 6
Nicotinate	3.5–5.5– 10.0

There was an approximate 1:2–5 ratio of blood vitamins between mother and neonate; the same ratio held when maternal hypovitaminemia existed. Vitamins A, B_6, E, and β-carotene were exceptions; vitamin B_6 paralleled each other, while the vitamin E and β-carotene ratios were reversed in favor of the mother: 4:1 and 7:1, respectively. Vitamin A values were slightly higher on the maternal side; when evidence of maternal hypovitaminemia A was present, the ratio was almost 2:1 in favor of the mother [7].

Most vitamins cross the placenta and accumulate in the fetus at greater concentrations than in the mother [7]. However, as mentioned, when the mother had hypovitaminemia the infant values fell below the mean of the population indicating that a fetus can be born with hypovitaminemia due to maternal hypovitaminemia. Several great differences in titers of fat-soluble vitamin between mother and infant were noted; compared with the mother, the vitamin A, E, and β-carotene concentrations were lower in infant blood whereas the water-soluble vitamin levels were higher. Vitamin increases in the fetus have not been satisfactorily explained. Perhaps the fetus needs more vitamins because of its more rapid metabolism and thus draws on the maternal circulation for vitamins, or perhaps the fetal blood rather than tissues acts as a storage depot. There may be another explanation as shown in the cases of ascorbic acid and riboflavin [6, 7]. Ascorbic acid exists in blood as dehydroascorbic acid and L-ascorbic acid; the placenta is freely permeable to dehydroascorbic but not to ascorbic acid. The fetus is supplied with only dehydroascorbic acid which it then converts to ascorbic acid; ascorbic acid and not dehydroascorbic acid then accumulates in the fetus. Riboflavin transport is similar: flavin adenine dinucleotide is found in maternal blood: free riboflavin in fetal blood. The placenta can convert the dinucleotide to riboflavin. Possibly modifications may occur in molecular structure during transplacental passage or in fetal tissue which thereby alter the permeability to vitamins on either side of the placenta. Thus, altered vitamin structure may determine vitamin passage and retention in the fetus.

The maternal-to-neonate (M:N) vitamin ratio emerges as an important indicator for identifying aberrations in vitamin diffusion across the placenta. A reversal of the ratio may indicate a blockage in placental vitamin transport or an incompetent placenta [6, 7]. We have observed this in a small number of pregnant diabetics in whom the normal M:N thiamin ratio (1:4) was almost always reversed (3–4:1) [7]. Among the subjects not ingesting vitamins there was strikingly high percentage of folate hypovitaminemia (71%) which was reduced (29%) when folate-containing supplements were ingested [7]. It is indeed the most common vitamin deficiency in the United States especially during pregnancy and is the most frequently recognized cause of megaloblastic anemia of pregnancy and infancy. Prevention of folate deficiency is important for normal pregnancy in view of the sequelae folate deficits have on the fetus, e.g., fetal malformation and death, megaloblastic anemia in both mother and infant, and impairment in neonate brain function. All reports agree that pregnancy increases the requirements for folates, and probably all the other water-soluble vitamins. Maternal hypovitaminemia will therefore be exaggerated during pregnancy, especially if vitamin supplementation is denied or is too low in concentration to meet the demands of the pregnant woman and the fetus. Increased avidity for vitamins by the fetus may be contributory to maternal hypovitaminemia [7].

Children (10–13 Years Old)

Because there is remarkably little information on the nutritional status of populations of young school children coming from diverse socioeconomic backgrounds, we surveyed 642 school children between the ages of 10 and 13 [8]. The nutritional status, clinical evaluation, dietary histories, and family background information were all obtained by a questionnaire. Each of the 642 children was examined and was found to be in good health; 29 % stated that

Tab. II.: Circulating vitamins as compared with protein intake

Substance	Percent below mean of total population	
	dietary protein above 38 g	dietary protein below 38 g
Vitamins		
Biotin	57 (53)[1]	75 (74)
Thiamin	56 (53)	86 (75)
Vitamin C	46 (51)	82 (78)
Vitamin B_{12}	40 (54)	25 (65)
Vitamin A	53 (46)	38 (62)
β-Carotene	42 (43)	38 (55)
Pantothenic acid	43 (47)	25 (50)
Vitamin E	46 (49)	38 (57)
Riboflavin	44 (51)	52 (50)
Nicotinic acid	48 (51)	48 (45)
Vitamin B_6	42 (49)	57 (56)
Folic acid	52 (49)	50 (51)
Lipids		
Triglycerides	56 (60)	13 (16)
Cholesterol	50 (50)	57 (64)

[1] Figures outside parentheses represent percent below mean taking oral vitamins; figures in parantheses represent percent below mean taking no oral vitamins.

they received a multivitamin preparation at home. This population consisted of children from Chinese, Black, Caucasian, and Puerto Rican families; the latter group formed the greater majority.

In our study, protein nutriture was arbitrarily considered inadequate if the protein intake, derived from milk, fish, poultry, vegetables, and eggs, was below 38 g; this represents approximately four-fifths of the US National Research Council's recommended daily dietary allowance of protein. 12% of the population studied here had an intake of less than 38 g; in this group 92% were appraised as having no signs of malnutrition although their calculated protein intake was less than 38 g. «Clinical» nutritional evaluation, without laboratory evidence, thus emerges as a poor indicator of nutritional adequacy in the absence of overt signs of nutritional deficiencies. Table II compares the percentage of the total population falling below the median of a specific circulating vitamin with the intake of protein, fortified or not with various commercially available oral multivitamin preparations. Such results permitted evaluation of the influence of vitamin intake upon circulating vitamin titers during inadequate protein intake and allowed judgment as to which analyses best correlated with inadequate protein intake. The vitamin patterns for the various groups studied [8] are:

a) Puerto Rican. This group comprised approximately 65% of the population studied. The children tended to show lower levels of thiamin, nicotinic acid, and folate, and higher levels of biotin, pantothenate, and vitamin E than the total population. Lowered folate and nicotinic acid levels marked approximately 60% of this group. Their diets were high in fats, milk, and cheese, low in citrus fruits and meat.

b) Chinese. This group comprised approximately 15% of the study population, and provided the most extreme upward movement from the mean values of the population; 94% were above the thiamin mean, 81% above the ascorbic acid mean, and 71% above the folate mean. Vitamin B_6, nicotinic acid, and vitamin B_{12} levels were also much higher. The Chinese were, however, lower in vitamin A, β-carotene, pantothenate, riboflavin, and vitamin E. Their diets were low in milk and cheese but high in fish, fruits, vegetables, and rice; the latter, highly fortified with thiamin, may have contributed greatly to the high proportion of 94% in this population with a titer above the thiamin mean for the total population.

c) Black. This group was approximately 10% of the population. Eighty-two percent of this group had vitamin B_{12} values above the mean of the total population; their folate, vitamin A and vitamin E levels were also higher than the mean for the entire study population. Approximately 68% of the Black population fell below the total population mean in thiamin, biotin, and pantothenate. Their diets were high in meat but low in milk and cheese.

d) Caucasian. This group was approximately 8 % of the population. Between 61–66 % of this group had higher levels of pantothenate, vitamin B_6, vitamin A, and vitamin E; their riboflavin and β-carotene levels were somewhat lower than those of the total population. Their diets were high in fats, fruits and starch-containing vegetables but low in green and yellow vegetables.

From these results [8], it can be concluded that various population groups have distinctive patterns of vitamin nutriture. If a diet is not deficient in protein, then vitamin values will be approximately within 50 % above or below the mean for the total population. In contrast, a diet deficient in protein, as noted in 12 % of this population, elicited gross deviations from the mean in some vitamin patterns. Inadequate protein intake led 74, 75, and 78 % of this population (none taking supplemental oral vitamins) to fall below the mean of the total population in levels of biotin, thiamin and ascorbic acid, respectively; oral multivitamin supplements did not lower the percentage falling below the mean. The percentage falling below the mean for vitamin B_{12}, vitamin A, β-carotene, vitamin E, and pantothenate was reduced considerably when the diet was fortified with oral multivitamins, indicating that multivitamin therapy will raise the circulating levels of these vitamins in subjects with protein-deficient diets. The deviations noted above were not evident with dietary intake above 38 g of protein. The riboflavin, nicotinic acid, vitamin B_6, and folate levels were not markedly affected by inadequate protein intake, nor by oral supplemental vitamins. As already mentioned, thiamin, biotin, and ascorbate fell considerably below the mean for the total population despite supplemented vitamin ingestion, indicating that adequate protein nutriture must be maintained to permit these vitamin titers to stay within the mean for the total population studied. It thus emerges that the combination of extremely lowered biotin, thiamin and ascorbic acid levels forms part of the pattern common to inadequate protein intake.

Elderly

Some type of vitamin deficiency frequently occurs in hospitalized populations in the United States, and such deficiencies are especially conspicuous among the elderly. Vitamin deficits in older individuals may be more widespread than the few available surveys have indicated. In addition, long-term subclinical malnutrition may be cumulatively injurious to the elderly. In geriatric populations aging may change nutrient intake, increase the need for specific nutrients, and interfere with absorption, storage, and utilization of nutrients. Persons older than 60 are prone to disorders that lead to vitamin deficiencies.

Older persons may need supplemental vitamin B_6, vitamin B_{12}, vitamin C, thiamin, and folic acid to compensate for poor absorption of these vitamins. This malabsorption may be exacerbated by a low intake of iron, which results in the decreased absorption of folic acid and vitamin B_{12} and thereby contributes to nutritional anemia. Circulating levels of vitamin C, vitamin B_6, thiamin, vitamin B_{12}, folic acid and pantothenate are known to decline with increasing age, although the causes for this decline are not well understood. The elderly are also prone to conditions that lead to hepatic and biliary insufficiency consequently resulting in poor absorption of fat-soluble vitamins. Table III shows some responsible factors that lead to vitamin malabsorption in the elderly.

Folate deficiency occurs frequently in persons more than 70 years of age and may contribute to the prevalence of anemia in this age group. Folate deficits may be related to many factors, e.g. malnutrition, malutilization, and most importantly, folate malabsorption. Folate deficiency itself may produce malabsorption resulting in further folate depletion. The etiology of the folate deficit remains unclear, but several explanations have been suggested.

One such explanation is based on the decreased intestinal secretion of mucus found to be associated with aging. This decreased mucus secretion may

Tab. III: Etiology of vitamin malabsorption in the elderly

Mechanical interference
  Extirpative surgery
  Enteritis
  Malignancy
  Intestinal blind pouch

Steatorrhea
  Sprue syndromes
  Chronic pancreatitis
  Antibiotic therapy

Infestations

be accompanied by decreased secretion of enzyme, especially of intestinal folate conjugase (pteroylpolyglutamate hydrolase), a γ-carboxypeptidase. Folate conjugase, which is secreted primarily by the small-intestinal mucosa, deglutamylates (deconjugates) folylpolyglutamates present in food. Folylpolyglutamates cannot be absorbed until deconjugation to monoglutamates has occurred. Folate absorption then takes place preferentially in the proximal jejunum, the probable site of most conjugase activity. Depletion of folate conjugase would correspondingly diminish absorption of food folates (e.g., folylpolyglutamate), thereby inducing folate deficiency.

In one study, low folate levels were detected in 40% of 93 elderly patients [9]. In 30% of this group, dietary folate deficiency appeared to account for anemia. Other investigators noted subnormal folate values in two groups of hospitalized geriatric subjects [10]. The diet in the two hospitals was presumably satisfactory, and the reason for this finding was unclear. Some investigators who have reported similar observations have attributed the high incidence of low-to-deficient folate levels to poor folate intake despite an adequate diet. Our own study suggests an alternative explanation [11]. Absorption of folates, vitamin B_6, pantothenate, and riboflavin from a natural source (yeast) was studied in 24 elderly subjects (age range, 73 to 101 years) as compared with 12 healthy younger subjects (ages 24 to 42 years). All absorbed the yeast's riboflavin, vitamin B_6, and pantothenate. Ingested folylpolyglutamates (the preponderant folates in yeast) proved to be a poor source indeed of folates for the elderly subjects, whereas synthetic folylmonoglutamate was good [11]. This observation was subsequently confirmed in old animals [12]. In the younger subjects, yeast was a significant folate source. Evidently folate deficits, so common in the elderly, reflect impaired ability to secure folate from ingested foods. The resultant folate deficit may induce changes in the small-bowel epithelium and enzyme secretion, which may further exacerbate folate malabsorption. Folate deficiency, common in the 70 and over age group, may contribute to the prevalence of anemia in them.

As mentioned, our findings indicate that older persons tend to manifest an impaired ability to digest food folylpolyglutamates. This impairment would eventually lead to a folate deficit, even though the folate requirement could normally be satisfied by the folylpolyglutamates in foodstuffs, which usually suffice, as well as by synthetic folylpolyglutamate as a folate source. Thus, the nutritionally adequate diet may not constitute a sufficient folate source in the elderly.

We have also evaluated the patterns of circulating vitamins in 473 elderly persons older than 60 years of age living at home or in nursing homes [13]. These patterns were compared with those in 204 healthy younger subjects 20 to 50 years of age. A multiplicity of latent vitamin deficits was found that could lead to impairment of health if left untreated.

Circulating levels of biotin, pantothenate, riboflavin, vitamins A, B_6, B_{12}, C, and E, folate, thiamin, nicotinate, and the carotenes were determined in these groups of subjects. Levels of biotin, pantothenate, riboflavin, vitamin A, vitamin E, and the carotenes were normal in both institutionalized and non-institutionalized elderly subjects.

Blood levels of thiamin, vitamin C, and vitamin B_{12} were, however, strikingly depressed in the non-institutionalized elderly, as compared with the institutionalized elderly subjects and the younger controls. Vitamins B_6 and nicotinate deficiencies were detected in 30% of the institutionalized elderly subjects. Both the institutionalized and the non-institutionalized elderly subjects showed depressed blood levels of folate and vitamin B_{12}. Vitamin supplementation had no marked effect on these deficits. The vitamins found to be deficient in the institutionalized subjects were (in descending order of frequency): vitamin B_6, nicotinate, vitamin B_{12}, folate, thiamin, and ascorbate. The pattern in the non-institutionalized elderly was: vitamin B_{12}, thiamin, ascorbate, vitamin B_6, nicotinate, and folate. In the elderly population as a whole, vitamin B_6, nicotinate, and vitamin B_{12} deficiencies (in that order) were most commonly detected.

In this study [13], deficiencies of thiamin, ascorbate, vitamin B_6, nicotinate, folate, and vitamin B_{12} prevailed in a high proportion of the elderly. These deficits existed despite the supposedly excellent diet of the institutionalized subjects. Vitamin deficiencies and other nutritional deficits might be expected among the non-institutionalized elderly, who may have inadequate knowledge of good nutrition or whose living situation may restrict the availability of an adequate diet. We were surprised, however, to detect severe hypovitaminosis in such a high percentage of institutionalized subjects, despite diets that were considered adequate by conventional standards. The vitamin most lacking in the elderly population, as compared with younger controls, was vitamin B_6. Our study confirmed that aging is associated with depressed vitamin B_6 levels despite an apparently good diet.

Nicotinate levels in the elderly have not been extensively surveyed. Our results [13] indicate that circulating nicotinate levels are often severely reduced in the older age group. In addition to biochemical abnormalities induced by low levels of nicotinates involving the nicotinate coenzymes (e.g., nicotinamide adenine dinucleotides), which mediate cell redox systems, nicotinate deficits can also depress folate titers despite adequate dietary folate intake. As demonstrated in animals and in patients with pellagra, nicotinate deficits can cause anemia by disrupting the biosynthesis of folate enzymes and normal ferrokinetics. This explanation may account for some of the anemias seen in nicotinate-deficient elderly persons. In human nicotinate deficiency (pellagra), nicotinic acid treatment increases circulating folate and iron levels independent of dietary intake and causes hemoglo-

bin levels to increase to normal with the concomitant disappearance of anemia [13].

The close metabolic relationship between folates and vitamin B_{12} is
demonstrated by the similar changes in the hematopoietic system and
epithelial cells resulting from the blockade of deoxyribonucleic acid (DNA)
synthesis produced by either deficiency in humans. Vitamin B_{12} values in older
persons are significantly lower than in younger age groups and decrease with
advancing age. Like blood folate levels, vitamin B_{12} levels in our study were
severely depressed in the elderly.

Mental deterioration is associated with vitamin B_{12} deficiency, and some investigators believe the decline in vitamin B_{12} with age to be associated with
senile dementia. This relationship, however, has been refuted. Yet the
possibility of a vitamin B_{12} deficiency should be considered in elderly patients
with neurologic disorders, mental confusion, or dementia of unknown origin.
The presence of megaloblastic anemia is not always a useful indicator of
vitamin B_{12} deficiency. Laboratory determination of the vitamin B_{12} status is
more informative.

A decrease in vitamin-binding sites with age and a resultant compromise in
vitamin storage may explain why vitamin deficiency promptly occurs after
withdrawal of supplementation. This explanation would account for the increased circulating levels of vitamins observed during the administration of
supplements. When the constant source is withdrawn, insufficiency of vitamin
reserves becomes apparent, as evidenced by decreased levels of circulating
vitamins and signs of vitamin deficiency. The level of circulating vitamins in
the elderly can be increased by increasing dietary intake but because a decrease
in dietary vitamin intake or vitamin supplementation promptly produces
the vitamin deficit present before supplementation, this increase is only
temporary. Thus, if vitamin binding is compromised, vitamin stores
remain depleted. Because younger individuals retain adequate vitamin reserves as a result of the presence of sufficient vitamin-binding sites, vitamin deprivation has a much lesser effect on the young. The increased
vitamin needs in the elderly may reflect (at least in part) a decrease in vitamin binding.

In the case of some vitamins, continual supplementation or flooding of the
vitamin-receptor sites may be necessary in order to protect against
hypovitaminosis. We evaluated the intramuscular administration of a bolus of
vitamins as a means of avoiding vitamin malabsorption and drug antagonism
from any cause [14]. The bolus contained larger amounts of vitamins than the
oral vitamin preparations and could supposedly saturate vitamin-receptor
sites in the tissues. Saturated receptor sites would then permit vitamins to leak

into the circulation, thereby making the vitamins available whenever needed for coenzyme activity.

As mentioned previously, the administration of an oral vitamin preparation for three to five months did not permit adequate circulating vitamin levels to be maintained in the elderly. As a result, hypovitaminosis developed. A single intramuscular dose of 10 mg of thiamin hydrochloride, 10 mg of riboflavin, 80 mg of nicotinamide, 70 mg of pyridoxine hydrochloride, 23.2 mg of calcium pantothenate, 0.2 mg of biotin, 100 mg of ascorbic acid, 5 mg of folic acid, and 1.0 mg of vitamin B_{12}, however, restored adequate blood vitamin levels, which were maintained for at least three months. Three months after a single intramuscular multivitamin injection, vitamin deficits were no longer detectable in 89–100 % of vitamin-deficient elderly. Intramuscular rather than oral vitamin supplementation thus appears to be an effective method for maintaining adequate blood vitamin levels in the elderly. The intramuscular route apparently promotes saturation of tissue stores with enough vitamins to meet the needs of the patient and thus obviates problems of vitamin malabsorption possibly related to drug interference or small bowel atrophy. Thus, vitamin saturation by intramuscular administration of multivitamins ensures that the binding sites available do become saturated with a maximum concentration of vitamins without relying on rate-limited vitamin absorption by the oral route.

Results achieved with intramuscular administration of vitamins provide a plausible answer to the question raised earlier as to why hypovitaminosis and associated clinical symptoms may exist despite oral vitamin supplementation. The small amounts of vitamins absorbed from oral preparations may be insufficient to saturate depleted tissues. Consequently, vitamins are rapidly depleted after discontinuation of oral supplements. Oral vitamin supplementation may not suffice to obviate existing hypovitaminosis in the elderly. Intramuscular administration of vitamins appears to be the method of choice for maintaining adequate vitamin levels in the elderly, for correcting existing hypovitaminosis, and for preventing depressed circulating vitamin levels.

References

1 BAKER, H, FRANK, O: In: "Clinical vitaminology: methods and interpretation", pp 1–238. Wiley, New York, 1969.
2 SCRIVER, C R: Vitamin B_6 deficiency and dependency in man. Am J Dis Childh *113*, 109–114, 1967.
3 THOENE, J G *et al:* Impaired intestinal absorption of biotin in juvenile multiple carboxylase deficiency. N Engl J Med *308*, 639–642, 1983.

4 Nutritional Anemias. Wld Hlth Org Tech Report Ser, pp 405–432, WHO, Geneva, 1968.

5 Kaminetzky, H A, Baker, H: Micronutrients in pregnancy. Clin Obstet Gynecol 20, 363–380, 1977.

6 Baker, H et al: Role of placenta in maternal-fetal vitamin transfer in humans. Am J Obstet Gynecol 141, 792–796, 1981.

7 Baker, H et al.: Vitamin profile of 174 mothers and newborns at parturition. Am J Clin Nutr 28, 59–65, 1975.

8 Baker, H et al: Vitamins, total cholesterol and triglycerides in 642 New York City School children. Am J Clin Nutr 20, 850–857, 1967.

9 Morgan, A G et al: A nutritional survey in the elderly: haematological aspects. Int J Vit Nutr Res 43, 461–471, 1973.

10 Girdwood, R H et al: Folate status in the elderly. Br Med J 2, 670–672, 1967.

11 Baker, H et al: Severe impairment of dietary folate utilization in the elderly. J Am Geriatr Soc 26, 218–221, 1978.

12 Kesavan, V, Noronha, J M: Folate malabsorption in aged rats related to low levels of pancreatic folyl conjugase. Am J Clin Nutr 37, 262–267, 1983.

13 Baker, H et al: Vitamin profiles in elderly persons living at home or in nursing homes, versus profile in healthy young subjects. J Am Geriatr Soc 27, 444–450, 1979.

14 Baker, H et al: Oral versus intramuscular vitamin supplementation for hypovitaminosis in the elderly. J Am Geriatr Soc 28, 42–45, 1980.

Herman Baker, PhD, Professor of Preventive Medicine, Community Health and Medicine, UMDNJ – New Jersey Medical School, 100 Bergen Street, Newark, NJ 07103, USA
Oscar Frank, PhD, Professor of Medicine, UMDNJ – New Jersey Medical School, 100 Bergen Street, Newark, NJ 07103, USA

Concept of Borderline Vitamin Deficiencies

K. Pietrzik

Institute of Nutritional Science, Department of Pathophysiology of Human Nutrition,
University of Bonn, Bonn, West Germany

Key Words: Vitamin deficiency stages · Borderline deficiency · Functional parameters ·
Folate · Cell malformation

Abstract: Malnutrition is a serious problem all over the world. But the reported incidence especially of vitamin deficiency is contradictory even in homogeneous population groups. The reasons for these differences in the assessment of the nutritional status is to be found in the lack of objective criteria. In this paper the sequence of events in the development of deficiency is described as there are several physiological changes between the stages of optimum vitamin supply and manifest clinical nutrient deficiency.

At first there is a lowering of body vitamin content to be found in different tissues. The next stage is characterized by reduced synthesis of vitamin metabolites followed by a depressed activity of vitamin dependent enzymes and hormones. The transit to the fourth step – characterized by morphological or functional disturbances – should no longer be ignored as it is important to prevent people from clinical symptoms (fifth stage) leading finally to death. From the health point of view the borderline vitamin deficiency is proposed to be represented by the transit from the third to the fourth stage.

With folate as an example it is demonstrated how to proceed in the establishment of biologically based functional parameters for the assessment of borderline deficiency. In this case morphological disturbances (hypersegmentation of neutrophilic granulocytes) are taken to characterize the borderline.

Introduction

Malnutrition is one of the most serious health problems all over the world. The problem of protein and energy malnutrition is very well known. Besides these the insufficient intake of vitamins, minerals and trace elements have not to be ignored any longer. Because there are many physiological changes between the stages of optimum nutrition and manifest nutrient deficiency, the reported incidence of nutrient deficiency varies widely. Especially the frequency of vitamin deficiency is absolutely contradictory even in homogeneous population groups [1].

The reason for these differences in estimating the vitamin status is often to be found in the lack of objective criteria. Since it is well recognized that some period of depletion of body stores precedes the manifestation of classical clinical symptoms of nutrient deficiency, nutritionists have elaborated sensitive diagnostic tests indicating different stages of deficiency. The problem to be solved in this context is to find out, up to which stage of vitamin depletion there is a physiological and biochemical adaptation. These events in the development of vitamin deficiency generally are of no concern in a healthy person. But, from the health point of view, it is important to know the *borderline* indicating the transit to pathophysiological symptoms of vitamin deficiency.

Sequence of Events in Vitamin Deficiency

The depletion for vitamin nutrients is a gradual process illustrated in Figure 1. An optimum vitamin intake in the amount of the RDA guarantees optimal health. In this context, for example, it guarantees mental and physical activity and immune resistence etc. Depending on the duration of severity of a deficiency, different stages of depletion will finally result in maximum disturbances, well known as the severe classical symptoms of vitamin deficiency diseases, leading to irreversible tissue damage and finally to death.

This pattern is not only valid for vitamins but for other essential nutrients as well. According to BRUBACHER [2] the questions to be answered are, on the one hand: What is the desirable level of nutrients or their metabolites or what is the activity of nutrient-dependent enzymes corresponding to optimal nutrient body stores? On the other hand it is also important to know the nutrient levels and their metabolites and nutrient dependent enzyme activities corresponding to the first metabolic, morphological or functional disturbances. From the health point of view, these early disturbances should no longer be ignored because, for example, in this case vitamin-dependent enzymes or hormones are reduced leading to unspecific symptoms related to mental behaviour.

From the practical point of view it is of less importance to know the statistic indices of vitamin levels based on a comparison with mean values of a healthy reference group. What is required are biologically and functionally based indicators of nutritional status as diagnostic tests to determine the efficiency of the whole organism to permit cells, tissues, organs and other systems to per-

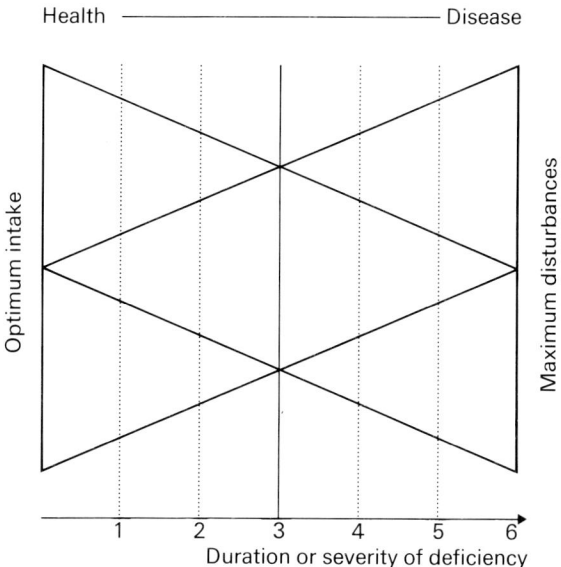

Fig. 1: Different stages of nutrient deficiency and the development of disturbances.

form optimally the intended, vitamin-dependent characteristical function. In this context cut-off points are needed indicating different stages of vitamin deficiency. In practical terms a borderline must be indicated to distinguish harmless physiological and biochemical changes from those relevant to the health point of view.

In Figure 2 the sequence of events in vitamin deficiency is shown. The nomenclature for the different deficiency stages has been given according to the literature [3-6]. It has been attempted on an international basis to standardize the nomenclature of the different deficiency stages. But till today, there is a lot of confusion in this regard and terms as suboptimal, marginal, subclinical, deficient etc. are often used synonymously. So long as there will be no standardization in nomenclature a detailed description of the pathophysiological events is needed in any case, otherwise the different results can never be compared with each other.

For practical purposes it might be helpful to objectify and simplify the nomenclature. That's why only three stages of vitamin deficiency (prelatent, latent, manifest) are listed additionally in Figure 2. The pathophysiological meaning of these three terms is summarized as well.

But to demonstrate all the different events in the development of a vitamin deficiency, at least six stages can be subdivided (Fig. 3). In this context it must be taken into account that our present knowledge of nutrition is insuffi-

Stage	Brin (3, 4)	Brubacher (5, 6)	Proposed simplified classification	Pathophysiological meaning
1	preliminary	} latent	prelatent	(lowering of vitamin concentrations in different tissues)
2	biochemical			
3	physiological	subclinical	latent	(lowering of metabolites and enzyme activity)
4	clinical	marginal	manifest	morphological and/or functional disturbances { subclinical symptoms / clinical symptoms
5	anatomical	} manifest		
6				

Fig. 2: Vitamin deficiency stages.

cient to define clear cut-off points for all stages in the case of each vitamin.

In the *first stage* of deficiency body stores are progressively depleted. This can be demonstrated by estimation of the vitamin concentration in certain tissues, for example blood. In this stage the decreased vitamin excretion in the urine is often regarded as the first sign. Though the supply of an essential nutrient becomes limited, the homeostatic regulation guarantees in a very early stage of deficiency «normal» blood levels.

In the *second stage* of depletion the urinary excretion of vitamin drops and vitamin concentrations in the blood and other body tissues are generally impaired. In this stage a diminished concentration of vitamin metabolites might be observed as well.

In a healthy person the first two stages are regarded not to be a problem as long as the vitamin supply and the requirement remain constant. But in the case of diseases (when the requirement increases), or if the supply drops, the following stages of deficiency will emerge.

Generally the *third stage* is characterized by a measurable diminished activity of vitamin-dependent enzymes. In some cases hormone concentrations might be reduced and physiological alterations may be observed. Unspecific symptoms such as general malaise, insomnia, loss of appetite, and other mental changes are the result of the continuous depletion of vitamin stores. Though immune response is reduced specific clinical manifestations are still absent. In case of limited vitamin intake this stage may be maintained over longer periods, but in case of extreme physiological or pathological conditions clinical signs will rapidly develop.

In the *fourth stage* the biological and physiological symptoms become more

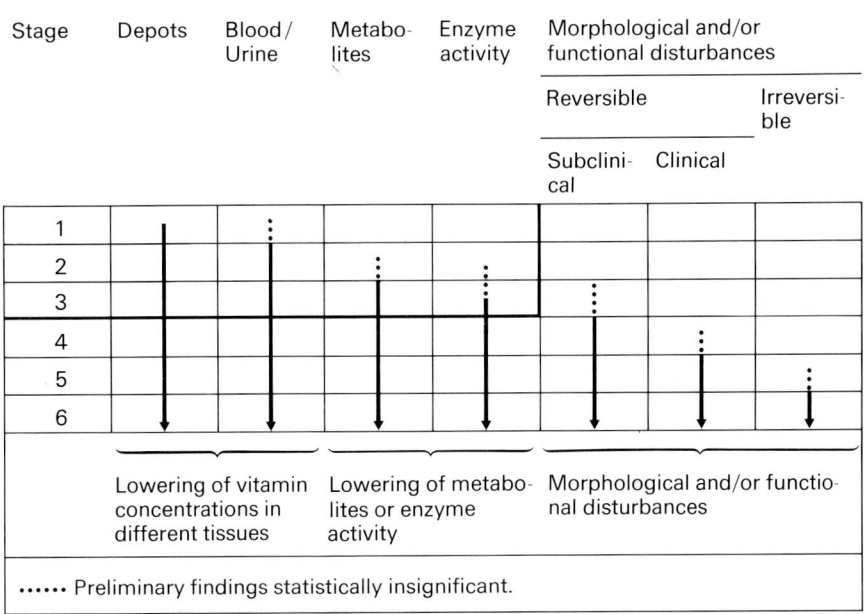

Stage	Depots	Blood/ Urine	Metabolites	Enzyme activity	Morphological and/or functional disturbances		
					Reversible		Irreversible
					Subclinical	Clinical	
1							
2							
3							
4							
5							
6							

Lowering of vitamin concentrations in different tissues · Lowering of metabolites or enzyme activity · Morphological and/or functional disturbances

•••••• Preliminary findings statistically insignificant.

Fig. 3: Sequence of events in vitamin deficiency.

severe exceeding the normal physiological deviation. Apart from that morphological or functional *disturbances* are observed. These disturbances might be corrected either by vitamin application in therapeutic amounts within a relatively short time or vitamin supplementation in the amount of (or exceeding) the recommended dietary allowances over a longer period. The time for the correction of the morphological disturbances depends on the life time of the cell system affected as malformation of cells is reversible in this stage.

Finally, in the *fifth stage* the classical clinical symptoms of vitamin deficiency will appear. Anatomical alterations characterized by reversible damage of tissues might be cured in general by hospitalization of the patients. In this stage, generally there is no selective deficiency of specific nutrients, in most cases there are deficiencies of several nutrients and a complicated dietetic and therapeutic regimen has to be followed.

If the deficiency stage continues or in the case of insufficient therapeutic supply the morphological and functional disturbances will become irreversible, finally leading to death.

Definition of Borderline Vitamin Deficiency

Knowing the sequence of events in vitamin deficiency one can imagine that from the health point of view, the third stage of deficiency should no longer be ignored, as extreme physiological situations or pathological conditions will rapidly lead to clinical symptoms and the vitamin deficiency will become manifest.

For practical purposes it is important to know a biologically based borderline to objectify a critical vitamin supply situation and to prevent people developing severe deficiency symptoms. In so far, the *transit from the third to the fourth stage has to be regarded as the borderline* in vitamin deficiency. In any case the third stage of vitamin deficiency is characterized by low levels of vitamins in blood, urine and tissues and by a low activity of vitamin dependent enzymes, metabolites or hormones, whereas in the fourth stage, besides these biochemical parameters, there is an impairment of metabolic or physiological functions leading to pathophysiological disturbances often combined with morphological changes. This border is not a fixed line, it surely depends on our actual knowledge of vitamin deficiency symptoms and their relationships to health. This means that in case of increasing knowledge of vitamin related health problems the border may shift to an upper stage. Obviously there is an essential need to objectify functional parameters for the assessment of the nutritional status indicating this borderline.

Assessment of Borderline on Example of Folate

With folate as an example it is demonstrated on the basis of our own findings how to establish the biologically based borderline for this vitamin. According to the literature it is very well known that the reported incidence of folate deficiency varies widely. On the one hand, folate deficiency is regarded to be the most common hypovitaminosis not only in developing countries, but throughout the world [7, 8]. On the other hand, there are numerous reports and reviews stating the folate status on the average to be acceptable. Only pregnant, or lactating women or chronic alcoholics should be regarded as vulnerable groups [9–11].

The reason for these differences in estimating the folate status is to be found in the lack of objective criteria. Generally, serum folate concentrations are taken for the estimation of the nutritional status and the so called «normal values» are based on mean values of the healthy «reference» population, and the deviation from these values is to be diagnosed as deficient. Moreover, there is no generally accepted guideline for normal serum folate levels. The lowest limit of the «normal» range to be found in the literature is 7 nmol/l and the highest limit reported in the literature is about 14 nmol/l. As serum levels are actually influenced by diet, this parameter is not a satisfactory indicator for the assessment of the nutritional status.

The problems concerning the interpretation of the blood folate levels are indicated in Figure 4. Serum folate levels of 250 persons are summarized in a logit log scale. Basing on the «normal values» with a range from 7 to 14 nmol/l the serum folate level alone has little clinical usefulness as a diagnostic test, particularly because the majority of the tested group has serum levels just in this range of critical clinical importance. If one is taking the lowest limit of the «normal» range only about 10% of the tested group are in a deficiency status. On the other hand, nearly 45% are in a deficiency range utilizing the highest limit of the «normal» range.

Because of this contrary classification it would be helpful to have a more direct estimation of the vitamin supply. In this context functional or morphological parameters have several potential advantages over statistic indices. As a result of the pioneering studies of Herbert [12] the sequence of biochemical and haematological events in the development of folate deficiency in man is known. We consider the neutrophilic segmentation as a biologically based indicator of folate deficiency in order to obtain a critical basis for an objective evaluation of the borderline, as morphological disturbances characterize the transit from the third to the fourth stage of deficiency.

The serum folate level may be influenced by changes in intake by way of diet. We could therefore expect that careful observation of the peripheral blood films for hypersegmentation would allow the early detection of folate deficiency long before the development of the more severe later changes. With this consideration in mind, it could be demonstrated that groups with relatively high mean values of serum folate levels (20 nmol/l, 14 nmol/l and 10 nmol/l) do not differ significantly in the segmentation of the neutrophilic granulocytes. The mean lobe average was calculated with 3.2. This means, that these different mean values down to 10 nmol/l are not combined with any morphological alterations.

But on the other hand, serum levels < 10 nmol/l correspond with an increasing lobe average indicative for an insufficient vitamin intake. And serum levels < 8 nmol/l differ significantly in neutrophilic hypersegmentation with a mean lobe value of > 3.6.

In Figure 5 the close correlation between low blood folate levels and neutrophilic hypersegmentation and vice versa is demonstrated.

Our studies indicate that hypersegmentation is associated with a low serum

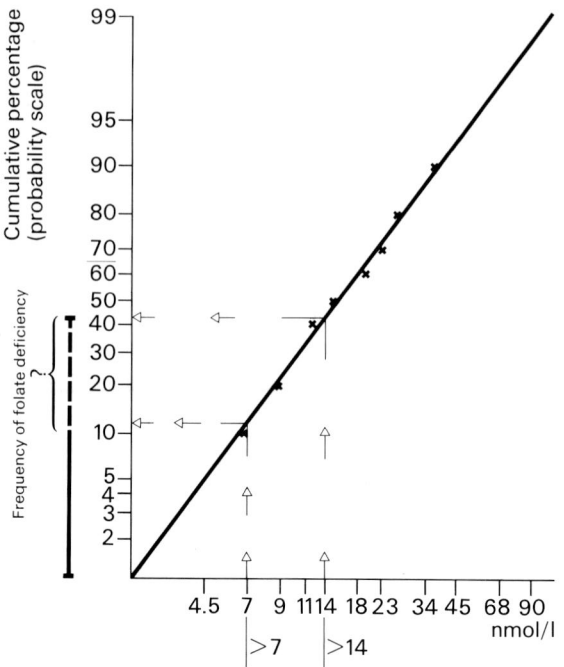

Fig. 4: Graphic analysis of means of 250 serum folate concentrations.

folate level in nearly all cases. Our results show that a serum folate concentration of > 10 nmol/l reflects a good folate status. On the other hand, an average lobe index of > 3.6 corresponds with serum levels indicating an incipient deficiency status.

According to these findings a serum folate level < 10 nmol/l has to be regarded as an early symptom in the development of folate deficiency. Serum levels lower than 8 nmol/l correspond with hypersegmentation and reflect the borderline deficiency.

In order to verify these criteria for the evaluation of the nutritional status of folate, we determined the serum folate and the erythrocytic folate concentration in an independent other group of volunteers.

As mentioned above, the serum folate level is actually influenced by diet and biological interactions. Because of this it is recommended to measure instead the erythrocytic folate level, measured instead, as this is thought to be a more accurate reflection of tissue folate levels. It has been established that a decreased red cell folate level, even in the face of high serum folate levels (actual fluctuation) is a more reliable parameter indicating folate depletion of the body.

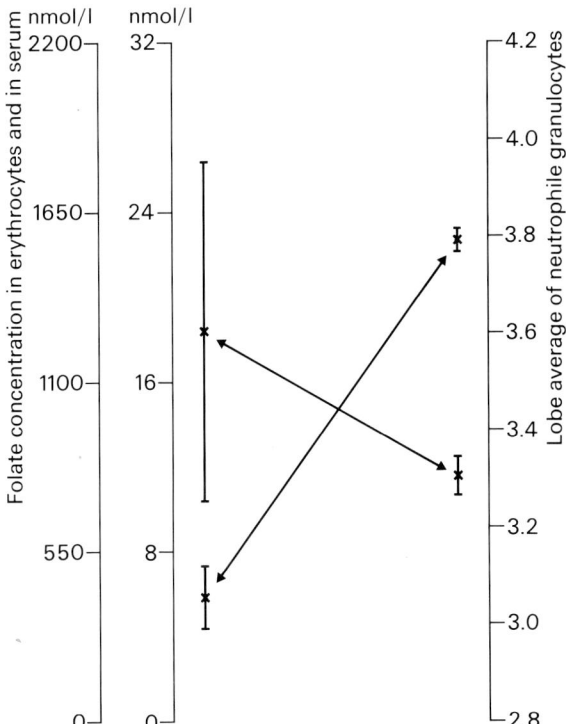

Fig. 5: Correlation between folate tissue concentration and morphological findings.

Our results demonstrate that decreasing erythrocytic folate levels of < 700 nmol/l are closely correlated with an increasing lobe average of > 3.2. Erythrocytic folate concentrations of < 550 nmol/l correspond highly significant with hypersegmentation of neutrophilic granulocytes exceeding 3.6 lobes in the average. We therefore suggest that the red cell folate levels of < 550 nmol/l as well as hypersegmentation (> 3.6) generally have to be regarded as an indicator of an insufficient folate status with a high risk of developing manifest megaloblastic anaemia [further details see 13–16].

Regarding these biologically based data as stated above it could be demonstrated that in the population group tested (250 apparently healthy industrial workers in West Germany) nearly 20% showed folate deficiency in a relatively progressed stage (fourth stage / morphological disturbances). According to the simplified nomenclature (see Fig. 2) this stage is termed «manifest folate deficiency» (Fig. 6). Another 10% showed a folate deficiency status marking the beginning of vitamin depletion. This indicates that

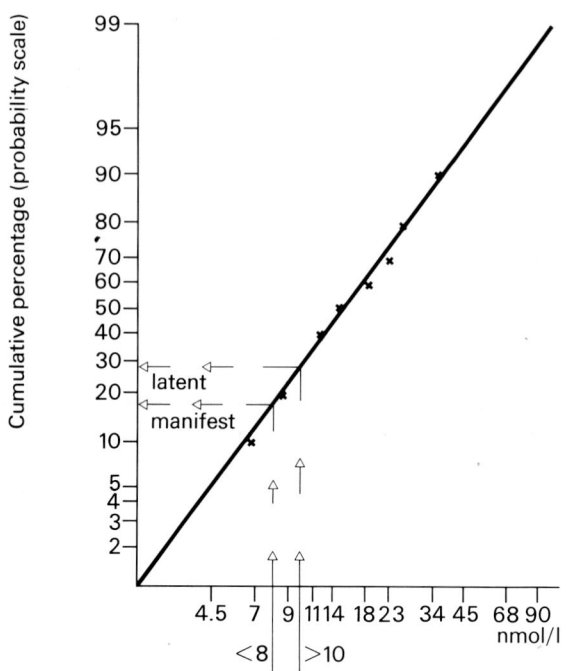

Fig. 6: Graphic analysis of means of 250 serum folate concentrations.

borderline vitamin deficiency is not only a problem in the population of developing countries but even in people in industrialized areas.

Moreover, it must be taken into account that hypersegmentation may be influenced by vitamin B_{12} deficiency as well. But cobalamin deficiency is a relatively seldom hypovitaminosis and if suspected (for example in the case of vegetarism, in chronic alcoholics or lack of intrinsic factor) vitamin B_{12} dependent deficiency symptoms should not be neglected.

Finally, the borderline based on hypersegmentation of neutrophilic granulocytes is only valid for healthy persons as in the case of infections the hypersegmentation is overlapped by unsegmented young neutrophilic cells coming directly from the bone marrow into the blood stream.

But for the estimation of a borderline folate deficiency in healthy persons the morphological changes in neutrophilic cells are regarded as a very useful biological indicator. The other events in the development of folate deficiency are summarized in Figure 7. It must be taken into account that in practice the sequence is dependent on analytical methodology (radioimmunoassay or microbiological methods), performance of loading tests (FIGLU), and tested tissue (cell malformation in bone marrow or peripheral blood films). Each

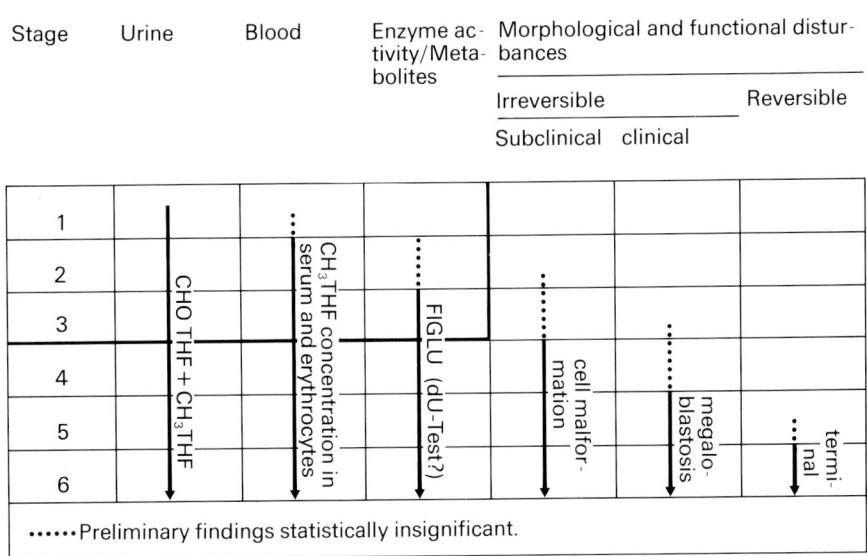

Fig. 7: Sequence of events in folate deficiency. CHO THF = Formyltetrahydrofolate
CH_3 THF = methyltetrahydrofolate; FIGLU = formiminoglutamic acid.

laboratory engaged in the assessment of borderlines has exactly to define its morphological or functional cut-off points to establish a clear basis for the comparison of results.

In one of our recent studies we set up the *different cut-off points* for blood folate levels estimated by *different commercial radioassays*. It could be demonstrated that in the case of method-adapted borderlines (concentrations) based on biological parameters (hypersegmentation) comparable results concerning the frequency of folate deficiency could be obtained [17, 18].

Concluding Remarks

In future there seems to be an obvious need to expand research in the field of functional assessment of nutritional status for up to this day a lot of the cut-off-points suggested as indicative of the borderline are simply based on the mean concentration of a given nutrient or on an individual biochemical parameter of a «reference» group.

Solomon *et al* [19] give a classification of functional indices of nutritional status as well as functional methods for appraising the nutritional status. Based on these biological parameters it might be possible to define objective borderlines not only for vitamins but for other nutrients as well.

The observations concerning the sequence of events in developing vitamin deficiency symptoms may change from time to time. Though there are many physiological changes between optimum nutrition and manifest nutrient deficiencies the assessment of borderlines indicating critical vitamin deficiency in a population group is of great importance to public health.

References

1 Ernährungsbericht 1980. Deutsche Gesellschaft für Ernährung e V, Frankfurt, 1980.
2 BRUBACHER, G et al: Borderline vitamin deficiency and the assessment of vitamin status in man. Ernährung/Nutrition 3, 4-9, 1979.
3 BRIN, M: Erythrocyte as a biopsy tissue for functional evaluation of thiamine adequacy. Am Med Ass 18, 762-766, 1964.
4 BRIN, M: Dilemma of marginal vitamin deficiency. Proc 9th Int Congr Nutr, Mexico 1972, vol. 4, pp 102-115. Karger, Basel 1975.
5 BRUBACHER, G: The notion of borderline vitamin deficiency. Vitamin Symposium, Greek Soc Nutr Food, Athens, May 1983.
6 BRUBACHER, G: Was versteht man unter subklinischem Vitaminmangel? In: SCHLIERF and WOLFRAM (eds) "Mangelernährung in Mitteleuropa". Wissenschaftliche Verlagsgesellschaft, Stuttgart, 1982.
7 KITAY, D Z et al: Neutrophil hypersegmentation and folic acid deficiency in pregnancy. Am J Obstet Gynec 104, 1163-1173, 1969.
8 HOFFBRAND, A V: The role of malabsorption in the development of folate deficiency. Clin Med 19, 19-22, 1972.
9 HIBBARD, B M, HIBBARD, E D: Neutrophil hypersegmentation and defective folate metabolism in pregnancy. J Obstet Gynaecol Brit Com 78, 776-780, 1971.
10 HIBBARD, B M, HIBBARD, E D: Anemia and folate status in late pregnancy in a mixed Asiatic population. J Obstet Gynaecol Brit Com 79, 584-591, 1972.
11 ROETZ, R, MERKER, H J: Zur Bedeutung der Folsäure für Schwangerschaft und Entwicklung des Menschen. Therapie Woche 22, 255, 1972.
12 HERBERT, V: Experimental nutritional folate deficiency in man. Trans Ass Am Phys 75, 307-320, 1962.
13 URBAN, G: Die Beurteilung der Folatversorgung verschiedener Bevölkerungsgruppen anhand biochemischer und haematologischer Messgrössen unter gleichzeitiger Berücksichtigung der Cobalamin- und Eisenversorgung. Thesis. Department of Agriculture, University of Bonn, 1980.
14 PIETRZIK, K et al: Biochemische und haematologische Massstäbe zur Beurteilung des Folatstatus beim Menschen. 1. Mitteilung: Beziehung zwischen Serumfolat und Segmentation der neutrophilen Granulozyten. Int J Vit Nutr Res 48, 391-396, 1978.
15 PIETRZIK, K et al: Biochemische und haematologische Massstäbe zur Beurteilung des Folatstatus beim Menschen. 2. Mitteilung: Vergleichende Messungen von Folat im Serum und in Erythrocyten. Int J Vit Nutr Res 48, 397-401, 1978.
16 PIETRZIK, K et al: Biochemische und haematologische Massstäbe zur Beurteilung des Folatstatus beim Menschen. 3. Mitteilung: Bedeutung der Formiminoglutaminsäureausscheidung im Urin im Vergleich zu anderen Messgrössen. Int J Vit Nutr Res 50, 261-266, 1980.
17 HÜMMELER, M, PIETRZIK, K: Angleichung der Beurteilungsmassstäbe für verschiedene Radioassays zur Folatbestimmung im Serum. Ernährungsumschau 30, 223, 1983.

18 HÜMMELER, M, PIETRZIK, K: Folate concentration in serum and erythrocytes estimated by different commercial radioassays - criterions to objectify borderlines. IV. European Nutrition Conference, Amsterdam, 1983.
19 SOLOMONS, N W, LINDSAY, H A: The functional assessment of nutritional status: principles and potential. Nutr Rev *41,* 33-50, 1983.

Prof. Dr. K. Pietrzik, Institut für Ernährungswissenschaft, Endenicher Allee 11-13, D-5300 Bonn, West Germany

Vitamin A Deficiency as a Factor in Nutritional Anemia

L.A. Mejía

Division of Nutrition and Health, Institute of Nutrition of Central America and Panama, Guatemala City, Guatemala

Key Words: Hypovitaminosis A · Anemia · Iron deficiency · Vitamin A · Iron interaction · Hematopoiesis · Vitamin A fortification

Abstract: Epidemiological and experimental studies in both humans and laboratory animals suggest that lack of vitamin A may be a contributing factor in the etiology of nutritional anemia. Human subjects depleted of vitamin A develop anemia which does not respond to iron treatment until their vitamin A status is improved. Chronic vitamin A deficiency in the rat also leads to anemia characterized by low levels of serum iron and elevated amounts of this mineral in the liver and spleen. The incorporation of radioactive iron (^{59}Fe) into erythrocytes is also diminished. Furthermore, preschool children with low serum retinol levels may have low levels of serum iron and a high concentration of serum ferritin. The short-term effect of improving their vitamin A status – for example, through sugar fortification with retinyl palmitate – is a decrease in serum ferritin and a significant elevation in serum iron, percent saturation of transferrin and total iron binding capacity. The available data indicate that there is a biological interaction between vitamin A deficiency and iron nutrition and metabolism.

Effect of Vitamin A on Hematopoiesis and Iron Metabolism

The existing reports on the effect of hypovitaminosis A on hematopoiesis reveal two lines of contrasting evidence. On the one hand the occurrence of anemia and on the other of polycythemia. Early reports of hematopoietic changes associated with vitamin A deficiency in either human, experimental animals or both, have appeared since 1922. Anemia was found to be associated with vitamin A deficiency by a variety of authors [1–9]. In contrast, other researchers observed elevated levels of hemoglobin and hematocrit [10–15]. All these early findings have been reviewed and discussed by Hodges et al [16], and there is now data available which may explain this discrepancy.

Recent Studies

In 1978 Hodges *et al* [16] reported an experiment in which vitamin A deficiency was induced by feeding diets deficient or low in vitamin A to eight middle-aged men who voluntarily participated. As expected, the concentration of serum carotene fell rapidly and the concentration of retinol fell slowly during the vitamin A depletion which varied in the different subjects from 359 to 771 days. Despite a daily intake of 18–19 mg of iron in their diet, the men gradually began to manifest a mild degree of anemia accompanied by low serum iron levels. It was observed that during the depletion period there was a simultaneous drop in the levels of both vitamin A and hemoglobin (Fig. 1). When the anemia became manifest, oral medicinal iron (310 mg/day) was given. It turned out that the iron treatment had little or no effect as long as there was a vitamin A deficiency. The subject presented in Figure 1 responded transiently to medicinal iron, but relapsed despite continued therapy. Soon after vitamin A repletion was started with β-carotene, he made a prompt and complete hematological recovery while continuing the same diet.

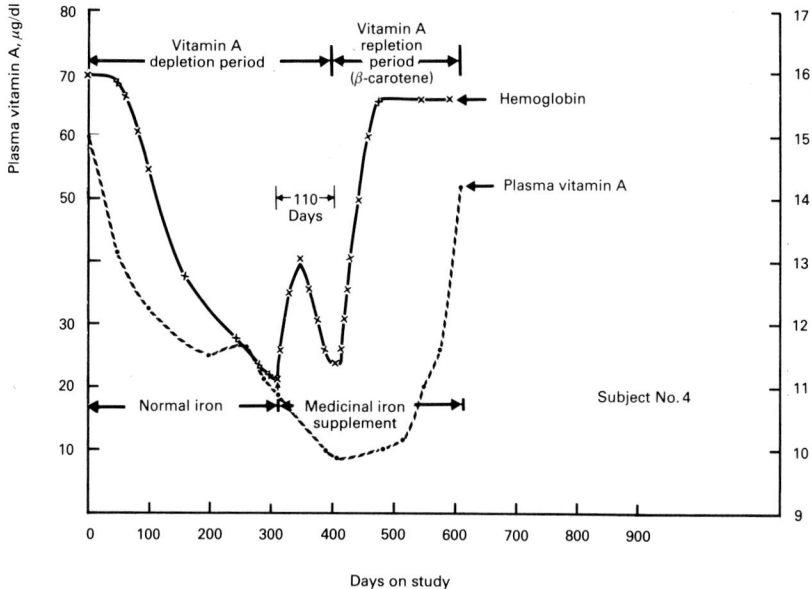

Fig. 1: Effect of vitamin A and iron supplements on plasma vitamin A and hemoglobin levels in a vitamin A depleted human volunteer [16].

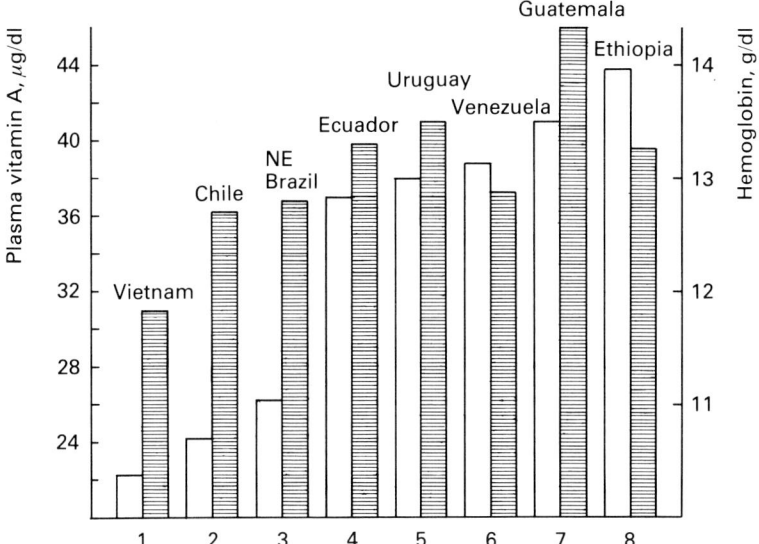

Fig. 2: Relationship of hemoglobin and plasma vitamin A as observed in several ICNND nutrition surveys (non-pregnant, non-lactating females 15–45 years of age) [16].

From the epidemiologic point of view it can be demonstrated not only that vitamin A deficiency and anemia coexist in some populations, but also that there is a significant association between plasma vitamin A and hemoglobin. This is demonstrated in Figure 2, showing a comparison between vitamin A and hemoglobin levels in a selected group of non-pregnant, non lactating females of reproductive age surveyed several years ago in several countries by the Interdepartmental Committe on Nutrition for National Defense (ICNND). In the countries examined, women with low vitamin A levels also had low hemoglobin values. In contrast, countries reporting higher vitamin A levels also showed higher hemoglobin levels.

In the Central American region, MEJÍA *et al* [17] have found significant correlations between plasma retinol and serum iron (Fig. 3). Children with low plasma retinol have low serum iron levels and those with high plasma retinol have high serum levels of iron. These correlations have been confirmed both in Indian children [18, 19] and in a group of elderly persons in Vienna [20].

Experimental animal studies have also shown that anemia may result from a lack of vitamin A [16, 21]. As illustrated in Figure 4, after approximately 40 days of feeding a vitamin A free diet to young adult rats, they exhibited lower hematocrit or hemoglobin levels than the control groups. At around 90 days, however, hematocrit and hemoglobin levels increased even reaching higher levels than those observed in the control groups. Isotopic dilution studies have

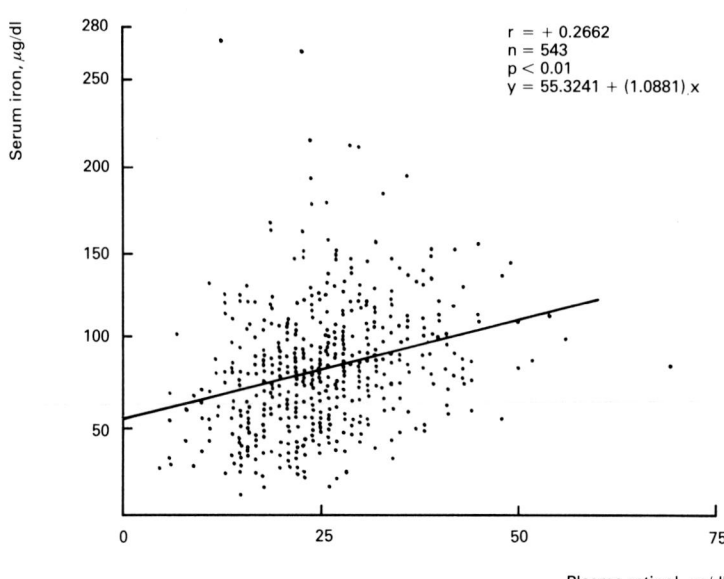

Fig. 3: Plasma levels of retinol versus serum iron in rural Central American children with
iron intake ≥ 12 mg/day [17].

shown that this phenomenon is due to a reduction in blood and plasma
volume which occurs when the vitamin deficiency becomes severe [22]. At this
stage, the anemia is masked by hemoconcentration. This may be the reason
why several investigators have failed to observe anemia in hypovitaminosis A.
When the anemia developed, these animals also showed a reduction in serum
iron and a concomitant elevation of the amount of iron in the liver. As illustrated in Figure 5 the concentration of liver iron began to increase in these
animals at approximately the same time when hematocrit levels became lower
than normal. Spleen iron also increased when the deficiency became severe.

These findings are supported by the radioisotope data presented in Table I
which shows a greater incorporation of ^{59}Fe in the liver and spleen of the
vitamin A deficient rats as compared with the control group [22]. All these
data indicate that in hypovitaminosis A there is a shifting of body iron
resulting in an elevation of iron stores and a decrease in plasma iron. Thus
iron becomes less available to the erythropoietic tissue for red cell formation.
In addition, it has been also demonstrated that in vitamin A deficient rats,
there is a lower incorporation of ^{59}Fe into erythrocytes, suggesting that in
vitamin A deficiency iron utilization for red cell formation is also impaired
[22].

Tab. I: Absorption of ^{59}Fe and specific activities of liver and spleen in experimental rats [22]

	Absorption, %	Specific activity, C/g tissue	
		liver	spleen
Control	43.9 ± 14.6^{a1}	242 ± 22.4^{a}	533 ± 97.2^{a}
Pair-fed	12.0 ± 12.8^{b}	180 ± 18.1^{a}	280 ± 77.3^{b}
Deficient	38.3 ± 6.7^{a}	552 ± 85.4^{b}	1217 ± 185.0^{b}

[1] Means $\pm$ SEM. Means with differing superscripts are significant
at $p < 0.005$.

Effect of Vitamin A Fortification

In Central America, nutrition surveys have revealed a high prevalence of hypovitaminosis A. Children in this region of the world have a low vitamin A intake, and the prevalence of serum retinol levels less than 20 µg/dl in rural children varied in the six countries from approximately 20 % in Nicaragua to 50 % in El Salvador. In an attempt to overcome this nutritional problem of the area, the Institute of Nutrition of Central America and Panama (INCAP) began a national vitamin A fortification program in Guatemala at the end of

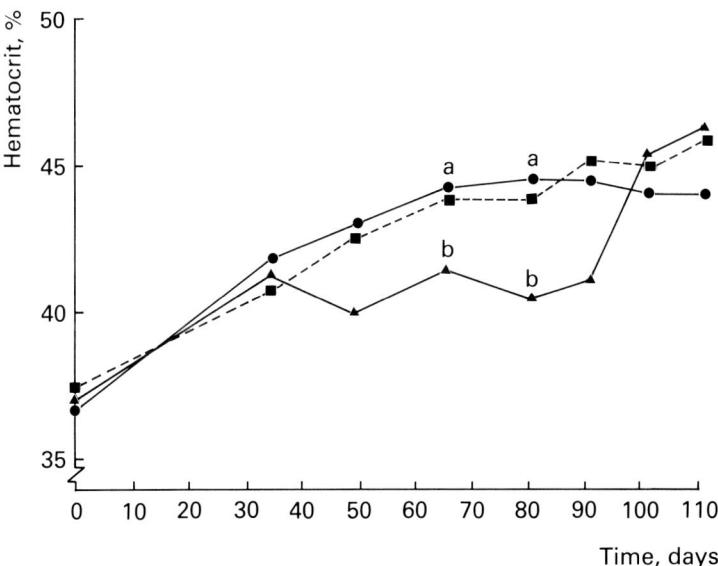

Fig. 4: Changes in the levels of hematocrit during depletion of vitamin A in the young adult rat [21]. Points bearing different superscript letters are significantly different at $p < 0.05$.
● = Control; ■ = pair-fed; ▲ = deficient.

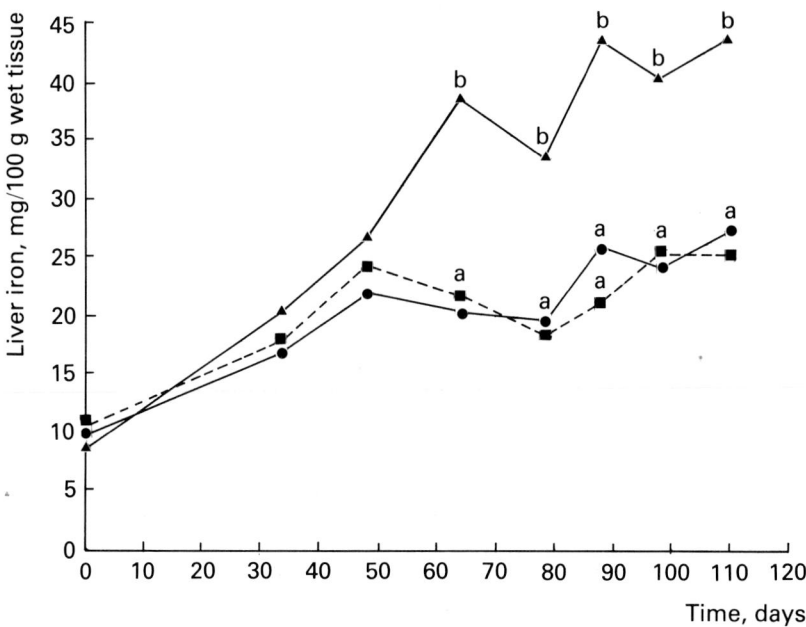

Fig. 5: Levels of iron in liver tissue of the young adult rat during depletion of vitamin A [21].
Points bearing different superscript letters are significantly different at $p < 0.05$.
● = Control; ■ = pair-fed; ▲ = deficient.

1975 using table sugar as the dietary vehicle. The concentration used was 15μg retinol equivalent (RE)/g sugar. The experimental design and methodology of this program and its evaluation have been published previously [23]. In summary, preschool children and lactating mothers from 12 small rural communities were studied for two years in five consecutive surveys; one prior to vitamin A fortification (Survey I), and four additional ones (Surveys II–V), at six month intervals after the intervention began. The dietary data revealed that in comparison with the pre-fortification survey, the implementation of sugar fortification resulted in a significant three-fold increase in the average daily intake of RE. As a result, there has been a highly significant reduction in the prevalence of low and deficient serum retinol levels in children. Similar results have been obtained in breast milk of lactating mothers. The average intake of iron, however, did not change throughout the two-year period of evaluation. This vitamin A program provided a unique opportunity to evaluate the effect of this single intervention on iron nutrition and metabolism at the population level. The results showed that vitamin A fortification alone had a positive effect on the iron nutriture of this population [24]. Figure 6

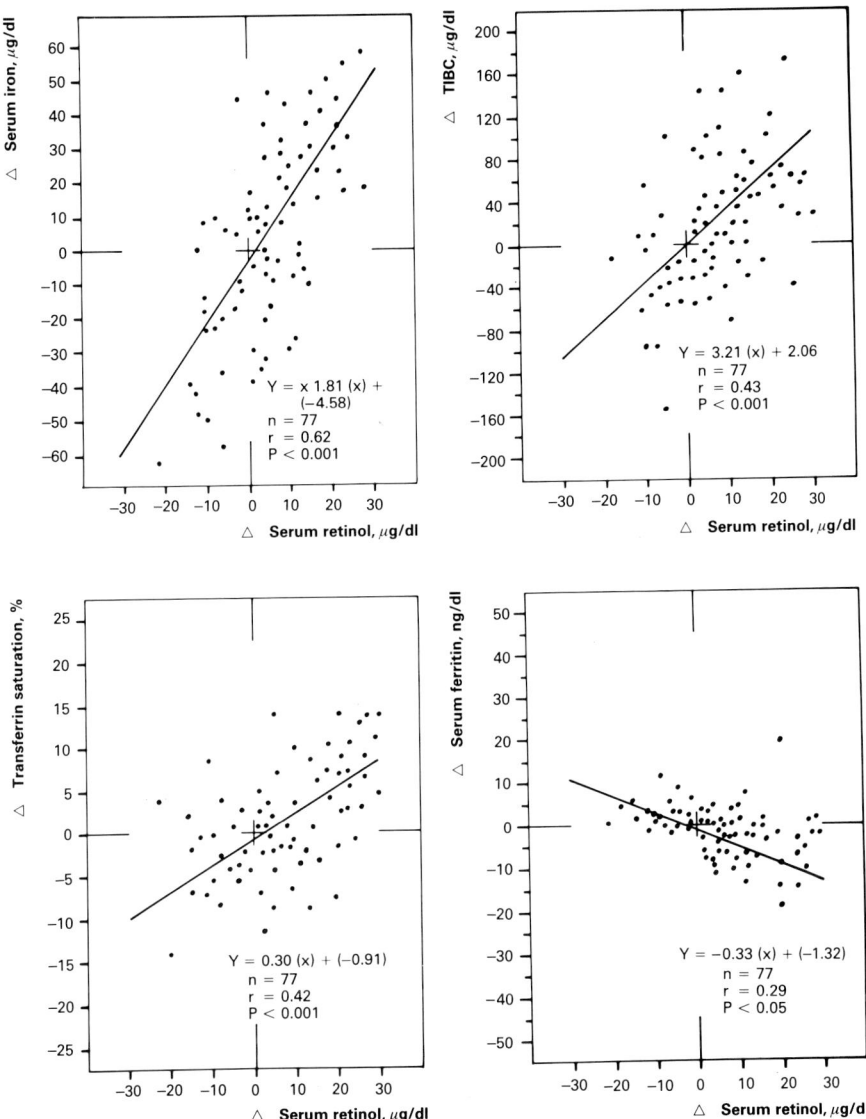

Fig. 6: Correlations between changes in serum retinol and changes in serum levels of iron parameters after six months of vitamin A fortification of Guatemalan children.
△ = Change [24].

shows the change observed in serum retinol in relation to changes in iron indicators in a group of pre-school children sampled in the basal survey and at six months after fortification began. In these children, there were significant positive correlations between the experienced change in serum retinol and changes in serum iron, total iron binding capacity (TIBC) and saturation of transferrin. In contrast, stored iron, as defined by serum ferritin levels, correlated negatively. These results suggest that vitamin A mobilized the stored iron into the circulation and also support previous observations in experimental animals. It is interesting to note that in these children, despite an increase in serum iron levels, there is also an elevation in TIBC suggesting that vitamin A could have affected the levels of the glycoprotein iron carrier, transferrin. However, a recent separate study has shown that this is not a direct effect of vitamin A, but rather an improvement on protein nutritional status probably mediated through this vitamin [25].

After a more prolonged intervention, the effect of vitamin A on iron nutriture changed particularly in relation to iron stores (Table II). When comparing, in a group of children, the distribution of cases by categories of levels of adequacy of iron indicators between the basal and the last survey, an overall improvement in the levels of iron indicators can be observed. This

Tab. II: Percent distribution of cases in surveys I and V by categories of iron parameters

	Survey I[1], %	Survey V[2], %
Serum iron, µg/dl		
< 50	43.1	25.5[3]
50–75	27.5	39.2
> 75	29.4	35.3
Serum TIBC, µg/dl		
< 250	5.9	2.0
250–350	37.3	49.0
> 350	56.9	49.9
ST, %		
< 15	39.2	27.5
15–20	33.3	33.3
> 20	27.5	39.2
Serum ferritin, ng/ml		
< 10	64.7	21.6[3]
10–20	23.5	58.8
> 20	11.8	19.6

[1] Basal survey.

[2] Two years after initiation of vitamin A fortification.

[3] The distributions are significantly different ($p < 0.05$ or better).

favorable effect was more marked in regard to the amount of stored iron. There was a lower prevalence of children with low serum ferritin levels in survey V than in survey I, prior to vitamin A fortification. Siimes et al [26] have shown that in healthy children the levels of serum ferritin remain constant from 6 months to 16 years of age; therefore, the observed favorable change in iron reserves cannot be attributed to the fact that the children were two years older at the end of the study. Most probably this elevation in iron stores observed after two years is due to an enhancement of dietary iron absorption triggered as a response to the initial depletion of iron reserves experienced after 6 months of vitamin A fortification, and in addition to a possible increment on hematopoietic utilization of this mineral. Since this was a retrospective study performed in stored blood serum samples, no hematological data were available.

Conclusion

Although further information about the impact of vitamin A nutriture on the hematological condition of given populations must be obtained, the existing data indicate that there is a metabolical interaction between vitamin A and iron nutrition. Through this relationship vitamin A deficiency may contribute to the occurrence of nutritional anemia, especially in areas where hypovitaminosis A is highly prevalent and endemic. When planning nutritional interventions, proper consideration should be given to this interaction.

References

1 Findlay, G M, McKenzie R D: The bone marrow in deficiency diseases. J Pathol 25, 402–403, 1922.
2 Wolbach, S B, Howe, P R: Tissue changes following deprivation of fat soluble A vitamin. J Exp Med 42, 753–781, 1925.
3 Koessler, K K et al: The relation of anemia primary and secondary to vitamin A deficiency. J Am Med Ass 87, 476–482, 1926.
4 Sure, B et al: The effect of avitaminosis on hematopoietic function. I. Vitamin A deficiency. J Biol Chem 83, 375–385, 1929.
5 Blackfan, K D, Wolbach, S B: Vitamin A deficiency in infants. A clinical and pathological study. J Pediatr 3, 679–706, 1933.
6 Frank, M: Beitrag zur Hämatologie der A-Avitaminose. Monatsschr Kinderheilk 60, 350–355, 1934.
7 Wagner, K H: Die experimentelle Avitaminose A beim Menschen. Hoppe-Seylers Z physiol Chem 264, 153–159, 1940.
8 US Department of Health Education and Welfare. Nutrition Survey of Paraguay, May–August 1965, pp 1–241. US Government Printing Office, Washington, 1967.

9   O'TOOLE, B A et al: Vitamin A deficiency and reproduction in Rhesus monkeys. J Nutr 104, 1513–1524, 1974.

10   McLAREN, D S et al: Xerophthalmia in Jordan. Am J Clin Nutr 17, 117–130, 1965.

11   McLAREN, D S et al: Biochemical and hematological changes in the vitamin A deficient rat. Am J Clin Nutr 17, 131–138, 1965.

12   NOCKLES, C F, KEINHOLZ, E W: Influence of vitamin A deficiency on testes, bursa Fabricius, adrenal and hematocrit in cockerels. J Nutr 92, 384–388, 1967.

13   AMINE, E K et al: Comparative hematology during deficiencies of iron and vitamin A in the rat. J Nutr 100, 1033–1040., 1970.

14   COREY, J E, HAYES, K C: Cerebro-spinal fluid pressure, growth and hematology in relation to retinol status of the rat in acute vitamin A deficiency. J Nutr 102, 1585–1593, 1972.

15   MEE, J M L, STANLEY, R W: Association between blood vitamin A and packed cell volume in dairy animals. Nutr Rep Int 9, 401–406, 1974.

16   HODGES, R E et al: Hematopoietic studies in vitamin A deficiency. Am J Clin Nutr 31, 876–885, 1978.

17   MEJÍA, L A et al: Vitamin A deficiency and anemia in Central American children. Am J Clin Nutr 30, 1175–1184, 1977.

18   MOHANRAM, M et al: Hematological studies in vitamin A deficient children. Int J Vit Nutr Res 47, 389–393, 1977.

19   JAGADEESAN, V, REDDY, V: Interrelationship between vitamins E and A: a clinical study. Clin Chim Acta 90, 71–74, 1978.

20   WENGER, R et al: Beziehungen zwischen dem Vitaminstatus (Vitamine A, B_1, B_2 und C), klinischen Befunden und den Ernährungsgewohnheiten in einer Gruppe von alten Leuten in Wien. Wien Klin Wochenschr 91, 557–562, 1979.

21   MEJÍA, L A et al: Clinical signs of anemia in vitamin A deficient rats. Am J Clin Nutr 32, 1439–1444, 1979.

22   MEJÍA, L A et al: Role of vitamin A in the absorption, retention and distribution of iron in the rat. J Nutr 109, 129–137, 1979.

23   ARROYAVE, G et al: Evaluation of sugar fortification with vitamin A at the national level. Sci Publ No. 384. Pan American Health Organization, Washington, 1979.

24   MEJÍA, L A, ARROYAVE, G: The effect of vitamin A fortification of sugar on iron metabolism in preschool children in Guatemala. Am J Clin Nutr 36, 87–93, 1982.

25   MEJÍA, L A, ARROYAVE, G: Lack of direct association between serum transferrin and serum biochemical indicators of vitamin A nutriture. Acta Vitaminol Enzymol 5, 179–184, 1983.

26   SIIMES, M A et al: Ferritin in serum: Diagnosis of iron deficiency and iron overload in infants and children. Blood 43, 581–589, 1974.

L. A. Mejía, PhD, Division of Nutrition and Health, Institute of Nutrition of Central America and Panama (INCAP), PO Box 1188, Guatemala City, Guatemala

Possibilities of Enriching Sugar with Micronutrients in Mexico

A. Chávez, A. Mata and J. Sandoval

Division of Community Nutrition, Instituto Nacional de Nutrición, Mexico City, Mexico

Key Words: Food enrichment · Micronutrients · Sugar · Vitamins · Iron

Abstract: A nutrition survey was implemented for the whole Peninsula of Yucatàn, and the results suggested the need to enrich the sugar with iron, niacin, vitamin A and ascorbic acid. At the same time several methodologies were developed, including systems of mixture, qualitative determinations of micronutrients in sugar, of iron and vitamins, in saliva and urine determinations and evaluations of the functional impact of some micronutrient deficiencies. A full coverage with enriched sugar of the Halacho district with 30000 inhabitants was attempted and a similar region, Maxcanu, was used as control. A random sample of 250 families in each region was intensively studied longitudinally. The most important program drawback consisted in the failure to adequately supply the experimental region with enriched sugar. This was due to administrative short-comings in the government organization in charge of sugar distribution. At best 68 % of the random samples of sugar taken from homes was enriched and contained on average 76 % of the expected concentration of nutrients. At the end of the evaluation period the sugar mixture started getting dark and having some mellification. Therefore the final evaluation, planned for the 18th month, was performed instead after 15 months.

Comparisons of blood determinations before and after the program in experimental vs control communities showed no significant differences. However, a subsample of 15 families to whom the program's personnel directly distributed the enriched sugar, controlling its intake, showed some improvements. In conclusion, due to administrative difficulties it was not possible to demonstrate a biological impact of the program. However, the research group considers that this type of program has great potential advantages, particularly in the case of Mexico where the government produces and distributes practically all the sugar in the market.

Antecedents and Justification

Micronutrient deficiencies in Mexico. From nutritional surveys carried out in 17 zones of the country between 1958 and 1964, it became evident that the Mexican diet among the rural and poor urban populations was lacking in calories and protein as well as in several micronutrients, especially niacin, vitamin A, and ascorbic acid [1]. Iron was present in sufficient quantity, but since it was supplied mainly with beans, its quality, and therefore its absorption, was poor [2].

From 1964 to 1970 several specific studies were carried out, and several epidemiological studies aimed at fixing more precisely the magnitude of the deficiencies and the repercussion on the health status [3]. A study based on an analysis of urine samples over a known period was carried out at that time, and it was among the school population throughout the whole country [4]. Also, experimental studies were begun in order to evaluate interventions and different types of methodology.

Regarding micronutrients, it was possible to define, although not with the desired precision, the main regions of deficiencies and the clinical manifestations that they caused: 1) It was clear that there was endemic pellagra on the Yucatán Peninsula, and sporadically in several other areas of the country, especially in the central region [5]. 2) The lack of vitamin A was more prevalent than had been believed; it gave rise to several clinical problems such as night blindness among preschool children in the arid regions of the North of the country, and xerophthalmia and blindness, especially on the Yucatán Peninsula [6]. 3) Anemia was the main specific syndrome of deficiency, and it included practically all the tropical areas of the country and some of the semi-arid areas in the North [7]. 4) The consumption of vitamin C was low, but it was possible to detect cases of clinical deficiency only in the mountains in the South. 5) The riboflavin deficiency was more or less generalized, with manifestations particularly among school children [8]. 6) The national survey of goiter showed improvement in relation to previous reports [9]. 7) Collecting information regarding the importance of deficiencies of zinc and fluor in some areas was begun.

The importance of deficiencies in micronutrients. From the beginning it was accepted that the nutritional problem of the country was protein-calorie malnutrition. Therefore, the value of interventions with micronutrients continues to be debated. Some specialists have insisted that if the calorie problem is not resolved, it is practically useless to work on a solution of the rest of the deficiencies. This opinion is the same as proposing that in the total diet, as is the case with the amino acids, there is a "limiting factor", which, if not corrected, makes it useless to treat secondary deficiencies.

The autors have always insisted that the contrary is rather frequently the case. Not only does each deficiency have its specific impact on health, and its correction an equally specific result, but, due to the interaction among nutrients, it is necessary to deal with the primary deficiency to understand and to resolve the secondary deficiencies.

Calorie deficiency is not always due directly to a quantitative lack of food; it is also due, and sometimes to a greater degree, to a qualitative factor. Specialists who worked in rural areas and who are familiar with the nutrition of the poor, will have noted that in most cases of dietary insufficiency there is some food in the house that becomes spoiled or is given to the animals. What these families need is appetite to eat more of the deficient and monotonous diet [10]. These people are often hungry despite stacks of tortillas in the house.

A diet of poor quality, based on a single cereal and, therefore, deficient in amino acids and micronutrients, may result in a series of physical compensations and adaptations reducing the functionality of the people and, consequently, their consumption of food. The fact is well known that when an anemic person is given iron, his appetite increases appreciably. This is also the case for other micronutrients.

Previous experiences with food enrichment. Regarding the problem mentioned above, there is the experience of enriching cooked maize with tablets containing soya before the maize is ground as well as with vitamins and iron. When the maize and the tablets are ground together to form the dough from which the tortillas are made, these tortillas are better balanced nutritionally. Most of the individuals consuming enriched products stated that they had a better appetite and therefore "were able to eat more tortillas".

In general, in spite of the fact that the programs of enrichment with micronutrients are theoretically feasible, practical experience has on the whole not been as positive as one would expect [11]. In this context it is instructive to consider the programs carried out in Central America where vitamin A was added to sugar. The evaluation of these programs was positive [12]. However, permanence and stability of the programs have not been achieved. The scientific evaluations of Viteri *et al* [13] and Layrisse *et al* [14] with iron EDTA in Guatemala and Venezuela have also shown beneficial effects. Nevertheless, it has not been possible to implement actions having a wider coverage.

In Mexico our field group has had some experience, almost all at an experimental level. For example, in one case, nicotinic acid was added as an enrichener during the grinding of maize in those areas where pellagra is endemic [15]; in other cases several nutrients were added together in tests on a community level. The results have been quite positive. This experience allows to support the idea that enrichment could be an effective weapon for the improvement of nutrition among the more marginal population groups.

Undoubtedly no program, even when working experimentally, can achieve 100 % of the expected impact. But even when the efficiency of a program may at times be limited, it has social importance. Indeed, in the matter of nutrition even small improvements can lead to significant results.

Technological possibilities of enriching sugar. For many years now there has been insistence on the possibility of using sugar as a vehicle for enrichment with micronutrients as in many countries, especially in Latin America, sugar reaches all social strata [16]. Frequently, as in the case of Mexico, sugar is consumed in a proportion inverse to income, greater amounts in lower than in higher income groups. The latter consume sugar primarily in industrialized products. Furthermore, and, of course, proportionally, more sugar is consumed by children than by adults.

The program of enriching sugar with vitamin A in Guatemala showed for the first time that it is technologically possible to reach the table of the needy population and produce a beneficial impact on its health [12].

It has been criticized that if the nutritional quality of sugar is improved, its consumption may increase and that this food, although enriched, is bad for health. This objection would be valid if the program were to publicize or promote the consumption of sugar, or if, as a consequence of the program, the consumption of sugar were to increase. But all the specialists who have worked in this area made it clear that sugar is used only as a vehicle; that is, the product is enriched in accordance with the quantity already consumed, and there is no expectation of increasing the quantity.

However, it would be important to show whether enrichment programs already carried out in Latin America have or have not resulted in a per capita increase in the consumption of sugar.

The Enrichment Program in Mexico

Participating organisms. In the case of Mexico several conditions are favorable to the enrichment of sugar. Most important is the fact that 90 % of sugar production is government controlled. For the management of the mills, the government created the National Commission of the Sugar Industry (CNIA). Unfortunately, another organization was separately formed for the distribution of sugar, UNPASA. (Recently, after this program, the CNIA and the UNPASA were merged to form a single company: Azúcar, S.A. [Sugar, Inc.]).

From the beginning, the project of enrichment of sugar was carried out by means of collaboration between these two organizations, the Mexican Food System (SAM), an industry created for the purpose of promoting enrichment of foods (Nutrimex), the office of Public Health of the State of Yucatán, and the National Institute of Nutrition, the technical organization in charge of evaluating results.

Yucatán Peninsula was chosen for the project because it is an area that, perhaps on a world-wide level, presents great problems regarding deficiency of micronutrients [17]. This phenomenon is basically due to the fact that since the end of the past century the Peninsula has changed its production of foods to a very peculiar monoculture, the cultivation of henequen (sisal). This is a cactus whose fiber was widely used in the United States to tie the bundles of wheat stalks produced as a result of agricultural mechanization. The population of Yucatán bruskly ceased to produce maize and beans and became salaried workers of very low income, without having been educated as to how to invest their money in a more balanced diet. As a consequence, from the end of the last century, Yucatán has been a region suffering serious nutritional deficiencies. It was the first place in the world where pellagra as well as kwashiorkor were medically reported.

Materials and Methods

Stages of the program. The entire program consists of four stages:

1) Verification diagnosis of nutrient deficiency on Yucatán Peninsula and standardization of the methodology and logistics of production, storage, and distribution.

2) Evaluation of the impact of enrichment in a geographic area of approximately 30 000 inhabitants compared with a control area.

3) Implementation of the program in the entire rural area of Yucatán Peninsula and an evaluation of the results by means of indirect and direct indicators.

4) Extension of the program to all the marginal areas of the country, especially the tropical regions.

This report will present only the information and results of the first two stages.

Work procedures. It was decided to undertake multiple enrichment using nicotinic acid, vitamin A, iron and vitamin C. It was believed that this was a necessary procedure considering the magnitude of the deficiency. Also, it is well known that there is an interaction between some of the micronutrients; for example vitamin C stimulates the absorption of iron from food. The concentrations used per 50 g sugar, that is, for the approximate daily per capita consumption, were 10 mg vitamin A palmitate (250 000 IU/g), 25 mg vitamin C, 12.5 mg niacinamide, and 40 mg ferric phosphate, which were later changed to 12 mg FeEDTA. This multiple enrichment was technologically possible at the laboratory level as well as at the pilot plant level.

A center of rural research was established in the community of Halachó, an experimental area, in order to evaluate the impact of the enrichment by means of the system of "before and after", particularly by measuring plasmatic levels of the nutrients and the urinary excretion of metabolites. A control area, Maxcanú, did not receive enriched sugar, thus permitting comparative studies.

In both areas the action was centered on small communities of about 1 000 inhabitants each, as the control of consumption and the taking of samples is easier in small communities. At the same time, it is in the small communities that the manifestation of deficiencies is more important and, therefore, changes are more apparent.

Initially, it was decided that Nutrimex, in its Guadalajara plant, would make the mixture; the Laboratorios Nacionales de Fomento Industrial (the National Laboratories for Industrial Development) would carry out the pilot tests on stability in regard to transportation and storage, simulating the conditions in Yucatán; UNPASA would distribute only enriched sugar in the area of Halachó and non-enriched sugar in Maxcanú; CNIA would finance and supervise the project; and the National Institute of Nutrition would take charge of local control, medical examinations, blood tests, and laboratory analyses. As will be mentioned later, this excessive fractioning of responsibilities proved to be the greatest problem when it came to evaluation.

Results of Phase 1: Creation of the Infrastructure

Confirmation of the diagnosis of deficiency in Yucatán. Regarding the results of Phase 1, a monograph was published by Mata *et al* [18], that although the Yucatán Peninsula had significantly improved its levels of nutrition as compared with what was found in the studies of 15 years ago, there still existed a sufficient basis for the enrichment program.

In order to confirm the deficiencies, a stratified sampling by regions was carried out in the so-called sisal, intermediate, and maize areas, in order to assess the magnitude of the current nutritional deficiency regarding vitamin A, vitamin C, niacin and iron. In addition, the consumption of sugar by age and sex as well as the clinical, biochemical and epidemiological characteristics of the population were studied.

Representative samplings were taken in 14 communities, and dietetic, clinical, laboratory and socioeconomic surveys were done. The study covered 2 248 persons.

The results gave proof of the poor nutritional state of practically the entire low income population on the Peninsula, but differing from the past. The sisal area was better than before as better than the maize area, while the latter was a little worse than previously.

Infant nutrition in the sisal area was equal to that of other marginal areas in the country, but it continued to be better in the intermediate and maize areas. In the maize areas the figures were found to be higher than in the rest of the country (Table I).

Regarding protein-energy consumption, average levels were not found to be as low as previously (Table II). This is due in part to the type of survey.

When the survey is not of the strictly quantitative type, it tends to overestimate the consumption of tortilla. However, this change in average, as was shown in other areas, is due to the fact that, when there is a greater cir-

Tab. I: Distribution of preschool age children according to the Gomez classification (%).

	Normal (110–91 %)	Grade I (90–76 %)	Grade II (75–61 %)	Grade III (60 % and less)
Area I (Sisal)	13.3	60.0	26.6	0.0
Area II (Intermediate)	17.9	48.7	30.7	2.6
Area III (Corn)	10.9	56.5	26.0	6.5
Total	13.8	55.4	27.7	3.1

Tab. II: Daily Energy and nutrient consumption (310 families from different areas of Yucatán, 1980)

	Energy, kcal	Protein, g	Fe, mg	Niacin, mg	Ascorbic acid, mg	Retinol, μg
Area I (Sisal)	2193	70.2	22.8	7.4	38.8	137.7
Area II (Intermediate)	1947	65.4	19.4	9.2	13.1	160.3
Area III (Corn)	2232	66.1	22.7	9.7	13.6	138.9
Total	2127	67.2	21.7	8.8	21.7	145.0

culation of money and a better offer of foods, only one sector can change while the majority remains the same. This is shown in Tables III–V. It can be seen that, regarding the consumption of niacin, half the population consumes very low quantities, while regarding vitamins A and C approximately 85 % of the population is in the same situation. These circumstances are the same as they were previously, and fully justify the enrichment program.

Tab. III: Niacin consumption in various areas (% distribution of 310 families according to the level of consumption)

	Consumption of niacin/day			
	9.9 mg or less	10.0–16.6 mg	16.7–23.4 mg	23.5 mg or more
Area I (Sisal)	45.0	41.6	11.6	1.8
Area II (Intermediate)	59.8	33.2	5.8	1.2
Area III (Corn)	61.1	35.9	1.5	1.5
Total	54.7	37.0	6.8	1.5

Tab. IV: Retinol consumption in various areas (% distribution of 310 families according to the level of consumption)

	Retinol consumption/day			
	300 µg or less	301–600 µg	601–900 µg	900 µg or more
Area I (Sisal)	86.3	10.7	2.3	0.7
Area II (Intermediate)	83.4	11.6	3.2	1.8
Area III (Corn)	89.0	7.2	3.8	1.2
Total	86.1	9.8	2.9	1.2

Tab. V: Ascorbic acid consumption in various areas (% distribution of 310 families according to consumption levels)

	Ascorbic acid consumption/day				
	20 mg or less	21–40 mg	41–60 mg	61–80 mg	81 mg or more
Area I (Sisal)	79.8	10.2	4.4	0.0	5.6
Area II (Intermediate)	82.8	10.8	2.3	1.7	3.0
Area III (Corn)	85.4	6.6	0.6	3.0	5.4
Total	83.2	8.3	2.2	1.3	5.0

Tab. VI: Frequency (%) of anemia in women (according to Ht, Hb, MCV)

	Area I (sisal)	Area II (intermediate)	Area III (maize)
At risk	14.4	11.6	14.5
Anemic	8.8	16.2	30.2
Total	23.2	27.8	47.7

Regarding iron, it is well known that in population groups on a vegetarian-type diet, especially beans, total consumption is of limited importance since absorption is low. The frequency of anemia was variable, from 9% in the sisal area to as much as 30% in the maize area (Table VI). This difference is due to the different levels of medical attention rather than to differences in ecology or diet. The population in the sisal area comes in under Social Security and thus receives free medical attention and medication. Besides, the Public Health Department has frequently distributed iron tablets to this population.

When special groups are considered, such as pregnant women and children in the second year of life, the frequency of anemia is higher. As much as 80 % show considerable deficiencies.

Regarding serum retinol it was found that, on an average, 25 % of the population had low concentration values. Almost half showed a clear deficiency (Table VII). The levels of urinary excretion of vitamin C and 1-N-methylnicotinamide showed a marked deficiency throughout the Peninsula (Table VIII). Of the population 27 % excreted very low levels. The problem is more important among women and preschool children.

Tab. VII: Serum retinol by age and sex (% population by levels)

	< 10 µg	10–20 µg	> 20 µg
Preschool children 18–60 months	23.2	33.3	43.5
Females 15–45 years	7.6	11.8	80.6
Males 15–45 years	5.7	9.1	85.2
Pregnant and lactating women	4.4	13.0	82.6
Total	10.2	15.7	74.1

Tab. VIII: Urinary excretion of N-methylnicotinamide and ascorbic acid (population with low values per age and sex)

	N-methylnicotinamide		Ascorbic acid	
	No. of cases	%	No. of cases	%
Preschool children 2–5 years	33	29.2	22	19.1
Females 15–45 years	37	30.4	31	25.0
Males 15–45 years	25	23.0	19	17.3
Total	95	27.9	72	27.3

Selection of the pilot area. The districts of Halachó and Maxcanú were selected because of their high frequency of deficiencies within the sisal area. The deficiencies were those of an intermediate area, that is, averages for the whole Peninsula, also they were similar to each other. They are located in the Southern part of the State of Yucatán, bordering on the State of Campeche. In both cases they are made up of the principal town of the country of about 6 000 inhabitants and several surrounding rural communities. In both areas a new nutritional, clinical and laboratory survey was done, and 250 rural families were chosen in each area for the evaluation process.

Operative coordination. The consumption of sugar per family was studied for an entire week. It was a little higher than for the Peninsula as a whole with 46.3 g/person/day, with a rather ample standard deviation of ± 16.7 g. In 95% of the cases consumption was higher than 15 g (Fig. 1).

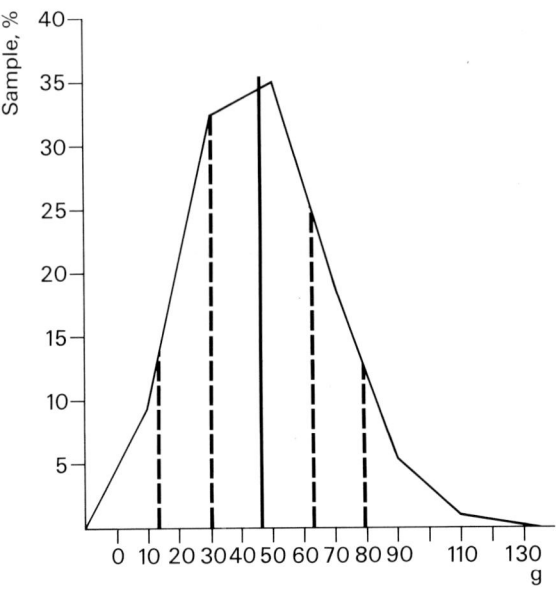

Fig. 1: Sugar consumption per person per day in rural areas of Yucatán (1982 survey).

A study was also made of the family habits regarding the use of sugar at home, the type preferred, its storage, its place of purchase and its utilization (Fig. 2). The levels of enrichment were planned on the basis of these findings.

In order to improve quality control of the industrial mixture, initially it was not made in the sugar mill but rather in the Nutrimex plant in Guadalajara. The sugar was then transported more than 2 500 km to a warehouse in Mérida, Yucatán, from where it was distributed to the corresponding area every two or three weeks.

The simulation studies of transport and storage carried out by LANFI as well as the analysis of the transported samples to the warehouse showed that the sugar was stable, that the concentrations of nutrients were acceptable; also, in various population samplings sensorial evaluations were made regarding its acceptance. These sensorial evaluation studies were also made with special panels with local groups specially trained for this purpose. The results of all these studies were positive [19].

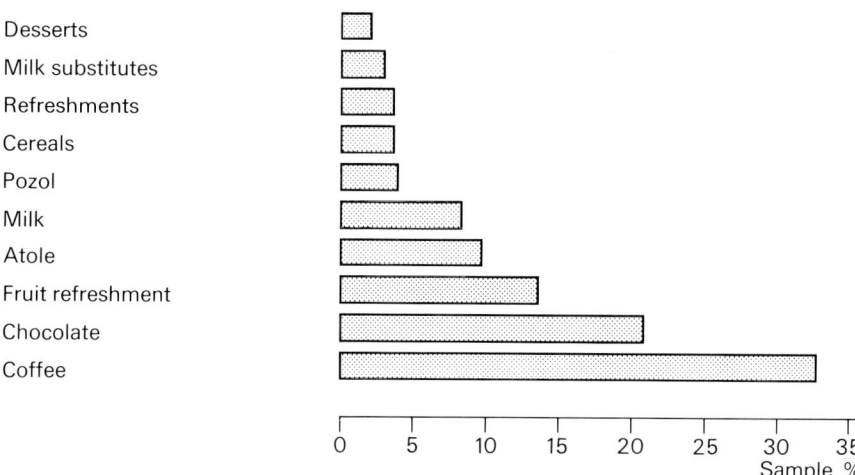

Fig. 2: Forms of sugar used in households in Yucatán (1982 survey).

Tests of stability of the nutrients in the sugar were made at different temperatures and at different times [19]. Studies of stability were also made of the samplings of urine, blood, and saliva that were taken. Similarly, studies were made regarding loss of nutrients in different culinary preparations, including some of availability. Thus, for example, it was found that there was practically no loss of nutrients in coffee. In chocolate and atole, however, there was a vitamin C loss of 17 and 28 %, respectively [19].

In the rural communities of Yucatán the people use sugar to prepare different desserts, for example, pineapple in sugar syrup, coconut loaf, and puddings. These were duplicated in the laboratory, using enriched sugar, in order to make different organoleptic tests.

Methodological developments. Taking previous experiences into account (INN of Mexico, INCAP of Guatemala and CONICYT of Venezuela), different technologies were developed for the determination of the nutrients to be added to the sugar and for the analyses of biological samplings [19]. Also developed were technologies of an industrial nature for the preparation of the premixtures (Roche Products, Inc.) and the techniques for the definitive mixture.

At the same time, studies were begun in the search for the best way to carry out the mixtures at the level of the production mills which supplied sugar to the Yucatán Peninsula.

Pilot projects were undertaken regarding distribution of the sugar to the localities involved, including cost estimates.

A manual of norms was drawn up concerning the process of fortification, the purpose of which was to ensure the availability of the normal as well as the enriched sugar to the communities. This manual was put at the disposition of the distributing companies. The logistics for the handling of the necessary volumes was developed, and a reserve storage was planned in order to avoid market fluctuations.

Samples of the sugar were taken for analyses at the levels of the pre-mixture plant, the enriching plant, the UNPASA warehouses, the local businesses, and of the families themselves. The total came to a little more than 2 000.

Evaluation of the Pilot Program

Longitudinal evaluation. The original pattern contemplated a longitudinal evaluation with an intermediate evaluation, and a final evaluation at the end of 18 months from the beginning of the program. We were aware of the fact that 18 months was a short term in function of the low dosages used in the sugar. But from the political point of view it was considered to be inacceptable to wait longer because there was some haste to make recommendations of a practical nature. In the event that the 18-month period showed some significant results, we would continue with the rural center of Halachó in order to make a later evaluation of Phase II (perhaps at the end of 30 months) as well as to have a center of operations for the administration and evaluation of Phase III.

The longitudinal evaluation was basically of the operative type. We wanted to have a control over the seasonal variations in the consumption of total foods, especially sugar, including the preferred forms. We also wanted an evaluation of the frequency of consumption of the enriched sugar. To this end, we designed specific procedures like qualitative methods to determine nutrients in sugar, a nutritional epidemiological study of the type of "systems of nutritional surveillance", the taking of biological samplings in alternate subsamplings, and the carrying out of some functional tests (vision in darkness and responses of physical exercise).

Seasonal variations in the consumption of the sugar was very evident – there was a difference of as much as 62.3 %. It was not known whether this difference was of a cultural type or whether it was due to problems of availability. Availability did suffer changes because in the middle of the program sugar became scarce throughout the whole country. The price of sugar rose sharply to as much as five times. Sugar did not reach Halachó during at least two periods of almost a month each period. Even though the program

(CNIA/UNPASA) presupposed that the supply was to be ensured in the experimental area as well as in the control area, in practice it was shown that this was not possible. The officials of the responsible organizations ceased to give sufficient attention to the evaluation of the enrichment program in the face of the sugar supply problem.

For many reasons the program suffered from serious inertia. It was not until three months after the program was begun that the enriched sugar began to appear in the rural homes. Six months later, hardly 32 % of the sugar consumed had added nutrients, and despite all our efforts, it was hardly possibly to go beyond the level of 50 % at the end of ten months. At this point, the National Institute of Nutrition took the system of distribution into its own hands but it did not succeed, at the end of 15 months saturation only reached 68 % of the sampling. Quantitative analyses at this time showed that the enriched sugar had only 76 % of the nutrient concentration expected.

It should be mentioned that, beginning with the tenth month of operation, the program also ran into economic problems. The CNIA ceased financing it, and the National Institute of Nutrition had to finish it alone.

Another important problem arose. The sugar samples stored in Yucatán were kept at a temperature of more than 30° C and a humidity of 70 %. Beginning with the fifth month, the sugar samples began to show changes. At first it was thought that this was due to some sacks having become humid. It later became clear that there was a change in coloration even in samples at the center. The sugar also underwent a certain mellification and agglutination. Several analyses proved that the mellification was due to changes in the vitamin C (the formation of ascorbates which brought on solubility) and possibly changes in niacinamide too.

Also the humidity affected the ferric iron that was used in the mixture, then there was more darkening of the sugar. Later, when FeEDTA was used, it also underwent changes of the same type after a period of two months.

Final evaluation. The above problems served to hasten the evaluation which, by no means, can be called final; it was made under conditions that were expected for an intermediate evaluation. It was made 15 months after the program was initiated but only 12 months after actual enrichment was begun, without having reached satisfactory level of saturation and with some changes in the quality of the sugar.

Still another complication was the presence of an epidemic of dengue. This had the greatest effect on the serum levels of vitamins A and C. Of the 150 children 73 % having low levels had only recently suffered from dengue.

Perhaps as a consequence of this situation, it was not possible to detect significant changes in biological values of any of the nutrients studied, before and after the program, and between Halachó and Maxcanú.

Longitudinal dietary surveys, using food composition tables and adding the expected fortification values, showed an important change in the level of micronutrient consumption (Tables IX, X). These values are theoretical, as enrichment, at the most, only reached 70 % of people and 70 % of the desired concentrations, giving just 50 % efficiency. Perhaps due this low efficiency and the short period of fortification, final evaluation of blood nutrient levels did not shown significant changes. As an example no changes were noted in several hematological values. Hb, ferritin and iron saturation index were about the same before and after. Some changes were shown in protoporphyrins (Tables XI and XII). No change was found in regard to vitamin deficiencies (Fig. 3).

Tab. IX: Retinol consumption changes in household diets in Yucatán 1981–82 (μg/day)

No.	Age, years	Retinol 1 July–Aug 81	Retinol 2 Nov–Dec 81	Retinol 3 Apr–May 82
Males				
20	2– 6	150	52	302
20	6–12	118	30	183
20	20–30	134	109	209
15	30–40	57	53	311
15	40–50	131	53	259
Females				
20	2– 6	90	48	147
20	6–12	103	48	230
15	20–30	123	103	231
15	30–40	101	71	282
15	40–50	43	62	144

Tab. X: Ascorbic acid (AA) consumption changes in household diets in Yucatán 1981–82 (mg/day)

No.	Age, years	AA 1 July–Aug 81	AA 2 Nov–Dec 81	AA 3 Apr–May 82
Males				
20	2– 6	3	4	23
20	6–12	7	15	12
20	20–30	6	8	18
15	30–40	3	5	21
15	40–50	17	19	22
Females				
20	2– 6	5	12	15
20	6–12	4	10	29
15	20–30	6	10	19
15	30–40	4	11	23
15	40–50	1	04	05

Tab. XI: Hematologic values in experimental communities prior to enrichment in Yucatán, June 1981

No.	Age, years	Hb, g/dl		Ferritin, ng/ml		Saturation index		Protoporphyrin, µg/dl RBC	
		x̄	SD	x̄	SD	x̄	SD	x̄	SD
Males									
25	20–30	14.6	1.5	45	35	28	10	301	169
23	30–40	14.8	1.2	58	30	28	07	308	150
25	40–50	14.8	0.9	51	42	28	08	308	118
36	50–70	14.5	1.3	57	37	29	13	272	93
Females									
34	20–30	13.2	.94	24	16	26	11	368	151
34	30–40	12.7	1.95	19	19	23	10	476	321
25	40–50	13.2	1.1	77	142	23	08	391	147
25	50–70	12.7	1.0	46	28	21	08	352	118

Tab. XII: Hematologic values in experimental communities after seven months of fortification in Yucatán, May 1982

No.	Age	Hb, g/dl		Ferritin, ng/ml		Saturation index		Protoporphyrin, µg/dl RBC	
		x̄	SD	x̄	SD	x̄	SD	x̄	SD
Males									
20	20–30	14.7	1.8	53	32	28	9	275	128
20	30–40	14.6	1.5	59	36	28	9	290	129
20	40–50	14.9	1.2	57	42	29	11	283	171
Females									
20	20–30	13.0	1.3	25	18	26	10	310	150
20	30–40	13.1	1.8	22	14	25	9	360	223
20	40–50	13.2	1.7	30	19	25	10	370	242

Beginning with the tenth month, when it was noted that there were difficulties in reaching the families through the regular commercial channels, the Nutrition Institute decided to make available directly enriched sugar (experimental) to 20 women in Halachó, by selling it at a low price. At the same time, normal sugar was sold to another 20 women in Maxcanú under the same conditions (control). Care was taken to assure that they ate 40 g/person/day.

As was expected considering the short time of supplementation, results showed no consistent changes in blood values. Therefore, some loading tests were designed of which an example is shown in Table XIII. When the study group received 30 mg of iron sulfate, urinary iron excretion was not different in the initial evaluation of the experimental and control groups, while after the fortification period the experimental group increased two times the urinary iron excretion, and the control group remained the same. This increase in urinary iron excretion may reflect saturation of the iron stores.

Before supplementation, June 1981   After supplementation, May 1982

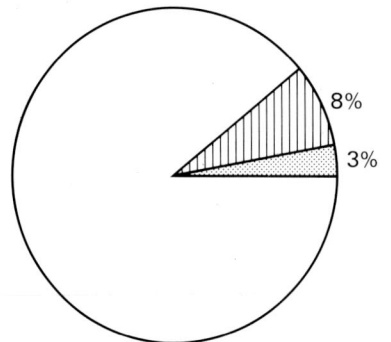
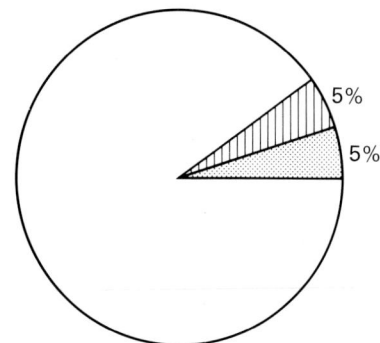

Fig. 3: Changes in the proportion of deficient population (≤ 10 μg/dl: dotted) and population at risk (10–20 μg/dl: hatched) as measured by serum retinol concentration.

Tab. XIII: Changes in urinary iron excretion in response to an oral load
(controlled supplemented subsample)

	Urinary excretion of iron, μg/g creatinine		t-test
	initial	final	
Experimental group (n = 20)			
$\bar{x}$	38	72	$p < 0.01$
Range	13–47	32–92	
Control group (n = 20)			
$\bar{x}$	37	39	NS
Range	14–59	16–49	

Comments and Conclusions

Unfortunately, it was not possible to arrive at definitive conclusions. Nevertheless, there is enough to be learned from this experience.

It is technically possible to enrich sugar with several micronutrients without changing their organoleptic qualities. However, it is necessary to solve the problem of the place where this is to be done. The dryer at the sugar mill seems to be the logical place. Curiously enough, though, perhaps because the dryer is made of steel, it removes the iron from the sugar. No satisfactory solution to this complication could be found.

In a new attempt, with FeEDTA, vitamin C may not be required. The problems of mellification and darkening under bad storage conditions and the possible involvement of vitamin C must be investigated further.

Administratively, there has been a large increase in the theoretical costs of the program. When the program was begun, direct costs of 9.1 pesos/person/year were calculated. As a consequence of the devaluation of the peso, the direct costs may be as much as ten times higher, thereby affecting the price of sugar for the consumer and other economic parameters.

The main problem of the program is logistic in nature. It is difficult that in such a long chain of responsibilities each one involved should comply with its individual obligation. In the case of the program in Yucatán, the main obstacle was distribution. Between the storage center in Merída and the stores in Halachó there seemed to be a distance that was almost impossible to overcome by the bureaucracy and the lack of responsibility of officials. This was especially true when sugar became scarce on the Peninsula.

The problem of storage is not easy to overcome because in Mexico the sugar milling period is from December to March. The sugar is then stored in tropical areas, to be sold during the following 12 months. Consequently, the average storage life is greater than the three or four months which, for our mixture, appears to be the point of maximum tolerance. The costs of better storage appear difficult to meet under the present situation.

Under the conditions in Mexico, known to us through the program, the enrichment of sugar seems to be possible only within a more responsible sociopolitical context, and this would imply a more decided policy – a virtual reconstruction of the patterns of sugar consumption. It would be necessary to produce a white, refined sugar for consumption in the cities and for the refreshment and candy industries. This sugar would be sold at a high price so as to control its consumption as well as to subsidize a darker but less humid sugar than the present so-called ''standard'' sugar. The latter sugar could be enriched and sold at a lower price in the rural areas and perhaps in the government stores in the poor urban areas. This would imply not only decision, but also educating the public as well as a change in the mentality of the bureaucracy that is charged with handling the sugar.

In this new situation, it would indeed be possible to resolve all the technical problems that might arise, but it would be necessary to restate the cost/benefit problem which has been mentioned. At this time the costs may be ten times greater than originally calculated, that is, near 100 pesos/person/year, and the benefit, according to the experience published in this report, appears to be less than expected. This is due to the time the program takes in saturating the people and, perhaps, to parasitosis and illness including greater loss in people.

One way in which the program could be made more beneficial would be to give the population an initial charge of iron and vitamin A so that later, with low dosages, the people can better maintain the level of reserves.

At the present time, the available systems for biochemically evaluating the impact of programs such as this one are not easy to interpret. Thus, for example, the seasonal variations in the serum retinol were much more marked than was expected, and the biochemical indicators were affected by other factors, such as in our case by dengue.

Skipping stages is not to be recommended; in spite of not having satisfactorily finished the second stage, the Institute of Nutrition would recommend beginning the third stage, that is, the enrichment of sugar in Yucatán. But this time it would be necessary to do the planning within a wider context, with a real change in the structure of sugar consumption on the Peninsula, a plan that would require an explicit obligation on the part of Azúcar S.A. to comply with its obligations and, of course, the implementation, too, of educational programs of ample coverage.

References

1   Chávez, A: Encuestas nutricionales en México. Publ División de Nutrición, México, 1963, 1976.
2   Pérez, H C *et al:* El problema nutricional del hierro en México. Rev Salud Públ Méx *13,* 71, 1971.
3   Pérez, H C *et al:* Recopilación del consumo de nutrientes en diferentes zonas de México. II. Consumo de vitaminas y minerales. Arch Latinoamer Nutr *23,* 292, 1973.
4   Chávez, A *et al:* Evaluación del estado nutricional por medio de la excreción urinaria de vitaminas. Arch Latinoamer Nutr *19,* 53, 1969.
5   Chávez, A, Pimentel, R A: Estudio epidemiológico de la pelagra en una comunidad rural. Bol Of San Pan *55,* 398, 1963.
6   Chávez, A, Hernández, M: Algunos datos para la prevención de la hipovitaminosis A en México. Bol Of San Pan *69,* 21, 1970.
7   Balam, G, Chávez, A: Frecuencia de anemia en algunas comunidades rurales del altiplano y de las costas. Rev Salud Públ Méx *8,* 225, 1966.
8   Pérez, H C, Chávez, A: La desnutrición en el medio rural Mexicano. Publ Div Nutr L-34. Instituto Nacional de Nutrición, México, 1976.
9   Maisterrena, A J *et al:* Nutrition and endemic goiter in Mexico. J Clin Endocrinol Metabolism *24,* 166, 1964.
10 Monroy, R, Chávez, A: Estudios sobre el enriquecimiento de la harina de maiz nixtamalizada con concentrados proteicos. Proc Soc Mex Nutr Endocrinol *6,* 283, 1966.
11 Arroyave, G: Fortificación de alimentos en los países en desarrollo. INCAP Publ E-819. INCAP, Guatemala, 1975.

12 Arroyave, G *et al:* Evaluation of sugar fortification with vitamin A at national level. IN-CAP Publ 384. INCAP, Guatemala, 1979.

13 Viteri, F *et al:* Iron fortification in developing countries. In: Nutrition in Health and Disease and International Development. Symp XII Int Cong Nutr, pp 345–354. Liss, New York, 1981.

14 Layrisse, M: Prevention of iron defficiency. In: Scrimshaw and Wallerstein (eds). Nutrition policy implementation, pp 89–97. Plenum Press, New York, 1982.

15 Madrigal, H *et al:* Estudios experimentales sobre la prevención de la pelagra. Publ Div Nutr, L-13. México, 1968.

16 Disler, P *et al:* Studies on the fortification of cane sugar with iron and ascorbic acid. Br J Nutr *34,* 141, 1975.

17 Carillo Gil, A: Historia de las enfermedades carenciales en Yucatán. Bruguera, 1964.

18 Mata, A *et al:* Diagnóstico de la deficiencia de nutrimentos en Yucatán y bases para un programa de enriquecimiento de azúcar. Publ Div Nutr, L-51. México, 1981.

19 Garcia Castro, I P E: Enriquecimiento de azúcar con micronutrimentos; Tesis profesional. Universidad La Salle, México, 1982.

Dr. Adólfo Chávez, Division of Community Nutrition, Instituto Nacional de Nutrición, Tlalpan 14000, México, DF, México

Iron Deficiency in Latin America
Causes and Prevention

M. LAYRISSE

Instituto Venezolano de Investigaciones Científicas, Caracas, Venezuela

Key Words: Iron absorption · Latin American diets

Abstract: Population surveys in Latin America indicate that iron deficiency is a public health problem in many countries especially in people belonging to the low socio-economic class. The prevalence and severity of this deficiency is increased in rural areas endemic for hookworm infection. Although the dietary iron intake is relatively high compared with values observed in Western countries, due to the low bioavailability of the iron in staple foods, Latin American diets do not meet the physiological requirements for men and even less those for women of reproductive age and those for children. The high prevalence of iron deficiency and the economic and cultural difficulties opposing a change in food habits suggest that national iron fortification programs are necessary in Latin American countries as the main measure to reduce and prevent iron anemia.

Prevalence of Iron Deficiency Anemia

The data indicate that iron deficiency represents a public health problem in Latin America. Anemia is found in approximately 40–80% of the people living in rural areas, where hookworm infection is endemic [1–3]. Its frequency may be as high as 30% in men and 80% in women. In urban and sub-urban areas, anemia is prevalent in the segments of the population vulnerable to iron deficiency. In infants during the first year of life it may be as high as 50%, in children between 15 and 57%, in adult women during reproductive age, between 15 and 30%, and in pregnant women it varies between 20 and 77% [4–14]. Although biochemical tests indicated in only some of these studies that anemia was due to iron deficiency, circumstantial evidence such as peripheral blood smears, MCHC values and the therapeutic trial indicated that iron deficiency was the principal cause.

It is of interest to mention the cooperative studies on the prevalence of nutritional anemia in seven Latin American countries. Samples were taken from pregnant women in the last trimester belonging to the lower socio-economic levels of the population, and from non-pregnant women and men belonging to the same socio-economic class (Table I) [15]. Iron deficiency anemia was present in 39% of pregnant women, 17% of non-pregnant women and 3% of men with the proportions of iron deficiency being 48, 21 and 3% respectively.

Tab. I: Prevalence of iron deficiency and iron deficiency anemia in Latin America

	Iron deficiency anemia, %	Iron deficiency, %
Men	3	3
Non-pregnant women	17	21
Pregnant women	39	48

The basic etiology of iron deficiency is an imbalance between the amount of iron absorbed and the amount required by the body to compensate iron loss and to form new tissues. Increased losses are associated with blood losses in menstruation as well as pathological losses including those associated with parasitic infection. In Latin America, hookworm infection is common from Mexico to the Northern part of Argentina. Due to either *Necator americanus* or *Ancylostoma duodenale,* this type of infection is prevalent in agricultural areas, especially on coffee plantations. Although the majority of the subjects showed only light infections, they may contribute to an increase in the prevalence of iron deficiency. For example, an infection of 1000 eggs/g feces (about 40 worms), which is considered a moderate subclinical infection by Public Health standards, causes an intestinal iron loss of the order of 1 mg iron/day in the case of *Necator americanus* and about 2 mg in *Ancylostoma duodenale* infections (Table II) [16, 17]. Even though about 10–40% of this amount of iron is reabsorbed by the intestinal mucosa [18], such a chronic loss eventually reduces iron stores and induces anemia, especially in the segment of the population vulnerable to iron deficiency.

Tab. II: Intestinal blood loss in intestinal parasitic infection

Parasite	Blood loss/ parasite, ml	Blood loss/ 1000 eggs, ml	Iron loss/ 1000 eggs, mg
Necator americanus	0.02–0.07	2.1	1
Ancylostoma duodenale	0.14–0.26	4.4	2
Trichuris trichiura	0.005	0.25	0.1

Trichuris trichiura infection also produces fecal blood loss, although less than that caused by hookworm infection [19]. Only heavy infections in children under 5 years of age may cause anemia. In a study carried out in the rural areas of Venezuela, where hookworm infection is endemic, it was found that 45 % of the individuals with an infection of more than 100 eggs/g feces were anemic, compared with only 30 % of the population, that was not infected or infected with less than 100 eggs/g feces. These data indicate that in these agricultural areas hookworm infection is a contributing factor to the development of iron deficiency, but it is not the only cause of the prevalence of this deficiency [1].

Iron Absorbed from the Diet

The amount of iron absorbed depends on the total iron intake, the bioavailability of food iron and individual absorption regulation. Surveys carried out in Latin America have shown that iron intake from the diet is of the order of 15-40 mg iron/person/day [20]; these data together with those studies of iron absorption using iron balance techniques, which showed that about 10-20 % of the iron intake from the diet is absorbed, provided strong grounds for the concept that diet does not play an important role in the development of iron deficiency. This concept which was universally accepted in scientific publications up to the sixties, was supplanted when the radioisotopic technique of MOORE and DUBACH [21] was introduced routinely in food iron absorption studies [22, 25]. This technique measures the iron absorption from food labeled with radioactive iron.

These studies showed that there is a wide range in absorption of vegetal iron, from about 0.5 % in rice to more than 7 % in wheat and soybeans, with intermediate values for maize and beans, that iron absorption from animal food such as beef meat and liver is about 3–4 times higher than the absorption from vegetable food and that iron absorption by iron deficient subjects with or without anemia is about 2–4 times higher than in normal subjects (Fig. 1).

Later contributions on this subject demonstrated that in the lumen of the gastrointestinal tract food iron and iron salts are organized in pools in terms of iron absorption [26, 28]. The absorption of iron from the heme pool (formed by hemoglobin and myoglobin) is not affected by vegetable foods, but its absorption is increased when ingested with proteins of animal origin such as meat or liver. The non-heme iron pool comes from vegetables, eggs, milk, ferric and ferrous iron salts. Its absorption is reduced by inhibitors present in vegetables, eggs and milk, and is increased by ascorbic acid and animal tissue

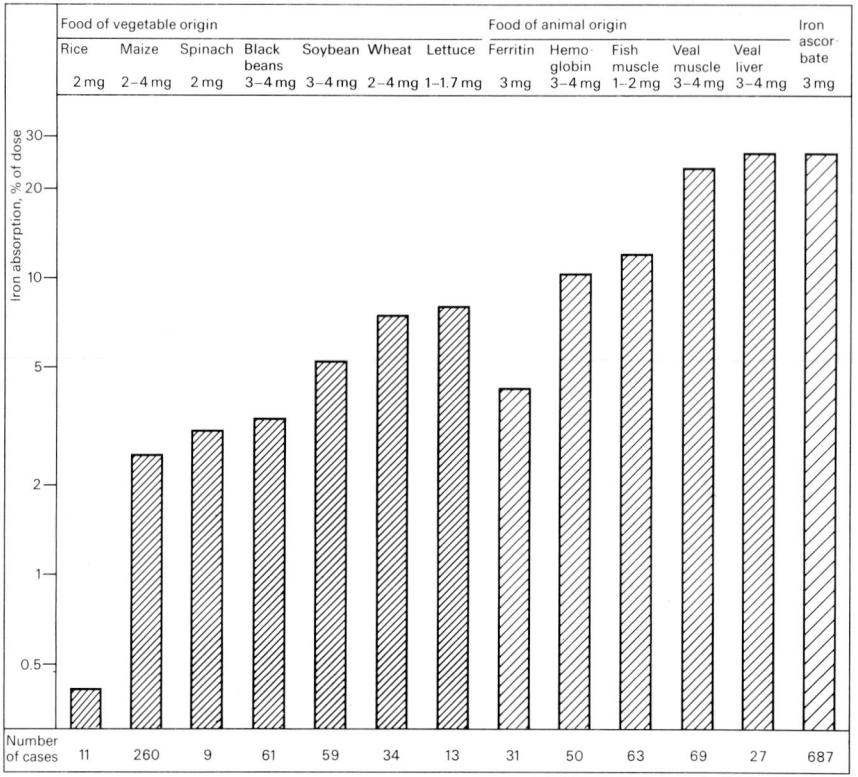

	Food of vegetable origin							Food of animal origin					Iron ascorbate
	Rice	Maize	Spinach	Black beans	Soybean	Wheat	Lettuce	Ferritin	Hemoglobin	Fish muscle	Veal muscle	Veal liver	
	2 mg	2–4 mg	2 mg	3–4 mg	3–4 mg	2–4 mg	1–1.7 mg	3 mg	3–4 mg	1–2 mg	3–4 mg	3–4 mg	3 mg

Number of cases: 11, 260, 9, 61, 59, 34, 13, 31, 50, 63, 69, 27, 687

Fig. 1: Mean iron absorption from vegetable and animal foods given alone and calibrated from the iron absorption of the reference dose of iron ascorbate.

proteins. Ferritin and hemosiderin may be considered as a subgroup of the non-heme iron pool; because of their tendency to polymerize their purified iron is not absorbed as well as vegetal iron, but their absorption is high when they are incorporated into meat or liver [29, 30]. The studies that identified these iron pools also demonstrated that the absorption of each iron pool during the ingestion of meals can be determined accurately by labeling a small amount of one of the iron compounds present in the appropriate pool. Thus, a labeled iron salt mixed with unlabeled vegetable food indicates the iron absorption of the total non-heme pool present in that meal, a small amount of labeled rabbit hemoglobin indicates the absorption of hemoglobin and myoglobin present in animal-derived foods, and a small amount of labeled purified ferritin that of ferritin and hemosiderin present in liver.

The revised concept of the iron pool and the simplification of the new technique to measure the iron absorption from the heme and non-heme pools present in a meal, allowed the measurement of the total iron available from a daily diet. These techniques were even more simplified using a reference dose of iron ascorbate as one of the absorption tests for a given diet [31]. From this the absorption of heme iron can be deduced, since there is a high correlation between the iron absorption from this salt and heme from meat, thus permitting the comparison of different dietary absorption rates.

Absorption from Diets

Two different methods have been used to determine the iron availability of a diet. One of them makes use of an average menu consisting of individual main foods that a population consumes over a period of 2–3 weeks [3]. The other utilizes a list of the total food intake of the population over several weeks. The various components are mixed, cooked and then administered as a pudding [32]. The last method has been demonstrated to be unphysiological since it does not take into consideration the different ways of preparing these foods which undoubtedly play an important role in the stimulation of the sensorial reflex during the different steps of digestion [33].

Since 1974, several studies have been published regarding the absorption from typical meals in the USA, Europe and Asia. These studies have shown the great variability in absorption, depending on the food contained in the diets, their preparation, and the subjects tested. They have shown great differences in iron absorption when a meal is ingested with a beverage such as tea, which precipitates the iron and reduces considerably the iron absorption, when a meal or part of a meal is prepared under acid conditions as occurs with sauerkraut or borsch [34] or when the mean contains a large amount of animal food such as meat, or fruit [25, 31, 34, 36].

The author has tried to find out the mechanism by which tissue animal protein increases the absorption of non-heme iron. He has demonstrated that cysteine is the only amino acid that increases the non-heme iron absorption in man. However, this effect was demonstrated only when cysteine was administered in capsules together with the food, since this amino acid is rapidly oxidized and transformed into cystine when mixed with the food before cooking [37]. Recent studies demonstrated that a parallel increase in the absorption of maize iron is obtained when comparable increased doses of either meat, cysteine of glutathione are administered with the vegetable food. However, since only a small amount of glutathione is present in meat, about 13–17 mg/100 g, it is probable that other cysteine-containing peptides are released from meat during digestion and these also facilitate the absorption of non-heme iron [38]. Further studies are being carried out in an attempt to clarify this point.

Iron Absorption from Latin American Diets

Only two studies have been carried out on Latin American diets; the first was published in 1974, based on three Venezuelan diets established by the Instituto Nacional de Nutrición in the Andean, Central and Coastal areas [31]. In order to compare these diets the iron absorption from each diet was calibrated according to the iron ascorbate absorption; they showed that the total iron absorption depends more on the composition of the diet than on the total iron intake. This coastal diet, in which only 9.5 mg iron was ingested showed the highest iron absorption, because fish was eaten at each meal (Table III). The total iron available in Andean and Central region diets, in normal subjects, was about 0.4 mg/day which is half of the physiological needs for adult men, and about 25 % of the needs in menstruating women. Although the nutrient contents of these diets refer to the whole family food consumption, including children and adults, the iron utilization is even lower for children in which the iron requirement is close to 1 mg/day. These data indicate that the population consuming the Andean and Central region diets are forced to become iron deficient in order to increase by a factor of two or three their iron absorption and thus prevent the development of iron deficiency anemia.

Tab. III: Iron absorption from Venezuelan diets

Regional diet	Energy, kcal	Iron content, mg		Total iron utilization		Bioavailable nutrient density, mg/1000 kcal
		non-heme	heme	normal	iron deficient	
Andes	1036	9.02	1.25	0.40	1.10	1.28
Central	1119	10.19	2.50	0.42	1.41	1.33
Coast	1351	9.36	0.09	0.82	1.62	0.77

The other absorption study was carried out in six Latin American countries under the auspices of the United Nations University and the laboratory of the IVIC in Caracas acting as reference center [39]. Typical diets from Salta, Argentina, São Paulo, Brasil; Santiago, Chile; Mérida, Yucatán State, México; Lima, Perú and Carabobo State, Venezuela, consumed by lower socioeconomic groups, were tested by the same method used for the Venezuelan diets. The total iron available from four out of the six diets for normal subjects did not meet the physiological iron requirements for male adults.

The nine iron absorption studies on these Latin American diets suggest that these diets, especially those consumed by the lower socio-economic segments of the population, which account for about 40–50% of the total population, play an important role in the development of iron deficiency and iron deficiency anemia. The low absorption from staple foods such as maize and beans, the inhibition of iron absorption by tea and coffee beverages, and the relatively small intake of animal food and fruits with each meal are responsible for the limited iron utilization from these diets.

Prevention of Iron Deficiency

Evidence has been accumulating to demonstrate that not only severe iron deficiency anemia is a health problem but also mild iron deficiency anemia and iron deficiency without anemia, because iron is an important nutrient for the function of the cells. It has already been demonstrated that this deficiency induces certain dysfunctions such as a reduction in the muscular working capacity [40, 41], reduction in the ability to maintain the body temperature [42–44], impairment of the immune response [45, 46], and impairment of the mental development in children [47].

There are three possible ways to prevent nutritional iron deficiency. One way would be to improve general sanitary conditions through measures such as the eradication of parasitic infections, and the substitution of iron-poor food for iron-rich food in terms of iron absorption. These measures take a long time, represent a great capital investment and cannot be expected to give spectacular results. Iron supplements, when correctly administered to vulnerable segments of the population, especially pregnant women and school children, represent another way of reducing iron deficiency. However this preventive measure is also costly, requiring full time personnel to supervise the administration of iron tablets.

The third alternative is the enrichment of a staple food with iron. In this respect we have to consider for each country or region a suitable food vehicle to be fortified with iron and the iron compound that could be used for each fortification program. The most suitable food vehicle is the one which a) is consumed by the total population or more specifically the segment of the population at risk, b) carries the least inhibitory substances of iron absorption and c) requires the least complicated food-enriching process. Table IV shows

Tab. IV: Iron absorption from ferrous sulfate mixed with various food vehicles

Food vehicle	Iron absorption, %		
	group A: ferrous sulfate + food vehicle (3–5 mg Fe)	group B: ferrous sulfate given alone (3–5 mg Fe)	ratio
Refined sugar cane	31.6	33.2	0.95
Sugar cane syrup	30.3	36.9	0.82
Sweet manioc	12.4	35.3	0.35
Milk	7.0	27.8	0.25
Wheat bread	7.7	49.3	0.16
Maize	2.7	32.9	0.08

Each value represents the mean of not less than 10 subjects tested.

the iron absorption from ferrous sulfate added to potential food vehicles for Latin America. The ratio between the iron absorption of the salt added to food vehicles and the iron absorption of the salt given alone shows that sugar contains practically no inhibitory substances for iron absorption while maize carries strong inhibitors, that reduce the iron absorption to 8 %. Wheat and milk also contain inhibitors, but less than maize. Other food vehicles are presently being used, such as common salt in India [48] and fish sauce in Thailand [49]. In the Latin American countries where the diets were tested for iron absorption, wheat seems to be the appropriate food vehicle for three countries, and sugar for another two.

Iron Compounds

Since 1941, the USA and England have enriched wheat flour with either reduced iron or ferric ammonium citrate but only proportionately iron loss during the refining process. There are several iron compounds that show the same percentage of iron absorption when they are used in iron fortification; they are reduced iron, ferrous sulfate, iron glycerophosphate, ferric ammonium citrate and ferric chloride. Since 1977, we have been studying the peculiar characteristics of Fe (III)-EDTA in comparison with ferrous sulfate when added to the same food vehicle. When ferrous sulfate is the fortification agent, iron absorption is inhibited by the chelating substances present in foods, whereas absorption from the EDTA complex is not affected by such substances. In addition, this iron complex exchanges iron freely with vegetal iron in the lumen of the gut and the absorption of both extrinsic and intrinsic iron is about twice as high as that expected using other salts under the same experimental conditions [50, 51].

There is a potential risk that NaFe-EDTA, a strong chelating agent, could react with other metals contained in food during digestion and provoke a nutrient deficiency. Recent studies have been carried out to clarify this problem by establishing the pathway of this compound from oral intake to elimination in urine and feces [52, 53]. These studies in man using the complex labeled with radioactive iron showed that the absorption follows the same pattern as any other ferric iron salt administered to fasting subjects, varying from 2 to 40 %, according to the iron status of the subjects. A small amount of the radioactive iron, less than 5 % of absorbed iron, is eliminated by the kidney in the form of Fe-EDTA. The studies in swine in which the complex was labeled with ^{55}Fe and ^{14}C, showed that as in man, about 2–25 % of the iron administered is absorbed and incorporated in circulating hemoglobin and about 5 % of absorbed iron is eliminated in urine. A different pathway was observed with the ^{14}C and ^{55}Fe measurement of the mucosal uptake, plasma turnover and kidney excretion of Na ^{55}Fe-EDTA-2-^{14}C indicates that ^{55}Fe is separated from the complex in the lumen of the gut before being taken up by the mucosa cells. The radioactive stool count showed that about 92 % of the ^{55}Fe administered is found in an insoluble form, probably as iron oxide. The chemical studies in humans and swine indicate that the EDTA complex is degraded in the lumen of the gut and not bound by any cation [54]. These results seem to indicate that the use of iron-EDTA as iron fortification does not represent a risk in terms of the development of any metal deficiency, and allowed the Venezuelan Nutrition Committee to introduce this complex in the national program of sugar fortification with iron.

The advances in the understanding of food iron absorption over the last 15 years, reviewed briefly in this paper, represent the ground work for the institution of national programs against iron deficiency. It is now possible to predict the bioavailability of the iron compound added to the food vehicle not only when eaten alone, but also when eaten with the regular diet, and from these results the amount of iron fortification necessary to effectively reduce the occurrence of iron deficiency anemia can be established.

Acknowledgments: Part of the studies presented here were intially supported by WHO and the Williams Waterman Foundation. In recent years it has been supported by the Consejo Nacional de Investigaciones Científicas y Tecnológicas, Caracas, and by the United Nations University.

References

1   LAYRISSE, M, ROCHE, M: Relationship between anemia and hookworm infection. Results of surveys of rural Venezuelan population. Am J Hyg 79, 279–301, 1964.
2   BLOCH, V, RIVERA, H: La enfermedad Uncinariásica en el Salvador. Arch Col Med El Salvador 19, 3–34, 1966.
3   VITERI, F E et al: Anemias nutricionales en Centro América. Influencia de infección por Uncinaria. Archos Latinoamer Nutr 23, 33–53, 1973.
4   PAEZ-PUMAR, E et al: Datos hematológicos e incidencia de parásitos intestinales en un grupo de niños estudiados en el Servicio de Nutrología. Archos Venezol Nutr 10, 145–158, 1960.
5   AGUERO, O, LAYRISSE, M: Anemias en obstetricia. Rev Obstet Ginecol Venezuela 20, 237–251, 1960.
6   LAYRISSE, M: The aetiology and geographic incedence of iron deficiency. In: XIth Congr Int Soc Haematol, pp 95–101, 1966.
7   LAYRISSE, M: Iron deficiency anemia in South America. In: Proc Western Hemisph Nutr Congr, pp 171–174, 1968.
8   GANDRA, Y R: La anemia ferropenica en la población de América Latina y el Caribe. Boletín Ofic Sanit Panamer, 1970: 375–383, 1970.
9   LORIS, A et al: Anemia nutricional III. Deficiencia de hierro en niños menores de 7 años de edad y de baja condición socioeconómica. Rev Invest Clin México 23, 11–19, 1971.
10 DIEZ-EWALD, M, MOLINA, R A: Iron and folic acid deficiency during pregnancy in Western Venezuela. Am J Trop Med Hyg 21, 587–591, 1972.
11 ROMERO-GARCÍA, F et al: Prevalencia de anemia y carencia de hierro, ácido fólico y vitamina B12 en una población aparentemente sanada o a 15 años procedente de medio socioeconómico débil. Sangre 25, 549–558, 1980.
12 STELLER, H C, HUONG, A Y: Epidemiología de la anemia en niños de edad preescolar y sus madres en El Salvador. Archos Latino-Amer Nutr 31, 679–697, 1981.
13 DIEZ-EWALD, M et al: Reserva de hierro en poblaciones de clase pobre en Maracaibo. Invest Clín 24, 69–82, 1983.
14 FOSI, M et al: Estudios hematológicos en la encuesta del Estado Carabobo del Proyecto Venezuela (submitted).
15 COOK, J et al: Nutritional deficiency and anemia in Latin America. A collaborative study. Blood 38, 591–603, 1971.
16 ROCHE, M, LAYRISSE, M: The nature and causes of hookworm anemia. Am J Trop Med Hyg 15, 1031–1102, 1966.
17 FARID, Z et al: Blood loss in pure Ancylostoma duodenale infection in Egyptian farmers. Am J Trop Med Hyg 14, 375–378, 1965.
18 ROCHE, M, PÉREZ-GIMENEZ, M E: Intestinal loss and reabsorption of iron in hookworm infection. J Lab Clin Med 54, 49–52, 1959.
19 LAYRISSE, M et al: Blood loss due to infection with Trichuris trichiura. Am J Trop Med Hyg 16, 613–619, 1967.
20 Interdepartmental Committee on Nutrition and National Defense of the United States (ICNND). Surveys in Northeast Brazil, Bolivia, Chile, Colombia, Ecuador, Paraguay, Peru and Venezuela. Reports of 1965, 1964, 1961, 1961, 1960, 1965, 1959, 1964, respectively.
21 MOORE, C V, DUBACH, R: Observation of the absorption of iron from food tagged with radioiron. Trans Ass Am Phy 64, 245–256, 1951.
22 LAYRISSE, M et al: Food iron absorption. A comparison of vegetable and animal foods. Blood 33, 430–443, 1969.
23 LAYRISSE, M, MARTÍNEZ-TORRES, C: Food iron absorption: iron supplementation of food. Progr Hematol 7, 137–160, 1971.
24 MARTÍNEZ-TORRES, C, LAYRISSE, M: Nutritional factors in iron deficiency. Food iron absorption. In: Clinics in haematol, vol 2, pp 339–352. Saunders, Philadelphia, 1973.

25 LAYRISSE, M, MARTÍNEZ-TORRES, C: Absorción del hierro a partir de los alimentos. Consejo Nacional de Investigaciones Científicas y Tecnológicas, Caracas, 1983.

26 COOK, J et al: Food iron absorption measured by an extrinsic tag. J Clin Invest 51, 805–815, 1972.

27 LAYRISSE, M, MARTÍNEZ-TORRES, C: Model for measuring dietary absorption of heme iron: test with a complete meal. Am J Clin Nutr 25, 401–411, 1972.

28 BJÖRN-RASMUSSEN, E et al: Food iron absorption in man. I. Isotopic exchange between food iron and inorganic iron salt added to food. Studies of maize, wheat and eggs. Am J Clin Nutr 25, 317–323, 1972.

29 LAYRISSE, M et al: Ferritin iron absorption in man. Blood 45, 689–698, 1975.

30 MARTÍNEZ-TORRES, C et al: Iron absorption by humans from ferritin and hemosiderin. J Nutr 106, 128–135, 1976.

31 LAYRISSE, M et al: Measurement of the total daily dietary absorption by the extrinsic tag model. Am J Clin Nutr 27, 152–162, 1974.

32 BJÖRN-RASMUSSEN, E et al: Food iron absorption in man. Application of the two-pool extrinsic tag method to measure heme and non-heme iron absorption from the whole diet. J Clin Invest 53, 247–255, 1974.

33 HALLBERG, L et al: Iron absorption from southeast Asia diets. II. Role of various factors that might explain low absorption. Am J Clin Nutr 30, 539–548, 1977.

34 HALLBERG, L: Bioavailability of dietary iron in man. Ann Rev Nutr 1, 123–147, 1981.

35 LAYRISSE, M et al: The effect of interaction of various foods on iron absorption. Am J Clin Nutr 21, 1175–1183, 1968.

36 HALLBERG, L et al: Dietary heme iron absorption. Scand J Haemat 29, 18–24, 1982.

37 MARTÍNEZ-TORRES, C et al: Effect of cysteine on iron absorption in man. Am J Clin Nutr 34, 322–328, 1981.

38 LAYRISSE, M et al: Effect of histidine, cysteine, glutathione and beef meat on iron absorption in man. J Nutr 114, 217–223, 1984.

39 ACOSTA AMAR, M et al: The iron absorption from typical Latin American diets (submitted).

40 VITERI, F E, TORUM, B: Anemia and physical work capacity. In: Garby, L (ed). Clinics in haematology, vol 3, pp 609–627. Saunders Philadelphia, 1974.

41 FINCH, C A et al: Iron deficiency in the rat. Physiological and biochemical studies of muscle dysfunctions. J Clin Invest 58, 447–453, 1976.

42 DILLMANN, E et al: Catecholamine elevation in iron deficiency. Am J Physiol 237, R297–R300, 1979.

43 DILLMANN, E et al: Hypothermia in iron deficiency due to impaired T_3 and T_4 conversion. Am J Physiol 239, R377–R381, 1980.

44 MARTÍNEZ-TORRES, C et al: Effect of exposure to low temperature on normal iron deficient subjects. J Appl Physiol 246, 380–383, 1984.

45 GROSS, R L, NEWBERNE, M: Role of nutrition in immunologic function. Physiol Rev 60, 260–264, 1980.

46 SOYANO, A et al: Effect of iron deficiency on the mitogen-induced proliferative response of rat lymphocytes. Int Arch Allergy Appl Immunol 69, 353–357, 1982.

47 LOSSOFF, B et al: Developmental deficits in iron-deficient infants. Effects of age and severity of iron lack. Pediat 101, 348–352, 1982.

48 NARASINGA-RAO, B S et al: Iron absorption in Indians studied by whole body counting. A comparison of iron compounds used in salt fortification. Br J Haematol 2, 281–286, 1972.

49 GARBY, L: Iron fortification from fish sauce in Thailand. Am J Trop Med Hyg 68, 467–476, 1974.

50 LAYRISSE, M, MARTÍNEZ-TORRES, C: Fe(III)-EDTA complex as iron fortification. Am J Clin Nutr 30, 1166–1174, 1977.

51 MARTÍNEZ-TORRES, C et al: Fe(III)-EDTA complex as iron fortification. Further studies. J Clin Nutr 32, 809–816, 1979.

52 MacPhail, A P *et al:* Factors affecting the absorption of iron from Fe(III)-EDTA. Br J Nutr
    45, 215–226, 1981.
53 Candela, E *et al:* Iron absorption by humans and swine from Fe(III)-EDTA. J Nutr *114,*
    2204–2211, 1984.
54 Camacho, M *et al:* In preparation.

*Dr. Miguel Layrisse, Director, Instituto Venezolano de Investigaciones Sientificas, Apartado
1827, Caracas, Venezuela*

Effect of Vitamin A on Visual Accuracy

D. WILSON, O.B. NETTO, A. SIMAO DA COSTA, A. STEINER,
M. DE FATIMA NUNES MARUCCI and M.C. BARBOSA

Department of Nutrition, University of São Paulo School of Public Health, National Institute of
Social Security, Municipal School Network, São Paulo, Brazil

Key Words: Vitamin A · Visual accuracy · Brazil · School children

*Abstract: Two comparable groups of 150 primary school children in a São
Paulo municipal school were studied to determine whether vitamin A supplementation in a subclinically deficient population can improve visual accuracy. One group received four daily doses of 50 000 IU vitamin A; the control group received nothing. All children were given the standard eyesight
screening test (Snellen table) at the beginning of the study and three weeks
later at its conclusion. The differences between the results of the two tests
were classified as: improvement (+ 20 %), no change (up to 10 %) or
deterioration (– 20 %).*

*The proportion of improved cases was significantly higher in the treatment
group than in the control group (p < 0.001). The proportion of unaltered cases
was significantly lower in the treatment group (p < 0.001). There was no
significant difference between the two groups in the proportion of
deteriorated scores.*

*In conclusion, it appears that vitamin A supplementation improved vision
in the treated group.*

Introduction

Special attention has been drawn to vitamin A deficiency in underdeveloped
countries by the prevalence of severe ocular lesions, i.e. xerophthalmia, which
can lead to blindness. In Brazil, many studies have been carried out [1–7],
especially in the states of São Paulo and Pernambuco, showing that the deficiency is most frequently subclinical. Xerophthalmia is far less common, and
severe lesions capable of causing blindness are practically non-existent.

Night blindness, another known manifestation of vitamin A deficiency, has
not been studied in Brazil as a mass phenomenon owing to the subjective
nature of the collected data, and a lack of suitable equipment.

The known importance of vitamin A in vision, for example, as a component
of rhodopsin in the rods of the retina, suggests that daytime visual acuity

might also be impaired by even a subclinical deficiency of vitamin A. However, an extensive literature search revealed no mention of such an observation. We sought to test this hypothesis in a study of school children in São Paulo.

Since poor eyesight is acknowledged as an important negative influence on children's scholastic performance, all municipal schools in the city of São Paulo subject their pupils to an eyesight screening test at the beginning of the year. We were able to time our study to take advantage of this annual screening procedure. However, we were limited by ethical considerations: for example, we could not suppress vitamin A intake in order to detect optical manifestations of deficiency, nor could we take blood from school children for determination of vitamin A levels. For this reason, we selected an indirect study method in which we measured the benefit of vitamin A supplementation by comparing the results of eyesight screening tests in a treated and an untreated group.

Materials and Methods

Study team. The study team comprised: two medical doctors, one an ophthalmologist, the other an internist in Public Health; a Public Health nurse; a teacher trained in health education; two nutritionists.

Study population. The study was conducted at a school drawing most of its pupils from the poorest socio-economic class in which, on the basis of our previous work, we would expect subclinical vitamin A deficiency to be highly prevalent. We conducted our study in conjunction with the annual eyesight screening tests.

All children of grades 1–4 were submitted to the routine eyesight tests, the results of which are used to refer pupils for ophthalmological care when necessary.

A sample of 150 children was drawn, using a randomization table. A second comparison group of 150 was then selected, matching for sex, age and eyesight test scores (binocular vision only). The children's group allocation was known only to the teacher and the public health service nurse, i.e. those conducting the eyesight tests were unaware of the group to which the children belonged.

Administration of vitamin A. The children in the treatment group received 200000 IU of vitamin A (Arovit®) orally, in four daily doses of 50000 IU. It was administered by the nurse and the teacher. The control group received nothing as a suitable placebo was not available.

Procedure. At the start of the study and three weeks later, children underwent eyesight testing. The results of the two examinations were recorded on separate cards so that, at the second examination, the examiners did not know the results of the first. At the end of the study all results were recorded on a third card to simplify processing.

Eyesight tests and evaluation criteria. Examinations were performed with the aid of a Snellen table, according to the specifications: well-lighted room; subjects' eyes 5 m away from the Snellen table. This table, although designed as a screening test providing a rather gross percentage grading, was thought sufficient for our purpose, since we were measuring not visual acuity per se, but changes in eyesight acuracy. Our criteria for change were correspondingly broad:
improved   = a positive difference of 0.2 (+ 20%)
unaltered   = a positive or negative difference of 0.1, or no difference (± 10%)
deteriorated = a negative difference of 0.2 (– 20%)

Statistical analysis. Inter- and intra-group differences between the scores of the 1st and the 2nd examination were analysed, using the significance test for proportions according to Bradford-Hill (A Short Textbook for Medical Statistics, Hodder & Stoughton).

Results

Table I shows the results obtained. The original number of 150 pairs (n = 300) decreased to 119 for reasons unrelated to the study itself. When a child of either group stopped attending, its pair was discarded from analysis.

Tab. I: Results after three weeks of vitamin A administration

	Vitamin A recipients		Control group	
	number	%	number	%
Improved	84	70.6	46	38.7
Unaltered	27	22.7	58	48.7
Worsened	8	6.7	15	12.6
Total	119	100.0	119	100.0

The significantly higher proportion of improved scores in the treated group compared with the control group (70 and 38.7 %), respectively; $p < 0.001$) suggests a positive effect of vitamin A on eyesight. Although 38.7 % of the control group improved, the proportion of those unchanged was significantly higher (48.7 %; $p = 0.05$). There was also a significant inter-group difference ($p < 0.001$) with regard to the proportion of subjects rated as unchanged. There was no significant difference between the two groups with respect to the proportion of subjects in whom vision deteriorated.

As expected in view of the total dose of vitamin A administered, there were no signs of hypervitaminosis A in the treated group.

Discussion

The significantly higher proportion of subjects with improved vision in the treated group strongly suggests a benefical effect of vitamin A supplementation. The improvement seen in 38.7 % of the control group was significantly less than in the treated group, and might have been attributable to other factors affecting the test results, such as a learning effect, difference in light (i.e. normal variation in natural light sources), and familiarity with the examiners. These influences, however, would not be sufficient to explain the significant improvement in the treated group.

Conclusion

Vitamin A supplementation significantly improved vision in a socio-economic group in which previous experience has shown vitamin A deficiency to be prevalent.

References

1 Batista, M: Considerações sobre o problema de vitamina A no Nordeste brasileiro. O Hospital *75,* 31–46, 1969.
2 Gandra, Y R: Inquérito sobre o estado de nutrição de um grupo da população de cidade de São Paulo. II- Investigações sobre a ocorrência de hipovitaminose A. Arq Fac Hig S Paulo *8,* 217–60, 1954.
3 Instituto Nacional de Alimentação e Nutrição. Hipovitaminose A no Brasil. Brasília, 1977.
4 Roncada, M J: Hipovitaminose A. Níveis séricos de vitamina A e caroteno em populações litorâneas do Estado de São Paulo, Brasil. Rev Saúde públ *6,* 3–18, 1972.
5 Roncada, M J *et al:* Hipovitaminose A em comunidades do Estado de São Paulo, Brasil. Rev Saúde públ *15,* 338–49, 1981.
6 Roncada, M J *et al:* Hipovitaminose A em filhos de migrantes nacionais, em trânsito pela capital do Estado de São Paulo, Brasil. Estudo clínico-bioquímico. Rev Saúde públ *12,* 345–50, 1978.
7 US Interdepartmental Committee on Nutrition for National Defense. Northeast Brazil nutrition survey: March–May, 1963: a report. US Government Printing Office, Washington, 1968.

Prof. D. Wilson, Universidade de São Paulo, Faculdade de Saúde Pública, Caixa postal 8099, 01255 São Paulo, S.P., Brazil

Metabolism and Function of Ascorbic Acid and its Metabolites

B.M. Tolbert

Department of Chemistry, University of Colorado, Boulder, Colorado, USA

Key Words: Ascorbic acid · Dehydroascorbic acid · Diketogulonic acid · 5-Ketoascorbitol · Metabolism: distribution, function

Abstract: The metabolism of ascorbic acid in higher animals can be considered as an oxidation-reduction cycle, two main metabolism/excretion processes, and a group of minor processes. The oxidation reduction cycle controls the ascorbate to dehydroascorbate (DHA) ratio which may either reflect or have some control over cell biosynthetic processes. One of the main metabolic processes is the excretion in the urine of six carbon metabolites derived from dehydroascorbic acid. This appears to be the major process in primates and to be common to all higher animals. This pathway is subject to limited control in which certain stresses, such as smoking, increase its rate. The rate of formation of these metabolites should be an excellent index of the nutritional status of ascorbate. The other main metabolic process is catabolism to CO_2 via DHA. A group of minor pathways include methylation, sulfation, and cleavage to oxalate in which ascorbic acid behaves as a catechol analogue.

The recognized roles of ascorbic acid include its function as a cofactor for mixed function oxidases, its role in iron metabolism and its role as a free radical scavenger. It seems likely that ascorbate is a precursor for other active forms of this vitamin, probably formed in the metabolic process leading to the six carbon urine products. The conversion of ascorbate to a 5-keto metabolite in animals and the postulated presence of a 5-keto intermediate in ascorbate metabolism in plants provides a basis for suggesting the existence of other forms of ascorbate that can function in the oxidation-reduction cycle. The high level of ascorbate in brain, adrenal and gonad tissues does not have a satisfactory explanation.

The molecular mechanism of transport and storage of ascorbic acid have been studied. Reduced ascorbate is probably transported and stored as the molecular ion. It seems unlikely that DHA can be transported or stored as the molecular species.

Introduction

The story of ascorbic acid metabolism and function is far from complete. It shares this dubious honor with the other reducing vitamin – vitamin E. Perhaps the incomplete understanding of the metabolism of these compounds arises from their roles in free radical reactions, or perhaps because their metabolic pathways seem to be complex. In any case, the lack of information has provided an exciting area for nutritional research and the innovation of new ideas.

Surely, ascorbic acid has multiple roles in biological systems. It functions as a generalized water-soluble oxidation-reduction system, and perhaps some of its metabolites function as co-factor of certain enzymes. Ascorbic acid is an excellent free radical scavenger forming a stable intermediate radical that holds cell biochemical processes safe from chemical damage. Lastly, ascorbic acid may function as a metabolic regulator, either directly or indirectly.

The metabolism of ascorbic acid in higher animals can be considered as follows: the oxidation-reduction cycle, two main metabolic processes and a number of minor processes. One of the main metabolic processes, the diketogulonate (DKG) pathway, was discovered shortly after the introduction of isotope tracer methodology and was extensively studied by Ashwell et al [1]. This process leads to catabolic degradation of the carbon skeleton of ascorbic acid to CO_2. The other process observed in the earlier studies was not defined until the early 70's and leads to the urinary excretion of ascorbic acid as a series of water-soluble metabolites, most of which are believed to have an intact carbon skeleton of ascorbate [2]. This pathway is called the dehydroascorbic acid pathway for reasons to be discussed later. Minor processes that result in methyl and sulfate derivatives are called here the catechol analogue pathway (Table I).

Tab. I: General classes of ascorbic acid metabolism

I Oxidation-reduction cycle
II Dehydroascorbic acid pathway – urine metabolites
III Diketogulonate pathway – CO_2 production
IV Catechol analogue pathways – urine metabolites

Not only are these pathways of considerable nutritional significance, but the tissue, subcellular location and control of enzymes involved in these processes are of more than passing interest. It is highly likely that some of these metabolites have functional roles. The distribution of ascorbic acid in tissues is anomalous in that this water-soluble vitamin is present in the highest levels in highly lipid tissues such as the brain, adrenals and ovaries.

The elucidation of ascorbic acid metabolism is a difficult chemical problem. Not only are many of the intermediates quite labile, but the isolation and identification of these carbohydrate derivatives and the characterization of the related enzymes have been difficult using classical biochemical procedures. New tools are now available for such studies, in particular high performance liquid chromatography (MPLC), carbon-13 nuclear magnetic resonance (NMR), modern mass spectrometry, and vastly improved methods of isolating membrane bound enzymes are available. These developments together with a continuing interest in this field should lead to general progress in this area. The well documented increase in ascorbic acid turnover in tobacco smokers must have a biochemical basis. It is likely that one or more neurological abnormalities may have an origin in genetic errors leading to modified ascorbic acid metabolism and function.

The Oxidation-Reduction Metabolism of Ascorbic Acid

Ascorbic acid undergoes an oxidation-reduction cycle that is probably mostly enzyme-mediated with only a few purely chemical processes. In this process (Fig. 2) ascorbic acid may be oxidized or reduced by way of the free radical intermediate, monodehydroascorbate ($As \cdot ^-$).

Enzymes that reduce dehydroascorbate (DHA) or $As \cdot ^-$ have been demonstrated in higher animal tissues and are probably common to all mammalian species [3]. The most important and abundant of these enzymes are glutathione reductases that catalyze this reaction. In turn this system is coupled to a NADPH reductase so that the reaction is linked to the activity of the pentose phosphate pathway (Fig. 1).

a) $As + [0] \rightarrow DHA + H_2O$
$DHA + G\text{-}SH \rightleftarrows G\text{-}SS\text{-}G + As$
$G\text{-}SS\text{-}G + NADPH \rightarrow G\text{-}SH + NADP$
$NADP + glucose\text{-}6\text{-}P \rightarrow NADPH + 6\text{-}P\text{-}gulonolactone$
$NADP + 6\text{-}P\text{-}gulonate \rightarrow NADPH + CO_2 + Ru\text{-}5\text{-}P$

b) $As + R \cdot \rightarrow RH + As \cdot ^-$
$2 As \cdot ^- \rightarrow DHA + As$
$As \cdot ^- + NADPH \rightarrow As + NADP$

Fig. 1: The major oxidation-reduction cycle (a) and the minor oxidation-reduction cycle (b). Abbreviations: As = ascorbic acid, DHA = dehydroascorbic acid, G-SH = glutathione, $As \cdot ^-$ = semidehydroascorbic acid radical.

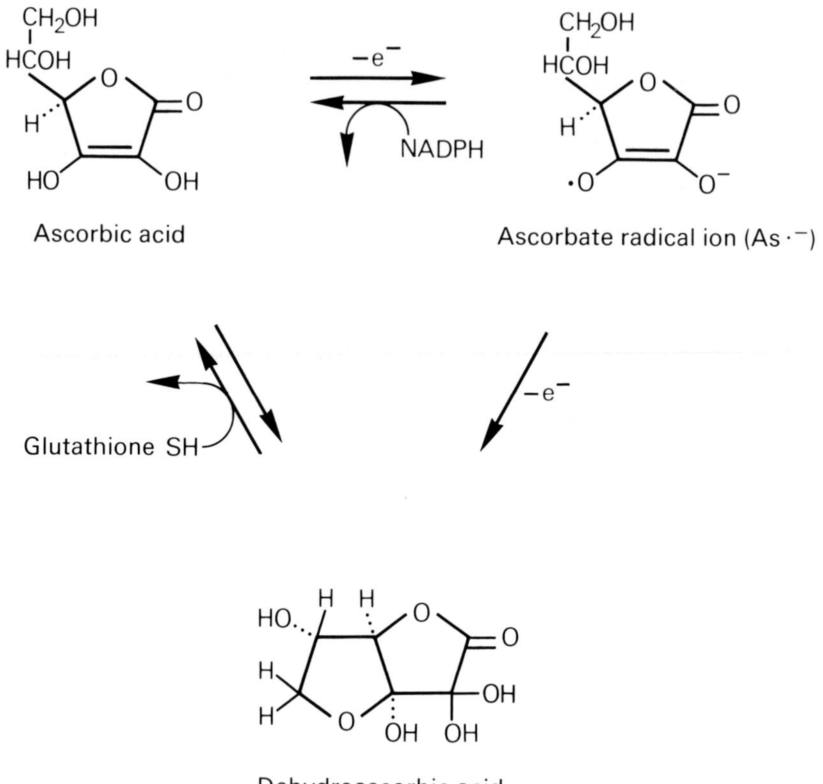

Fig. 2: The oxidation-reduction cycle.

As·⁻ is present at low concentrations in most tissues, and is commonly observed in electron spin resonance studies of whole cells or cell organelles. It is a remarkable radical in that it does not react rapidly with either oxygen, amino acids, nucleic acids or alcohols [4]. It can be formed by the rapid reaction of carbon and oxygen radicals with ascorbate, with the exception of molecular oxygen itself. The long lived As·⁻ radical reacts rapidly with itself to give DHA and ascorbate or it may be reduced by the enzyme system discovered by STAUDINGER et al [5, 6].

The ascorbate:DHA ratio has been a center of attention in ascorbic acid studies in recent years [7, 8]. First, this ratio must have a finite value. If the DHA concentrations in biological systems were zero, the driving force, $\triangle$G', for related reactions would be either infinitely large or small. This, however, is thermodynamically not reasonable. Recent measurements of this ratio in blood by new and improved methods give values of about 0.65:0.35 [7, 8]. Some early measurements yielding the ratio in 0.90:0.10 were considered as too high for blood ascorbate, but may be a value reasonable for tissue ascorbate. The estimation of this ratio, however, has been difficult due to methodological problems, since most of the work done by a differential diphenylhydrazone (DNPH) colorimetric procedure has a large error and is lacking specificity. It is now possible to measure this ratio by HPLC differential assay that is specific or by improved colorimetric methods [9]. Older data on this ratio need to be redetermined. This ratio may correlate better with physiological effects than actual levels of ascorbate [10].

The ascorbate:DHA ratio is controlled by the relative rates of oxidation and reduction in this cycle. The reduction of DHA is indirectly dependent on the NADPH:NADP ratio, which in turn is important in many biosynthetic pathways. Thus the ascorbate/DHA ratio may either reflect the biosynthetic vigor of cells or it may be involved in the control process [11]. The glutathione oxidized-reduced ratio is also presumed regulatory in nature. It is important to note that a primary biochemical effect of massive doses of ascorbic acid may change the ascorbate:DHA ratio. This may be a salutory change.

Enzyme processes producing significant amounts of DHA in higher animals are not known. Ceruloplasmin, a copper containing enzyme, has ascorbate oxidase activity, but the activity is minor and it probably is not a major producer of DHA, which may be produced by reversal of the glutathione:ascorbate reductase system, or by hydroxylase enzymes. Most workers in this field have presumed that DHA is formed by a non-enzymatic process.

Neither a blood ascorbate transport protein nor a cellular ascorbate binding protein have been reported, although some search has been made for such systems. It is therefore presumed that ascorbic acid is present in blood and cell fluids as the free monomeric ion. The problem is with DHA. This compound is rapidly hydrolyzed to 2,3-DKG at high and low pH and these results were confirmed by our group [12]. There is a window of stability at pH 2-4. At pH 7 DHA is rapidly hydrolyzed to DKG. Since these rate measurements are inconsistent with significant levels of DHA in blood of primates, it seems likely that there is a protecting system for DHA. Amino acids, polyamines or lysyl residues in proteins could serve this role by the formation of Schiff base complexes (Fig. 3).

These compounds would be very resistant to lactone hydrolysis. Schiff base complexes of DHA and bases have been studied on a chemical level [13]. Such compounds are also formed as intermediates in the browning reaction where ascorbic acid and amino acids are heated together. Schiff bases form readily between DHA and pyridoxamine, one of the forms of vitamin B_6, and between DHA and amino acids at pH > 8.

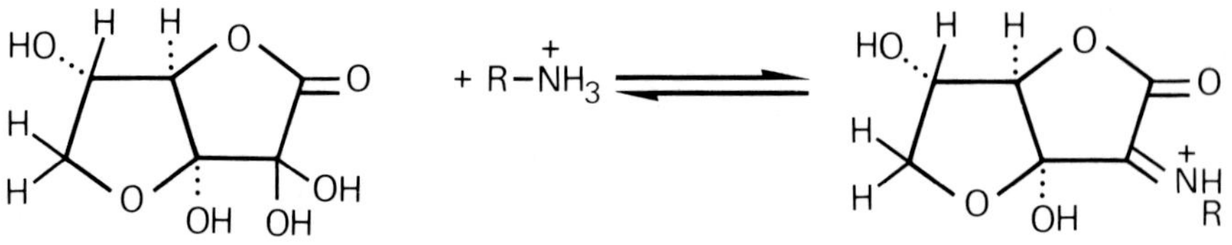

Dehydroascorbic acid

Fig. 3: Schiff base complexes of dehydroascorbic acid.

Metabolism of Ascorbate to Urinary Products: The Dehydroascorbic Acid Pathway

In primates, including man, the major fate of the metabolism of the ascorbate pool is a series of water-soluble carbohydrate-like compounds. Most of the compounds appear to have the intact carbon skeleton of ascorbic acid because the same chromatographic profile of metabolites is observed whether (1-^{14}C) ascorbate or (6-^{14}C) ascorbate is used in the studies. Three of these compounds were isolated and one was characterized by a combination of (^{1}H) and (^{13}C) NMR, mass spectrometry, and chemical behaviour [14]. The proposed structure for this compound is given in Figure 4.

The other compounds isolated have chromatographic properties similar to those of this compound. 5-Ketoascorbitol and the other metabolites did not have significant UV absorbance above 220 nm, which is again characteristic of carbohydrates. There are probably 9–12 of these compounds in human urine, of which 3 make up about 70% of the total [14]. These compounds are also found in rat, mouse and guinea pig urines.

5-Ketoascorbitol could be formed by a rather simple series of biochemical reactions starting with dehydroascorbic acid (Fig. 5). At present there is not much information available on 5-keto derivatives and metabolites of ascorbic acid. ANDREWS and CRAWFORD [15] have synthesized 5-ketoascorbic acid by a

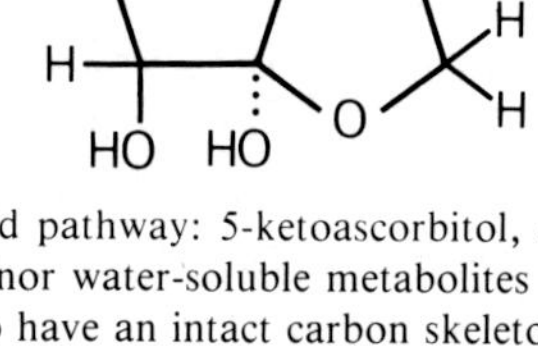

Fig. 4: The dehydroascorbic acid pathway: 5-ketoascorbitol, an ascorbate urinary metabolite. Three major plus at least six minor water-soluble metabolites are present in urine of primates. Most appear to have an intact carbon skeleton of ascorbate.

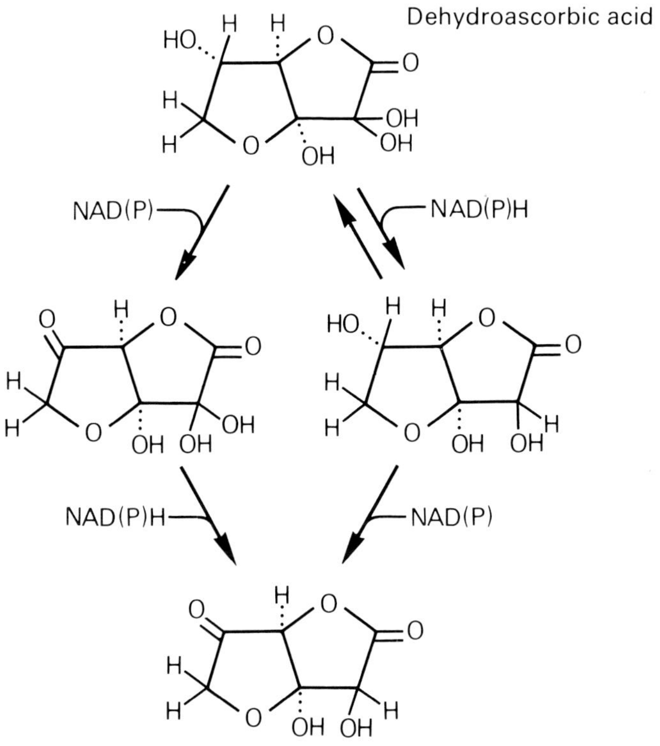

5-Ketoascorbitol

Fig. 5: Proposed pathways for the formation of 5-ketoascorbate.

series of reactions shown in Figure 6. The 5-ketoascorbic acid is mostly present as the hydrated form. It rapidly racemized at carbon C_4, leading to an exchange of the hydrogen at carbon C_4.

There are several tracer studies of ascorbic acid metabolism supporting the concept that the formation and the excretion of 5-keto metabolites are a significant process in higher animals. In 1967, TOLBERT et al [16], measured the excretion of tritium in man after ingestion of $(4-^3H)$ ascorbic acid. 32 % of the tritium was excreted as ^3H_2O, and the remainder as organically bound tritium. Since carbon catabolism to CO_2 is not a significant process in man, this metabolic pathway could not be explained on the basis of known biochemical steps.

In 1976, TOLBERT et al [17] reported on the metabolism of $(6-^3H)$ ascorbic acid in the macaque monkey under conditions where negligible amounts of ascorbate are catabolized to CO_2 (Fig. 7). About 43 % of tritium was found to

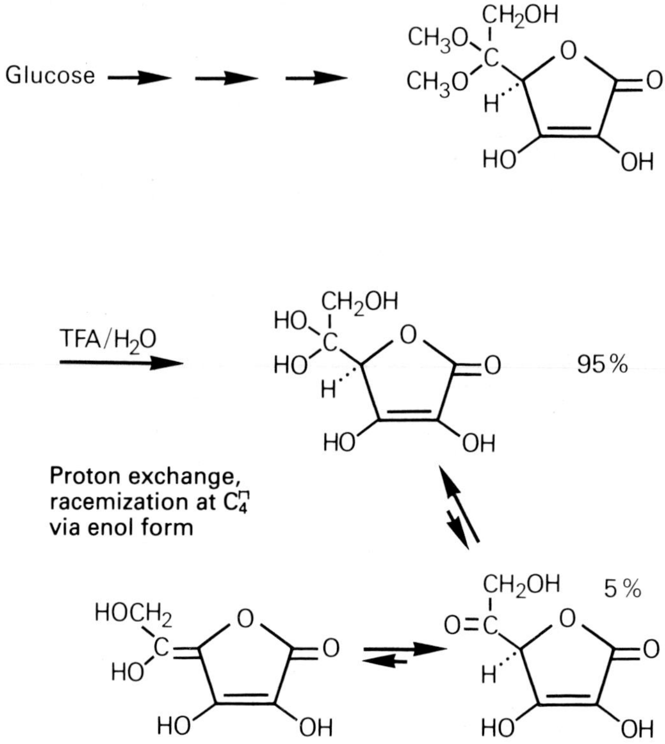

Fig. 6: 5-Ketoascorbic acid: synthesis and properties; according to Andrews and Crawford [15].

be excreted as water, and the remainder as organically bound tritium. This was postulated to originate from a C_6 oxidation process, but further studies failed to show either a saccharoascorbic acid metabolite or other C_6 oxidized metabolites.

The excretion of tritium water and organically bound tritium both followed the half time indicating that the turnover of both the organic metabolite pool and the tritium water pool was short compared with that of the ascorbate pool. The water turnover is about 7 days. Therefore catabolism leading to water must have been a process with a 20-day half time, which is the turnover time of the ascorbate pool itself. The body water is in secular equilibrium with the ascorbic acid pool tritium.

5-Keto metabolites of ascorbate have the potential for both 6H and 4H-exchange through an enol tautomer. These studies support the fact that a minimum of about 40% of the metabolism of ascorbate in primates follows a 5-keto metabolic process. Harkrader [14] estimated 5-ketoascorbitol to represent 35–40% of urinary ascorbate metabolites in primates.

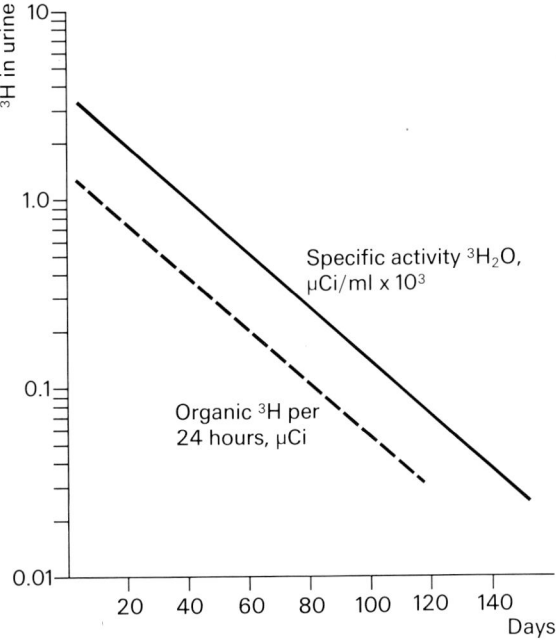

Fig. 7: Urine excretion of ${}^3H$ after injection of (6-${}^3H$) ascorbate in a monkey. ——— = Labeled water; — — — = labeled organic compounds. According to Tolbert *et al* [17].

Ascorbic Acid Metabolites via DKG

A major metabolic pathway in most higher animals except primates leads to oxidation of the carbon skeleton of ascorbate to CO_2. Most of these studies have been made with (1-${}^{14}C$) ascorbic acid and the carbon C_1 appears very rapidly as CO_2 in common experimental animals such as mice, rats and guinea pigs. These animals also have significant quantities of a liver enzyme that hydrolyzes DHA to 2,3-DKG [18], which has no vitamin activity, cannot be re-converted to ascorbic acid, and is itself rapidly catabolized to CO_2 [19]. A review of the literature shows that in carefully controled experiments in primates and man there is a very low rate of CO_2 excretion from the ascorbate pool compared with urinary excretion [20].

Because the DKG pathway (Fig. 8) is not present to any extent in primates it seems likely that none of the metabolites of this pathway has an essential role in ascorbic acid functions. This seems to be rather a disposal pathway – part of the mechanism whereby excessive blood and tissue levels of ascorbate are prevented.

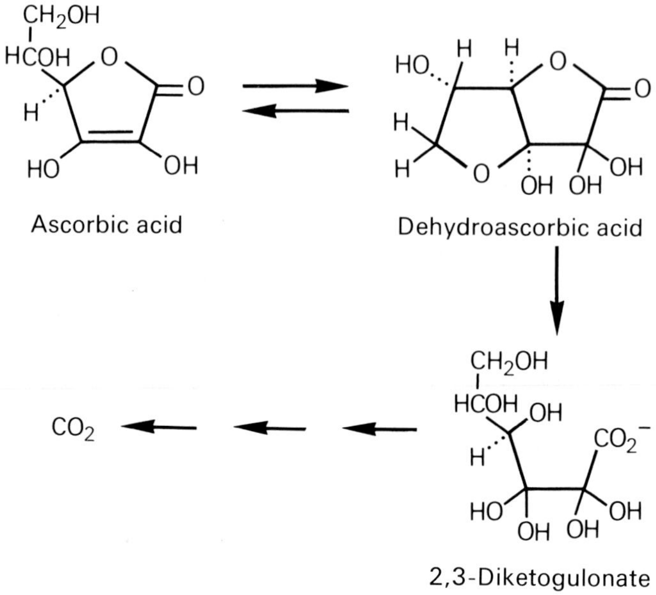

Fig. 8: The diketogulonate pathway: ascorbic acid metabolism to CO_2.

The concept that excessive ascorbate levels in tissues are physiologically undesirable is supported by the elaborate control system for ascorbate. Ascorbate levels in tissues, as for instance in the brain or the eye, are regulated by 1) a saturating transport system in the gastro intestinal system in some animals, 2) an efficient kidney excretion process above a certain blood level, 3) an induction system to improve this excretion in prolonged high intake situations, 4) a CO_2 catabolism system in many animals – although its regulation has not been studied, 5) a saturable transport system into tissues from the blood, and 6) a feedback control system on one of the ascorbate synthesis enzymes itself, namely on gulonolactone oxidase, in those animals that produce ascorbate. This DKG pathway was studied extensively, and further work on this process is not likely to lead to more insight concerning the function and nutritional requirements in man. However, it would be interesting to know if this pathway is operative in bats which require vitamin C, but have a long hibernation phase. These animals may have developed a conservation system of the ascorbic acid body pool different from primates, even as fish have developed a different system.

Catechol Analogue Pathways

Small amounts of ascorbic acid are excreted as ascorbate-2-sulfate [2], as 2-O-methylascorbate, and as oxalate. Because these metabolites are observed in primates, as well as in other animals, they are presumably not products of the DKG pathway which does not appear to exist in primates. This conclusion is contrary to the common postulate that DKG is the precursor of oxalate. It seems more likely that oxalate is formed by a dioxygenase attack on ascorbate itself. The latter reaction would be analogous to the metabolism of o-catechols (Fig. 9) in which a deoxygenase reaction results in a carbon-carbon cleavage reaction to give two dicarboxylic acid groups [21]. Baker [22] observed labelled oxalate excretion in human scurvy subjects long after blood ascorbate levels had fallen below reliable detection levels.

Under these conditions the major ascorbate pool in man is present in the neurotissue. Thus, the most likely site for oxalate production is the brain. There is no evidence that this is an essential pathway, and it could again be the result of fortuitous mimicry of the catechols by ascorbic acid.

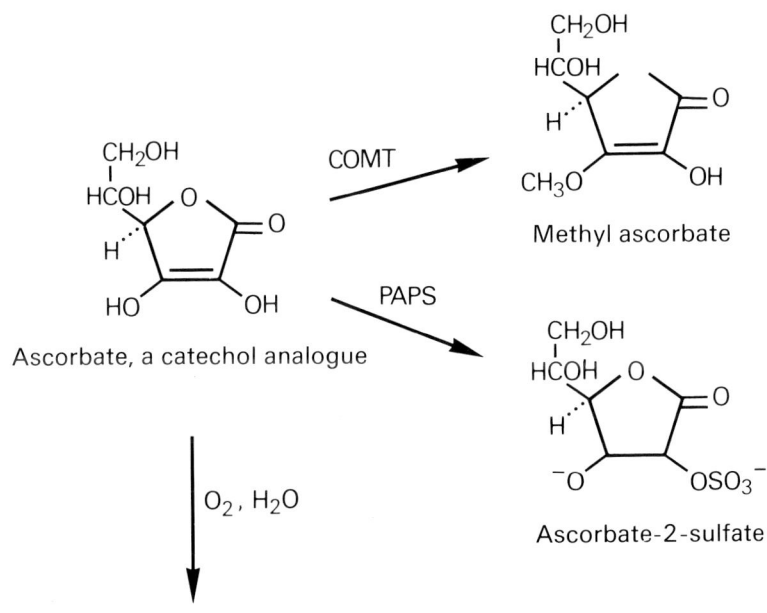

Fig. 9: The catechol analogue pathways. Abbreviations: COMT = catechol O-methyltransferase; PAPS = adenosine-3' phosphate-5' sulphatophosphate.

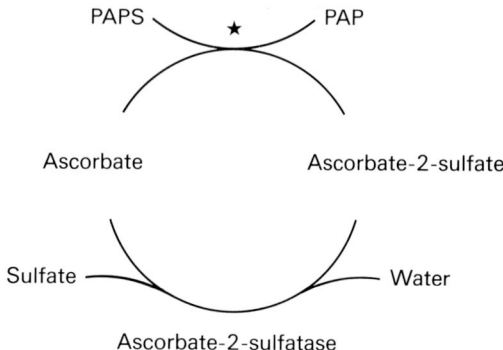

Fig. 10: The ascorbate-sulfate cycle (enzyme process not yet demonstrated).

At intervals reports of high oxalate excretion are published for subjects on a high ascorbate intake, but the results are variable. Oxalate absorption by the gut is fairly efficient, so if ascorbate were catabolized to oxalate by the intestinal flora one might expect absorption and urinary excretion of oxalate. This may be a likely source of oxalate formation.

Ascorbic acid is an analogue of the catechols and should be subject to methylation and sulfation by enzymes lacking sufficient specificity to prevent this process. Ascorbate is methylated by catechol-O-methyl transferase using S-adenosylmethionine as the methylating agent. Again it is likely that it is a brain enzyme. It does not seem reasonable to attach any direct physiological importance to these compounds in man. Ascorbate sulfate is interesting though because it appears to be a major storage form of ascorbic acid in many fish (Fig. 10) [23, 24]. In primates, there is no significant absorption of ascorbate sulfate, and the ascorbate sulfate formed is promptly cleared by the kidneys [25].

The fact that ascorbic acid is an analogue of the catechols is probably of more than coincidental importance in cell physiology. Reduced ascorbic acid has the potential to act as a metabolic regulator of the catechol enzymes by competitive inhibition, and it can form the same type of metal complexes with copper and iron as have been studied for the catechols. The intricate control of ascorbate levels in higher animals, including man, may well occur because high levels of ascorbate can seriously interfere with the catechol metabolism, but not because of its oxidation-reduction properties.

Ascorbic Acid Transport, Cellular Distribution and Storage

The localization of ascorbic acid in specific tissues has been a feature of this compound's history almost since its discovery. Radioautographic studies with carbon-14 labelled ascorbic acid clearly showed the extent of this distribution [26]. Tissue distribution data given in Table II (column 2) are from a report by Hornig [26]. The third column in this table contains data collected in the early 1970's using either carbon-14 or C_4 tritium labelling. Note that the chemical assay results of Hornig and the radioactivity assays agree closely. Thus there is not a large pool of metabolites of ascorbate other than DHA, and nominally it is considered part of the ascorbate pool. This distribution pattern of ascorbic acid shown in Table II is characteristic of higher animals most of which make ascorbic acid biosynthetically. The distribution, per se, is not needed for storage of ascorbate as in primates. It is possible that part of the storage of ascorbic acid in primates with their long time to develop scurvy is related to the large brain size. Most of the conservation of ascorbic acid in primates must stem from the absence of the DKG pathway. Even taking this into account the ascorbate requirement of man is almost an order of magnitude lower than that of the guinea pig. If one assumes the absolute minimum daily dietary requirement for ascorbic acid in a 200 g guinea pig to be 0.5 mg, and that 25 % thereof is metabolized by the DKG pathway to CO_2, then the resulting essential requirement/kg would be 0.625 mg, an amount about 10 times the essential minimum requirement in man: 0.07 mg/kg. Perhaps the DHA pathway in man is more efficient in conserving essential intermediates such as the postulated 5-keto compounds.

Tab. II: Distribution of ascorbate in rats [26]

Tissue	Ascorbate, mg/100 g	Carbon-14[1]
Adrenal	280–400	1000
Spleen	40– 50	243
Brain	35– 40	135
Gonads	25– 30	150
Liver	25– 40	44
Lungs	20– 40	106
Kidneys	15– 20	50
Heart	5– 10	24
Muscle	5	16

[1]Comparative values with (1-^{14}C) ascorbic acid. Similar values were observed with (4-^{3}H) ascorbic acid.

Ascorbic acid is subject to both active and passive membrane transport [27]. DHA seems to be transported by a simple diffusion process because of its solubility in lipid membrane systems. Two mechanisms are normally proposed by which ascorbate is held in high concentrations in specific tissues. One is that a specific transport system for ascorbate is responsible for the concentration system. The other is that DHA is transported, then reduced to ascorbate and thereby held in the cells. Neither of these systems can explain the remarkable retention of ascorbate in man or primates on a scurvy producing diet. Under these conditions blood ascorbate levels rapidly fall to near zero, but ascorbate is retained in specific tissues. There must be a certain level of DHA in these tissues; it seems very unlikely that all the ascorbate is present in the reduced form. What then is preventing diffusion of DHA and rapid depletion of ascorbate in the storage tissues? There is the probability that DHA is not present free but rather as a complex, perhaps a Schiff base complex. The working properties of DHA make it difficult to do *in vitro* binding studies between this compound and proteins or other amino compounds. In a recent paper, Schmidt *et al* [28] note "that *in vivo* metabolism of ascorbic acid might not involve dehydroascorbic acid". This observation is consistent with the chemical behaviour of ascorbate, but it is more likely that there is no significant concentration of *free* DHA in vivo at any time.

The vitamin C activity of DHA was estimated to be about 70%. Because of the difficulty in the preparation and administration of DHA and the possibility of substantial GI system loss by hydrolysis to DKG, 70% is probably a minimum value. Absorbed DHA is probably as effective as ascorbate in nutritional needs. As long as DHA is in the acidic environment in the stomach it is protected from hydrolysis – once in the blood it must either be protected as a complex or absorbed into the erythrocytes where it is reduced, as suggested by Hornig *et al* [26]. This is a very reasonable suggestion, but the process cannot be rapid, otherwise the very different tissue distribution of radioactivity after (^{14}C) DHA administration vs (^{14}C) ascorbate administration would not have been observed [24, 29].

Ascorbic Acid Functions

Bates [30] has recently reviewed the functions of ascorbic acid in man (Table III). The functions were grouped as follows: as a mixed function oxidase cofactor; as a metal ion metabolism cofactor; and as a free radical scavenger.

Tab. III: Some functions of ascorbic acid

I	*Cofactor for mixed function oxidases*
	Prolyl hydroxylase
	Butyrobetaine hydroxylase ⎱ carnitine [31, 32]
	Trimethyllysine hydroxylase ⎰
	Dopamine hydroxylase (norepinephrine)
	Cytochrome P-450 function
	Cholesterol hydroxylase (bile acids)
	Other hydroxylases
II	*Cofactor for metal ion metabolism*
	Iron transport and mobilization
	Copper metabolism
III	*Free radical scavenger*
	Direct reaction with R·
	Reaction with peroxyl radicals

   Both the molecular action as well as the enzyme role of ascorbate in mixed function oxidase reactions were described, or at least postulated. In most cases ascorbic acid serves as a reducing agent to maintain a metal ion in a reduced or active form. In general these enzymes are not sensitive to the stereochemistry of ascorbic acid, since its optical isomers work as well. Ascorbate is involved in many of these systems to explain all of the gross physiological effects of scurvy: neurological abnormalities, connective tissue weakness, physical and mental lassitude, and sudden death from heart failure.

   Even so, most specialists in ascorbic acid biochemistry have reservations that this is not the whole story, and that other roles remain to be found. The ubiquitous presence of L-ascorbic acid in all the eucaryotic systems that were studied and its absence in procaryotes is one unexplained factor. The lack of specificity for L-ascorbic acid in enzyme systems does not justify the rather specific requirement for L-ascorbic acid as a vitamin unless the 5-dehydrogenase forming enzymatically the 5-keto compounds is steriospecific and essential. Both of these seem likely. Most of the roles mentioned above do not seem so unique or important that the requirement for this vitamin should have been retained over all eucaryote history. Loewus [33] demonstrated the presence of complex ascorbic acid metabolic pathways in plants that probably involve a 5-keto intermediate and Harkrader [14] showed the presence of a 5-keto metabolite of ascorbic acid in primate urine. Therefore, it is believed that the presence of a 5-keto form of ascorbic acid in both plants as well as animals is more than a coincidence, and that the retention of the carbon C_5 metabolism in all the evolutionary steps between plants and higher animals is a teleological argument for an essential role of this metabolism.

Earlier several of the possible metabolism forms were shown which may be considered in connection with a 5-ketoascorbic acid oxidation-reduction cycle. An intriguing aspect of this cycle is that the keto intermediate could be bound to the enzyme as a Schiff base through a lysyl residue (Fig. 11).

This structure would then provide a reductive ene-diol ring on a moving arm that could be oxidized at one enzyme subunit and re-reduced at another subunit. The analogy for this mode of operation was developed with a number of co-enzymes in the past decades. These include the carboxylation process in biotin-containing enzymes and the acyl carrier protein function in fatty acid biochemistry. If the ketoascorbic acid served a one electron reduction process, the free radical could be retained and recycled or reduced. A Schiff base binding of an active coenzyme to the enzyme is not nearly as stable as the amide link of biotin, so it is possible that these enzyme complexes are rather labile and that substantial amounts of the intermediate are lost and excreted in the

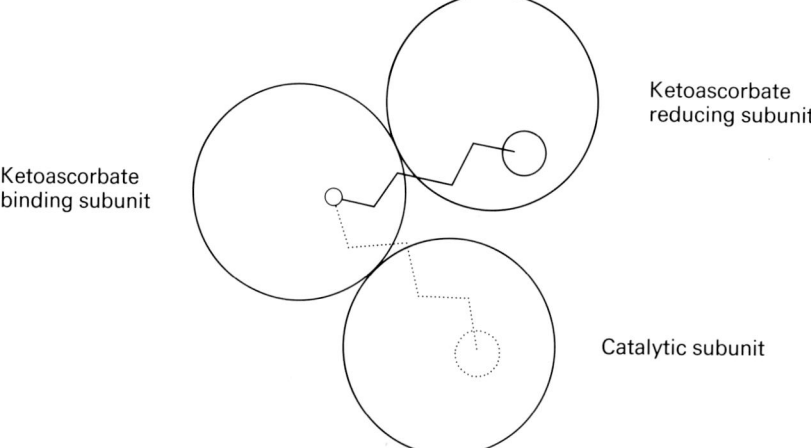

Fig. 11: Proposed 5-ketoascorbate acid cycle.

urine as 5-ketoascorbitol or similar compounds. The presence of an activated form of ascorbic acid would help to explain many difficulties in interpreting experiments carried out to elucidate the metabolism of ascorbic acid. In low concentrations 5-ketoascorbitol would have been difficult to detect, especially since these compounds respond to both the dinitrophenylhydrazine and dichloroindophenol assays of ascorbic acid. The key to future study is by the use of high performance liquid chromatography, which allows the distinction between rather similar carbohydrates.

References

1   ASHWELL, G et al: Metabolism of ascorbic acid and related uronic acids, aldonic acids and pentoses. Ann NY Acad Sci 92, 105–114, 1961.
2   TOLBERT, B et al: Chemistry and metabolism of ascorbic acid and ascorbate sulfate. Ann NY Acad Sci 258, 48–69, 1975.
3   FOYER, C H, HALLIWELL, B: Purification and properties of dehydroascorbate reductase from spinach leaves. Phytoch 16, 1347–1350, 1977.
4   BIELSKI, B: Chemistry of ascorbic acid radicals. In: SEIB and TOLBERT (eds) Am Chem Soc Ser, vol 200 "Ascorbic acid: chemistry, metabolism, and uses", pp 81–100. American Chemical Society, Washington, 1982.
5   STAUDINGER, H et al: Role of ascorbic acid in microsomal electron transport and the possible relationship to hydroxylation reactions. Ann NY Acad Sci 92, 195–207, 1961.
6   SCHULZE, H U, STAUDINGER, H: Untersuchungen zur Lipoidabhängigkeit der NADH: Semi-dehydroascorbinsäureoxidoreduktase. Hoppe-Seyler's Z Physiol Chem 352, 309–317, 1971.
7   TOLBERT, B M, WARD, J B: Dehydroascorbic acid. In: SEIB and TOLBERT (eds). Am Chem Soc Ser, vol 200 "Ascorbic acid: chemistry, metabolism, and uses", pp 81–100. American Chemical Society, Washington, 1982.
8   BANERJEE, S: Physiological role of dehydroascorbic acid. Indian J Physiol Pharmacol 21, 85–93, 1977.
9   SPACKMAN, D H: The analysis of ascorbic acid and dehydroascorbic acid in the mouse by a rapid fluorometric micro method. Fed Proc 42, 2179, 1983.
10 MARTIN, G R: Studies on the tissue distribution of ascorbic acid. Ann NY Acad Sci 92, 141–147, 1961.
11 GONZALEZ, A, BRECHT, P: Total and reduced ascorbic acid levels in rin and normal tomatoes. J Am Soc Hort Sci 103, 756–758, 1978.
12 VALISEK, J et al: On the behaviour of L-dehydroascorbic acid in aqueous solution. Coll Czech Chem Commun 37, 1465–1470, 1972.
13 SEKILY, M et al: Reactions of the 3-oxime 2-phenyl-hydrazone and mixed bishydrazones of dehydroascorbic acid: conversion into substrated triazoles and pyrazolinediones. Carbohyd Res 59, 141–149, 1977.
14 HARKRADER, R J: Isolation and characterization of ascorbate metabolites from primate urine. PhD Thesis. University of Colorado, Boulder, 1979.
15 ANDREWS, G C, CRAWFORD, T: Recent advances in the derivatization of L-ascorbic acid. In: SEIB and TOLBERT (eds). Am Chem Soc Ser, vol 200 "Ascorbic acid: chemistry, metabolism, and uses", pp 59–79. Washington, American Chemical Society, 1982.
16 TOLBERT, B et al: Metabolism of L-ascorbic-4-^{3}H acid in man. Am J Clin Nutr 20, 250–252, 1967.

17 Tolbert, B *et al:* C-6 oxidation of ascorbic acid: a major metabolic process in animals. Biochem Biophys Res Commun *71,* 1004–1009, 1976.
18 Kagawa, Y, Takiguchi, H: Enzymatic studies on ascorbic acid catabolism in animals. II. Delactonization of dehydroascorbic acid. Biochem J (Tokyo) *51,* 197–203, 1962.
19 Baker, E M *et al:* Respiratory catabolism in man of the degradative intermediates of L-ascorbic-1-^{14}C acid. Proc Soc Exp Biol Med *113,* 379–383, 1963.
20 Tillotson, J A: Ascorbate metabolism in the trained monkey. Int J Vit Nutr Res *48,* 374–381, 1978.
21 Hayaishi, O *et al:* Oxygenases: Dioxygenases. In: Boyer (ed). The enzymes, vol XII, 3rd ed; pp 119–189. Academic Press, New York, 1975.
22 Baker, E *et al:* Metabolism of ascorbic acid in experimental human scurvy. Am J Clin Nutr *22,* 549–558, 1969.
23 Tucker, B W: Studies on vitamin C metabolism in rainbow trout. PhD thesis. University of Washington, Seattle, 1983.
24 Tucker, B, Halver, J: Distribution of ascorbate-2-sulfate and distribution, half-life and turnover rates of 1-^{14}C ascorbic acid in rainbow trout. J Nutr *114,* 991–1000, 1984.
25 Machlin, L *et al:* Lack of antiscorbutic activity of ascorbate-2-sulfate in the rhesus monkey. Am J Clin Nutr *29,* 825–831, 1976.
26 Hornig, D: Distribution of ascorbic acid, metabolites and analogues in man and animals. Ann NY Acad Sci *258,* 103–118, 1975.
27 Siliprandi, L *et al:* Na + -dependent electroneutral ascorbate transport across brush border membrane vesicals from guinea pig small intestine. Biochem Biophys Acta *552,* 129–142, 1979.
28 Schmidt, K *et al:* Studies on the metabolic conversion of ascorbate. Int J Vit Nutr Res *53,* 77–86, 1983.
29 Hornig, D, Hartmann, P: Kinetic behaviour of ascorbic acid in guinea pigs. In: Seib and Tolbert (eds). Am Chem Soc Ser, vol 200 "Ascorbic acid: chemistry, metabolism, and uses". pp 293–316. American Chemical Society, Washington, 1982.
30 Bates, C J: Function and metabolism of vitamin C in man. In: Counsell and Hornig (eds) "Vitamin C", pp 1–22. Applied Science, London, 1981.
31 Henderson, L M *et al:* Mammalian enzymes of trimethyllysine conversion to trimethylaminobutyrate. Fed Proc *41,* 2843–2847, 1982.
32 Broquist, H P: Carnitine biosynthesis and function. Fed Proc *41,* 2840–2842, 1982.
33 Loewus, F A: Carbohydrate interconversions. Ann Rev Plant Physiol *22,* 337–364, 1971.

M. Tolbert, PhD, Department of Chemistry, University of Colorado, Boulder, Colorado 80309, USA

Vitamin C and Smoking: Increased Requirement of Smokers

D.H. Hornig and B.E. Glatthaar

Department of Vitamin and Nutrition Research, F. Hoffmann-La Roche & Co., Ltd., Basle, Switzerland

Key Words: Vitamin C/Ascorbic acid· Effect of smoking · Impaired vitamin C status · Daily vitamin C requirement · Increased by smoking

Abstract: Numerous studies on the vitamin C status of smokers and non-smokers revealed smokers with vitamin C intakes comparable to non-smokers to have a substantially impaired vitamin C status. This suggests that smokers have an increased risk of marginal vitamin C deficiency should the intake of vitamin C be diminished, since smokers' vitamin status is closer to a borderline vitamin C deficiency than that of non-smokers. Reasons for the impaired vitamin C status in smokers such as altered food intake, differences in absorption of vitamin C, or utilization of vitamin C as a detoxifying agent of smoke components are discussed.

Investigations with labelled vitamin C have demonstrated smokers to have a significantly increased metabolic turnover compared with non-smokers; smokers excrete a higher amount of vitamin C in the form of metabolites. Evidence suggests that smokers have a somewhat reduced absorption capacity for vitamin C when compared to non-smokers. As a consequence smokers require a 40 per cent higher daily intake than non-smokers to maintain a comparable vitamin C status. A daily intake of 140 mg of vitamin C for smokers and 100 mg for non-smokers is considered to be adequate to cover the basic physiological requirement. The impaired vitamin C status of smokers is therefore mainly determined by the altered vitamin C turnover caused by smoking. Possible consequences of a lowered vitamin C status on the general health of the individual are discussed.

Introduction

Cigarette smoking involves both pharmacological and physiological determinants. High on the list of the broad range of toxic components contained in cigarette smoke are nicotine, tar and carbon monoxide. The constant exposure to these medical villains subjects smokers to increased risk of arteriosclerosis, cardiovascular and pulmonary heart diseases, chronic bronchitis, emphysema, lung cancer, fetal damage and to other negative consequences [1].

Cigarette smoking produces a variety of biochemical abnormalities. There is evidence that nicotine is addicting, and the smoker needs to keep nicotine or one of its active metabolites at some optimal level [2]. A consistent parameter for a physiological alteration in cigarette smokers has been described to be their vitamin C status. Numerous reports show that the cigarette smoker needs more vitamin C each day than the non-smoker. These findings include some merely empirical observations as well as others based on experimental evidence. However, they all imply that there is a clinically important relationship between smoking and vitamin C utilization. In the absence of detailed knowledge about the mode of action of vitamin C and its metabolism, these results do not yet lend themselves for an easy explanation of the underlying reasons.

Review of the Literature

Early observations. As early as 1672, Maynwaring hinted in a "Discurs that tobacco is the cause of scurvey" at the possible connection between smoking and vitamin C.

In 1939, Strauss and Scheer [3] reported in a study of 30 presumably non-smoking healthy subjects, men and women aged 18–40 years, that smoking cigarettes resulted in a marked reduction of urinary ascorbic acid excretion after a 200 mg dose of vitamin C. In 1941, Harmsen [4] determined poor levels of vitamin C in the plasma of smokers. In addition, the aggravating effects on the vitamin C status of persons exposed to prolonged warming of their meals and increased work load were observed. Reif [5] described experiments indicating nicotine to accelerate the oxidation of ascorbic acid *in vitro*. Venulet [6] listed the following organs and functions in smokers prone to damage due to the worsened vitamin C supply: brain accompanied by psychological alterations, heart and vascular system, stomach and digestive tract, pituitary and adrenals, liver, kidney and spleen, muscles, as well as other systems. On the whole, resistance in general would be lowered because of the lack of enough vitamin C, the toxic effects of tobacco smoke notwithstanding. Venulet and Danysz [7] found lower vitamin C levels in the milk of women who smoke than in that of non-smokers. These authors suggest that lack of this vitamin may be harmful to the fetus and later to the infant. They also demonstrated that vitamin C concentration was higher in milk of women who stopped smoking than in women who received vitamin C supplements.

Calder et al [8] attempted to verify the observation of McCormack [9] that one single cigarette destroyed 25 mg of vitamin C in the body. They were unable to show that the level of the vitamin in the plasma is reduced in smokers and non-smokers who smoked one cigarette every half-hour over a period of six hours and smokers who smoked 19–25 cigarettes in six hours. However, looking at the level of ascorbic acid in the plasma and leucocytes of 91 non-smokers, 83 smokers puffing 14 cigarettes or less daily and 31 smokers consuming 15 cigarettes or more daily, highly significant differences were detected between non-smokers and smokers (Table I). The authors pointed out that these variations were not due to a larger intake of vitamin C among the non-smokers, therefore, there seemed to be a relationship between long-term smoking and vitamin C levels in the blood.

Brook and Grimshaw [10] compared 54 healthy men and 84 healthy women and found plasma and leucocyte vitamin C concentrations of the men to be significantly lower than those of the women. For non-smokers there was a significant decline in the plasma vitamin C concentration with increasing age in both sexes while the leucocyte concentrations did not change with age. Conversely, cigarette smoking was found to lower significantly both the plasma and the leucocyte vitamin C concentrations (Table I).

Tab. I: Compilation of reports on plasma vitamin C concentrations of non-smokers and smokers. Number of subjects investigated as given in brackets.

Vitamin C plasma concentration, mg/l				Reference
Non-smokers		smokers		
9.1 ± 0.4	(91)	5.2 ± 0.7	(31)	8
6.2 ± 0.7	(32)	4.4 ± 0.6	(22)	10
1.8 ± 0.1	(34)	1.3 ± 0.2	(18)	11
7.8 ± 3.8	(80)	5.1 ± 3.7	(96)	13
9.6		8.3		14[1,2]
5.9		5.3		14[1,3]
8.8 ± 2.7	(10)	6.9 ± 2.6	(12)	15,16
6.0 ± 0.5	(14)	4.2 ± 0.6	(14)	18
13.2 ± 0.7	(12)	13.2 ± 0.7	(7)	43

[1] Number of subjects and SD not given.
[2] High professional persons.
[3] Good to medium social level.

Recent investigations. The years after 1970 saw a host of papers from several countries dealing with the effect of smoking on the vitamin C status of smokers. Albanese *et al* [11] investigated methodological aspects of vitamin C concentration determinations in plasma and leucocytes. Although they confirmed the findings of earlier reports they called for the application of more systematic approaches involving longitudinal investigations, decisive protocols and accurate chemical procedures for measurements of necessary metabolites in available body fluids in order to gain a thorough understanding of the biochemical relationship between cigarette smoking and vitamin C metabolism, nutrition and pharmacology. Kevany *et al* [12] studied white cell ascorbic acid and serum cholesterol levels in relation to smoking habits in 41 middle aged males from Ireland. Ascorbic acid levels were significantly lower in smokers. There was also a significant correlation with serum cholesterol levels in smokers but not in non-smokers suggesting vitamin C to be possibly a limiting factor in cholesterol catabolism in smokers.

McClean *et al* [13] measured morning plasma and leucocyte vitamin C concentrations in 178 healthy men aged 17–68 years in New Zealand. While smokers among the youngest age group (17–29) had significantly lower vitamin C levels than non-smokers, the difference among those of the oldest age group [60–69] was not that marked, but in all cases smokers had lower levels (Table I). In the total population the differences in plasma vitamin C concentrations were in the means 22 % lower in smokers than in non-smokers. In leucocyte ascorbate concentrations the means differed by 32 %.

In Brazil, Hoefel [14] analysed 712 blood samples of habitual smokers for vitamin C levels. Data from persons belonging to poorer economic and social classes were excluded since their vitamin C values were below normal limits. The residual 482 subjects were divided into two groups, again according to social and economic conditions. The average ascorbic acid levels were lower in smokers, with a more marked difference in female subjects (Table I). These observations were explained by way of the action of nicotine on the cells of the adrenal glands and the liberation of catecholamines in their active, circulating form whose biosynthesis requires ascorbic acid.

Keith and Driskell [15] studied 12 cigarette smoking and 10 non-smoking healthy male volunteers (25–38 years) while at rest, during, and after various lung function and technical exercise tests. Plasma vitamin C levels were significantly lower for smokers although ascorbic acid intakes for the two groups did not differ much (Table I). Treadmill workload for non-smokers was significantly greater than for smokers. Also lung function, resting and exercise metabolism appeared to be impaired in an otherwise healthy group of smokers as compared to non-smokers. In a follow-up study [16], the same volunteers performed lung function and treadmill exercise tests over two periods of three weeks' duration while taking either ascorbic acid (300 mg daily) or placebo tablets in a random, double-blind cross-over design. Differences were more evident between smokers and non-smokers than between the ascorbic acid or placebo treatments. Plasma vitamin C levels of smokers and non-smokers were significantly increased by the ascorbic acid supplementation. Non-smokers tended to have lower postexercise systolic blood pressure and lactic acid values, but higher oxygen consumption during the ascorbic acid treatment than during the placebo while smokers also exhibited lower blood lactate levels. Moreover, since great individual variation was observed with regard to the measured responses, the overall effect of supplementary vitamin C is difficult to assess.

In a recent investigation from India, SULOCHANA and ARUNAGIRI [17] examined 50 volunteers of age between 20 and 30 years. Each subject was given 200 ml of water after 12 hours of fasting. One hour urine was collected and each participant then smoked five cigarettes within 45 min to one hour. Again one hour later, urine was collected. Urinary ascorbic acid excretion before and after smoking five cigarettes was determined. In all 50 urines collected after smoking, the ascorbic acid content was elevated above the control levels, on average by 18 %, resulting in an increased loss of vitamin C from the body. Since the collection of both urine samples was performed after 12 hours of fasting, the dietary influence on the excretion of ascorbic acid was believed to be eliminated and the increased excretion of ascorbic acid was therefore exclusively assigned to the immediate effect of smoking five cigarettes. These authors do consider cigarette smoking as one of the causative factors in vitamin C tissue depletion leading to an increased risk of getting arteriosclerotic lesions and associated diseases.

Results from nutritional surveys. Against the background of a large number of reports demonstrating the connection between smoking and impaired vitamin C status of smokers, the need for well-controlled studies resulted in careful assessments by PELLETIER [18] using data from the Nutrition Canada National Survey. The median serum vitamin C level of cigarette smokers was found to be about 30 % lower than that of non-smokers. For those smoking over 20 cigarettes a day, however, the median was 40 % lower than that of non-smokers. PELLETIER also found that when non-smokers and smokers were saturated with vitamin C, they became desaturated at the same rate when fed a diet low in vitamin C. This observation suggested that there was no impairment in the smokers' metabolism of vitamin C. Since statistical treatment of the data confirmed that lower vitamin C intakes were not responsible for the smokers' lower blood ascorbic acid levels, PELLETIER suggested that impaired vitamin C absorption may be one of the causes for the observed differences between smokers and non-smokers [18].

In Switzerland, RITZEL [19] looked at 4053 healthy employees of the Basle metropolitan area that included 3403 men and 650 women between 20 and 75 years of age. 1874 male subjects did not take any vitamin preparations. Table II gives the relationship between cigarette consumption and vitamin C status. Close to 90 % of the non-smokers showed a satisfactory vitamin C status ($\geq$ 4 mg/l). With increasing numbers of cigarettes consumed, the proportion of insufficiency regarding the vitamin C status rose, and only somewhat more than 60 % of the smokers (more than 30 cigarettes daily) were found to have a satisfactory vitamin C status. The negative correlation between cigarette consumption and plasma vitamin C level was confirmed by the results of the 650 female participants in this study.

Tab. II: Cigarette consumption and effect on plasma vitamin C concentration in male subjects: according to RITZEL and BRUPPACHER [19]

Daily cigarette consumption	Number of subjects	Plasma vitamin C concentration of $\geq$ 4 mg/l, %
None	1058	89.5
1– 5	157	91.1
6–10	127	81.9
11–20	399	80.2
21–30	100	71.0
30	33	63.6

On the other hand, cigarette smoking had no influence on the vitamin C status of 551 male participants who consumed regularly vitamin preparations containing vitamin C; practically all of these participants had a satisfactory vitamin C status ($\geq$ 4 mg/l), even when smoking more than 20 cigarettes daily. According to RITZEL [19], fruit consumption seemed to be more or less independent from smoking. The effect of the toxic components in the inhaled smoke was suggested to be the major cause leading to an insufficient vitamin C status rather than altered food habits.

Results from animal studies. In order to verify the findings from human studies and to explore the sequelae of vitamin C deficiency aggravated by tobacco smoke, several studies with experimental animals (mainly guinea pigs) were carried out.

HUGHES *et al* [20] worked with guinea pigs receiving a controlled dietary intake of ascorbic acid. The effects induced by inhalation of experimentally produced cigarette smoke for periods of up to 20 min each day on growth, vitamin C metabolism and organ weights were recorded. Growth rate was significantly depressed by the smoke treatment, but individual organs were not affected to the same extent. Already after 4 days' exposure to smoke a significant reduction in the vitamin C content of the adrenals was seen. After 18 days marked adrenal hypertrophy accompanied the lowered vitamin C levels. Also the lungs showed a smoke-induced hypertrophy.

Keith and Pelletier [21] administered daily defined doses of ascorbic acid (2 mg/100 g body weight) orally and nicotine (0.66 mg daily) subcutaneously to male guinea pigs on an ascorbic acid free diet. At the end of 2 weeks a radioactively labelled dose of ascorbic acid was given. The tissue distribution of ascorbic acid in the nicotine treated animals was different from the saline-injected control animals. The results indicated a delayed absorption of ascorbic acid in the presence of nicotine.

Leuchtenberger [22] exposed hamster lung cultures to tobacco smoke to investigate the effects of L-cysteine and vitamin C. Abnormal growth and malignant transformation could be inhibited or even be reversed. An increase of lysosomes after L-cysteine or vitamin C pointed to the possible importance of lysosomes in protecting the cultures against enhancement of carcinogenesis by smoke components.

Although rats are capable of synthesizing vitamin C, Chen and Chow [23] observed a lowering of vitamin C plasma levels upon exposing the animals to tobacco smoke (120 puffs/exposure/day) over a period of 3 and 7 days. Sufficient intake of vitamin E appeared to aid in maintaining plasma vitamin C at a higher level.

Cyanide has long been regarded as a respiratory-tract toxicant of cigarette smoke. Sprince *et al* [24] examined the possibility that ascorbic acid owing to its carbonyl group could act as a protectant against cyanide toxicity by way of cyanohydrin formation. Pretreatment of rats with oral doses of ascorbic acid gave good protection (90% survivors) against LD 90 oral doses of sodium cyanide. This result implies a simple chemical explanation for the increased need of smokers for vitamin C.

Faltot *et al* [25] suggested the carbon monoxide component of cigarette smoke as a possible explanation for the increased requirement of vitamin C of smokers. An increase in the carbon monoxide concentration of expired air resulted in a decrease in urinary ascorbate excretion in human subjects.

In a preliminary report, Wang *et al* [26] recently communicated that their data obtained from guinea pigs did not allow to conclude whether vitamin C supplements ameliorated the toxic effect of nicotine, but vitamin C deficiency appeared to aggravate small airway changes induced by nicotine.

Requirement of Vitamin C in Man

Requirement of non-smokers. A comprehensive review of research on the requirement of vitamin C of man has recently been compiled by Irwin and Hutchins [27]. Conclusions have been derived mostly from blood or plasma levels, from urinary excretion of ascorbic acid, or from investigations of the minimal intake of vitamin C to prevent the appearance of any scorbutic symptoms. Other approaches have been the saturation of the body with vitamin C and estimation of the need from the urinary response to high intakes. As a result of the various methods to assess the status of vitamin C in man, the estimates of the daily requirement of this vitamin differ considerably [27].

Only the availability of labelled ascorbic acid made it possible to use a kinetic approach and allowed estimations of half-life, turnover and body pool size of vitamin C in man. Several studies have been published dealing with vitamin C requirements which were not limited to determine solely the minimal intake necessary to prevent the appearance of vitamin C deficiency symptoms [28–30]. The study by Kallner et al [30] demonstrated that a daily intake of about 100 mg of vitamin C can be considered as adequate for healthy *non-smoking* male subjects in order to cover the basic physiological requirement of this vitamin. This investigation revealed several important results: the total body pool of vitamin C was found to be increased to a value of about 20 mg/kg body weight maintaining a plasma vitamin C concentration of between 8–9 mg/l. This finding confirmed earlier observations postulating "saturation" of the vitamin C body pool at a magnitude of approximately 1500 mg [31, 32]. Kallner et al [30] further showed that a plasma level of 8–9 mg/l corresponds to a total daily turnover of 60 mg of vitamin C. The total turnover represents the sum of the metabolic turnover (elimination of metabolites derived from vitamin C) and renal turnover (elimination of unchanged vitamin C via kidneys) and reflects the actual absorbed amount of the ingested vitamin C. The metabolic turnover was shown to level off at about 40–50 mg/day. This amount of daily metabolites necessitates a total daily turnover of about 60 mg of vitamin C (Fig. 1). In an earlier investigation by Kallner et al [33] it was demonstrated that vitamin C is incompletely absorbed even in physiological doses (up to 180 mg) (mean 84 %, range 78–88 % of intake). Thus, losses of up to 20 % may occur during the absorption process.

In considering all these data, Kallner et al [30] suggested that a recommended daily intake of vitamin C should be about 100 mg for healthy non-smoking male subjects. It was argued, however, that this dose range may not necessarily exclude any benefit of larger intakes of vitamin C.

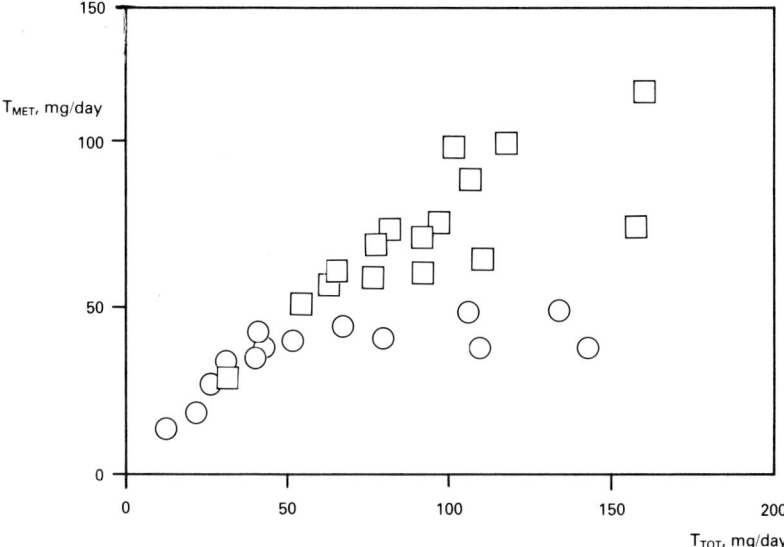

Fig. 1: Metabolic turnover of metabolites from vitamin C (T_{MET}) as function of total turnover of vitamin C (T_{TOT}) in non-smokers (O) and in smokers (□) according to Kallner *et al* [34].

Requirement of smokers. Since smokers have to be considered as a group having considerably lowered plasma and leucocyte vitamin C levels when compared with non-smokers, smokers have an increased risk of becoming marginally deficient in this essential nutrient. Using the same experimental set-up and kinetic approach as in non-smokers, the influence of smoking on the vitamin C status in man was investigated [34]. In brief, the experiment with smokers was as follows: 17 smoking male volunteers (chronic cigarette smokers for many years consuming more than 20 cigarettes a day) without any history of disease or abnormal biochemical tests were instructed to stay on a diet essentially devoid of ascorbic acid for an equilibration period of 3 weeks. They were supplemented with various amounts of ascorbic acid (1 × 30 mg up to 4 × 45 mg daily). After achievement of steady state conditions with regard to plasma ascorbate levels a single oral dose of (1-^{14}C) ascorbic acid was given. The time course of radioactivity in plasma and urine was followed, and the experimental data were treated by kinetic principles. The results obtained can be summarized and compared with data from non-smokers as follows (Table III):

Tab. III: Overview on results obtained from studies on the kinetics of vitamin C in man; according to Kallner *et al* [30, 34]

	Non-smokers	Smokers
Saturation of metabolic turnover, mg metabolites	40–50	70–90
Required total turnover, mg	60	90–100
Absorbed intake of up to 180 mg, %	84 (78–88)	76 (63–80)
Required daily vitamin C intake, mg	100	140
Size of body pool, mg vitamin C/kg body weight	20	20
Plasma vitamin C concentration, mg/l	8–9	8–9

– The renal handling of vitamin C is the same in smokers and non-smokers.
– There are only small differences in the absorption of vitamin C (smokers: mean 76%, range 63–80% intake; non-smokers: mean 84% range 78–88% of intake).
– The half-life of ascorbic acid in smokers is shorter at low plasma ascorbate concentrations than for non-smokers indicating that a smoker with low ascorbate plasma levels has a higher risk to come into a marginal vitamin C deficiency than non-smokers on termination of ascorbic acid intakes.
– The metabolic turnover is significantly different in smokers and non-smokers. In non-smokers the metabolic turnover approaches saturation at about 40–50 mg/day, whereas in the smoker group the results indicate a levelling off at about 70–90 mg/day (Fig. 1). To reach this level in smokers a total turnover of about 90 mg/day is required, which is related to an ascorbate plasma concentration of 9 mg/l. Therefore, a plasma ascorbate concentration of at least 9 mg/l should be aimed at.

Kallner *et al* [34] suggested that the total turnover is the physiologically optimal turnover at which the total amount of metabolites from ascorbic acid (metabolic turnover) approaches saturation. This would be for smokers at a total turnover of approximately 90 mg of vitamin C daily compared to that of non-smokers with 60 mg vitamin daily. Taking into account the incomplete absorption of vitamin C following oral administration and the variability of the individuals, the daily recommended intake for smokers is suggested to be 140 mg of vitamin C (non-smokers 100 mg).

For these reasons it is apparent that the requirement of smokers is increased by 40 mg/day or 40% compared to that of non-smokers. This increased requirement is mainly caused by a significantly enhanced metabolic turnover. The reduced ascorbic acid status of smokers found and confirmed by a large number of investigators is therefore not only due to altered dietary habits induced by smoking, but is mostly determined by the altered vitamin C turnover caused by smoking.

Thus, smokers represent one of those population groups, not necessarily regarded as being sick, which do have an increased requirement of essential nutrients, such as vitamin C. Other groups such as social drinkers, women on oral contraceptives, persons on long-term drug therapy etc, should also be assessed as 'risk groups', since they may require larger intakes of essential nutrients to match the daily need for optimum physiological functioning.

Consequences of a Low Vitamin C Status

It is obvious that one of the major problems facing nutrition today is whether low blood and tissue levels of a variety of the micro-nutrients which are essential to man, such as vitamins, constitute a threat to the health and well-being of the individual. The problem is even more complicated, since assuming they do, these effects are either small or very difficult to assess, but result in pathological alterations only after months or even years of nutritional deficiency. Smokers definitely are considered to have a reduced vitamin C status. The significance of reduced plasma vitamin C levels, concomitant with impaired vitamin C body reserves, has been documented in many studies during the recent years. From clinical and biochemical investigations in controlled vitamin C intake studies, guidelines for the interpretation of plasma vitamin C levels have been derived. In the National Survey of Canada in 1973 three risk categories were introduced. The Committee on Standards and Data Interpretation designated a high probability that vitamin C malnutrition exists as a high risk, an average probability that malnutrition is present or developing as a moderate risk, and a low probability that malnutrition exists as a low risk.

For vitamin C a high risk has been defined to exist for all age groups below a plasma level of 2 mg/l, a moderate risk of getting vitamin C deficiency has been observed in the age group up to 19 years between 2–6 mg/l, and aged over 20 years between 2–4 mg/l. A low risk of vitamin C deficiency is to be expected above 6 mg/l or 4 mg/l respectively, depending on age groups (35). From a public health point of view a low risk status is desirable. Guidelines comparable with those used in the National Survey of Canada in 1973 were suggested by the Interdepartmental Committee on Nutrition for National

Defense of the USA (ICNND). Levels of less than 1.0 mg vitamin C/1 were considered as deficient, levels from 1.0–1.9 mg/1 as low, while levels of 2.0 mg/1 and above were termed "acceptable" [36].

The question one should be concerned with when low levels of vitamin C are prevalent as e.g. in smokers is to what extent such a marginal vitamin C deficiency may compromise the health of these subjects. Thus, the crucial question to be answered is: are there symptoms, specific or unspecific, in those subjects with a moderate or great risk of vitamin C deficiency that could clearly be attributed to the lack of vitamin C, and will there be an improvement of health in these subjects when the borderline vitamin C deficiency status is normalized by either an adapted diet or supplementary vitamin C. It will, therefore, be attempted to scrutinize available investigations in order to assess whether a marginal vitamin C status may be of any consequence with regard to optimum health. Several of such investigations will be highlighted briefly.

In reviewing 300 consecutive cataract operations in India, JAIN et al [37] found a highly significant relationship of black cataract and smoking. Black cataract has been associated with arteriosclerosis which is a characteristic feature of senile cataract. It starts in the nucleus and spreads slowly to the entire tissue and is accompanied by the deposition of a yellow pigment which may develop into a brown or black colour. Of the 300 cases, 158 were males and 142 females. Of the 184 smokers, 28 had black cataract whereas of the 116 non-smokers only 3 were affected. Since smokers have low plasma levels and body stores of ascorbic acid, the authors suggest that the lowered ascorbic acid level in the lens may accelerate the oxidation of nuclear amino acids leading to deposits of pigments in the lens.

Most N-nitroso compounds tested in animals proved to be carcinogenic. Since nitrogen dioxide, which was estimated to constitute as much as 50% of the nitrogen oxide content of tobacco smoke, is a potent nitrosating agent particularly at alkaline pH values, N-nitrosamine formation can occur from amines in the unburnt tobacco. In view of the reported range of 145–1000 ppm of total nitrogen oxide content of tobacco smoke, a substantial amount of N-nitrosamines could be generated in the smoke. Some N-nitroso compounds were already identified as constituents of tobacco smoke [38].

Ascorbic acid is capable of inhibiting the formation of nitrosamines, therefore, use has been made either of salts of ascorbic acid or mixtures of such salts with ascorbic acid itself. Tobacco was treated with such mixtures within the range of 10–14 mg per cigarette containing about 1 g tobacco. In fast puff tests it was found that the formation of nitrogen dioxide was reduced by about one third of the controls by this measure [39]. These findings demonstrate that vitamin C apparently is not only important in the body to combat the negative side-effects of smoking, but also essential to remove dangerous components from the tobacco smoke itself.

Graham et al [40] carried out interviews with 374 male patients who had cancer of the larynx and 381 controls with diseases other than of the digestive or respiratory systems and other than neoplasm. A high risk was found to be associated with smoking as well as alcohol ingestion, both conditions causing a reduced vitamin C status. Low amounts of vitamin A and C doubled the risk. One of the reasons cited may be inhibition of formation of carcinogenic nitrosamines brought about by administration of vitamin C. Similarly, vitamin A is suggested to inhibit a variety of chemical carcinogens that promote tumour growth.

Sprince [41] in a series of papers pointed to acetaldehyde, a key intermediary metabolite of ethanol and contained in appreciable amounts in tobacco smoke, which is 10–30 times more toxic than ethanol. Acetaldehyde was listed by the US Surgeon General's Report as a suspected contributor to the health hazards of smoking and it may act by way of depleting tissues of catecholamines. Ascorbic acid has been found to provide protection against the toxicity of acetaldehyde, acrolein and formaldehyde and possibly against other toxic components of tobacco smoke.

Milochik [42] reviewed the current knowledge about the interactions between tobacco smoke containing a large number of noxious chemicals and the activity of enzymes involved in the metabolism of xanthines, vitamins and a variety of drugs. Selective enzyme stimulation or inhibition appear to be responsible for clinically significant effects. Vitamin C represents just one of many compounds whose metabolism is affected by tobacco smoke.

Kevany et al [12] investigated the hypothesis whether smoking in man by reducing the vitamin C status might limit the conversion of cholesterol to bile acids and increase cholesterol levels. It could be demonstrated in the investigated limited size of the subpopulation that vitamin C levels and serum cholesterol concentrations are significantly correlated in smokers but not in non-smokers. These authors suggest that ascorbate may be a limiting factor in cholesterol catabolism in smokers, but stressed the need for additional studies on the effect of vitamin C on cholesterol levels and bile acid excretion in depleted smokers.

Yeung [43] investigated 38 healthy female university students aged 19 to 26 years, and divided them into four groups depending on whether they smoked cigarettes and/or used oral contraceptives. It was found that cigarette smoking slightly increased the levels of vitamin A, triglycerides, and cholesterol while oral contraceptives significantly increased the plasma lipids. The effects of cigarette smoking and oral contraceptives were additive, whereas neither had any significant influence on plasma vitamin E and C. It was pointed out that the subjects used in these studies were healthy young adults, and that the dietary intake of vitamin C by the subjects in all four groups was well above 100 mg/day. Thus the lack of difference in the plasma vitamin C levels observed among the four groups of probands probably reflected the high dietary intake of vitamin C.

In a recent review [44] the available evidence on the impact of marginal vitamin C deficiency was compiled. Low vitamin C plasma levels or a reduced vitamin C status were reported to be associated with changes in capillary fragility [45], with signs of fatigue and lassitude, and impaired biosynthesis of carnitine [46]. Crandon et al [47] reported wound healing to be affected by low plasma vitamin C levels. A recent investigation demonstrated that patients with infected corneal ulcers have significantly lowered vitamin C leucocyte concentrations. These patients were therefore considered to have lowered aqueous vitamin C levels and to be more at risk of developing a corneal vitamin C deficiency at a time of an insult than healthy persons [48]. A higher incidence of hemorrhagic ocular pathologies (hemorrhagic clouding of the vitreous, central vein thrombosis, apoplectic glaucoma) was reported to be associated with low vitamin C levels [49].

The physical working capacity measured as oxygen consumption per kg of body weight was found to be correlated with serum iron, and vitamin C and riboflavin nutritional status. A statistically significant improvement was found when in an intervention study 20 mg vitamin C, 2 mg riboflavin, and 2 mg pyridoxine were taken daily over 12 weeks [50].

Schorah et al [51] have shown that mothers giving birth to lighter babies have a higher incidence of leucocyte ascorbate concentrations of less than 20 $\mu g/10^8$ cells than mothers giving birth to normal weight babies. This suggests that adequate nutrition near term is probably one of the factors determining the size of the newborn. In their study, Schellenberg et al [52] investigated 753 women on the relationship of vitamin status to pregnancy outcome. Women who experienced premature births were found to have significantly lower folate levels and those with stillbirths were found to have significantly lower plasma vitamin C levels. Vitamin C levels were on average low with 4.3 mg/l in the general population. This observation is of special interest, since Sexton et al [53] recently reported on a three-year study in 935 women on the effect of smoking on pregnancy outcome. The percentage of low birthweight infants was lower in the intervention group (special assistance to stop smoking) than in the control group (no assistance to stop smoking). In an earlier study by Yaffe [54] it was shown that mothers who smoke during pregnancy deliver smaller babies, have a greater incidence of premature delivery, and an increased incidence of abortion, stillbirths, and neonatal deaths.

Recent evidence suggests that smoking contributes significantly to the higher accumulation of trace elements, such as cadmium and copper, in the body [55, 56]. From animal experiments it is evident that vitamin C actively interferes with the detoxication and elimination of these compounds from the organism and that it is protective against many of the adverse effects of cadmium [57, 58]. Thus, a lowered vitamin C status such as in smokers may lead to a reduced capacity of detoxifying these transition metals.

References

1 US Department of Health, Education, and Welfare Public Health Service: The health consequences of smoking, 1975.
2 Schachter, S: Pharmacological and psychological determinants of smoking. Ann Int Med 88, 10–114, 1978.
3 Strauss, L H, Scheer, P: Über die Wirkung des Nicotins auf den Vitamin-C-Haushalt. Vitaminforschung 9, 39–48, 1939.
4 Harmsen, H: Der Vitamin-C-Blutspiegel des Krankenpflegepersonals im jahreszeitlichen Verlauf und in der besonderen Abhängigkeit von Ernährung, Arbeitseinsatz und Nikotinmissbrauch. Dtsch Med Wschr 29, 790–794, 1941.
5 Reif, G: Versuche über das Verhalten von Nikotin und Coffein gegen Ascorbinsäure. Biochem Z 315, 310–319, 1943.
6 Venulet, F: Raucherschäden durch Ascorbinsäureverlust. Med Klin 49, 259–262, 1954.
7 Venulet, F, Danysz, A: Effect of tobacco smoking on the vitamin C content of human milk. Pediat Polska 31, 811–817, 1955 (C.A. 51, 8977, 1957).
8 Calder H J et al: Comparison of vitamin C in plasma and leucocytes of smokers and nonsmokers. Lancet i, 556, 1963.
9 McCormick, W J: Ascorbic acid as a chemotherapeutic agent. Arch Pediat 69, 151–155, 1952.
10 Brook, M, Grimshaw, J J: Vitamin C concentration of plasma and leukocytes as related to smoking habit, age, and sex of humans. Am J Clin Nutr 21, 1254–1258, 1968.
11 Albanese, A A et al: An improved method for determination of leucocyte and plasma ascorbic acid of man with applications to studies on nutritional needs and effects of cigarette smoking. Nutr Rep Int 12, 269–288, 1975.
12 Kevany, J et al: The effect of smoking on ascorbic acid and serum cholesterol in adult males. Irish J Med Sci 144, 474–477, 1975.
13 McClean, H E et al: Vitamin C concentration in plasma and leucocytes of men related to age and smoking habits. NZ Med J 83, 226–229, 1976.
14 Hoefel, O S: Plasma vitamin C levels in smokers. Int J Vit Nutr Res Suppl 16, 127–137, 1977.
15 Keith, R E, Driskell, J A: Effects of chronic cigarette smoking on vitamin C status, lung function, and resting and exercise cardiovascular metabolism in humans. Nutr Rep Int 21, 907–912, 1980.
16 Keith, R E, Driskell J A: Lung functions and treadmill performance of smoking and nonsmoking males receiving ascorbic acid supplements. Am J Clin Nutr 36, 840–845, 1982.
17 Sulochana, G, Arunagari R: Smoking and ascorbic acid (vitamin C) excretion. Clinician 45, 198–201, 1981.

18 PELLETIER, O: Vitamin C and tobacco. Int J Vit Nutr Res, suppl *16*, pp 147-169, 1977.

19 RITZEL, G, BRUPPACHER, R: Vitamin C and tobacco. Int J Vit Nutr Res, suppl *16*, pp 171-183, 1977.

20 HUGHES, R E *et al:* Some effects of experimentally-produced cigarette smoke on the growth, vitamin C metabolism and organ weights of guinea pigs. J Pharm Pharmacol *22*, 823-827, 1970.

21 KEITH, M O, PELLETIER, O: The effect of nicotine on ascorbic acid retention by guinea pigs. Can J Physiol Pharmacol *51*, 879-884, 1973.

22 LEUCHTENBERGER, C, LEUCHTENBERGER, R: Protection of hamster lung cultures by L-cysteine or vitamin C against carcinogenic effects of fresh smoke from tobacco or marihuana cigarettes. Br J Exp Path *58*, 625-634, 1977.

23 CHEN, L H, CHOW, C K: Effect of cigarette smoking and dietary vitamin E on plasma level of vitamin C in rats. Nutr Rep Int *22*, 301-309, 1980.

24 SPRINCE, H *et al:* Protection against cyanide lethality in rats by L-ascorbic acid and dehydroascorbic acid. Nutr Rep Int *25*, 463-470, 1982.

25 FALTOT, P *et al:* Etude comparative de l'ascorburie des fumeurs et non-fumeurs. Bord Med *1*, 1387-1389, 1968.

26 WANG, N S *et al:* Vitamin C deficiency aggravates small airway changes induced by nicotine in guinea pigs. Am Rev Resp Dis *119*, 368, 1979.

27 IRWIN, H, HUTCHINS, B K: A conspectus of research of vitamin C requirements of man. J Nutr *106*, 821-879, 1976.

28 HORNIG, D: Requirement of vitamin C in man. Trends in Pharmacol Sciences *3*, 294-296, 1982.

29 SAUBERLICH, H E: Vitamin C status: methods and findings. Ann NY Acad Sci *252*, 438-450, 1975.

30 KALLNER, A *et al:* Steady-state turnover and body pool of ascorbic acid in man. Am J Clin Nutr *32*, 530-539, 1979.

31 BAKER, E M *et al:* Metabolism of ascorbic $-1-^{14}$ C acid in experimental human scurvy. Am J Clin Nutr *22*, 549-558, 1969.

32 BAKER, E M *et al:* Metabolism of ^{14}C- and ^{3}H-labeled L-ascorbic acid in human scurvy. Am J Clin Nutr *24*, 444-454, 1971.

33 KALLNER, A *et al:* On the absorption of ascorbic acid in man. Int J Vit Nutr Res *47*, 383-388, 1977.

34 KALLNER A B *et al:* On the requirements of ascorbic acid in man: steady-state turnover and body pool in smokers. Am J Clin Nutr *34*, 1347-1355, 1981.

35 Nutrition Canada National Survey. Information Canada, Ontario, 1973.

36 Interdepartmental Committee on Nutrition for National Defense. Manual for Nutrition Surveys; 2nd ed. US Government Printing Office, Washington, 1963.

37 JAIN I S *et al:* Black cataract – a smoking hazard. Bull Postgraduate Inst Med Education Res Chandigarh *16*, 9-11, 1982.

38 WALTERS, C L: The influence of ascorbic acid on the formation of N-nitrosamines in foods, drugs, cosmetics and tobacco. In: COUNSELL and HORNIG (eds) "Vitamin C (ascorbic acid)", pp 199-213. Applied Science, London, 1981.

39 Hoffmann-La Roche AG. Tobacco containing ascorbic acid or erythorbic acid and their salts to reduce nitrogen dioxide and nitrosamine content of smoke. US Patent 442 990 (15.02.1974).

40 GRAHAM, S *et al:* Dietary factors in the epidemiology of cancer of the larynx. Am J Epidemiol *113*, 675-680, 1981.

41 SPRINCE, H: Ascorbic acid, sulfur compounds, and anti-adrenergic agents as protectants against acetaldehyde toxicity, implications in alcoholism and smoking. Br J Alcohol Alcoholism *16*, 5-9, 1981.

42 MILOCHIK, J A: The effect of smoking on drug metabolism. Can J Hosp Pharmacy *34*, 144-149, 1981.

43 Yeung, D L: Relationship between cigarette smoking, oral contraceptives, and plasma vitamins A, E, C and plasma triglycerides and cholesterol. Am J Clin Nutr *29,* 1216–1221, 1976.

44 Hornig, D: Impact of marginal vitamin C deficiency. J Jap Soc Clin Nutr *3,* 127–141, 1982.

45 Eddy, T P: A study of the relationship between Hess tests and leucocyte ascorbic acid in a clinical trial. Br J Nutr *27,* 537–542, 1972.

46 Hughes, R E: Recommended daily amounts and biochemical roles – the vitamin C, carnitine, fatigue relationship. In: Counsell and Hornig (eds) "Vitamin C (ascorbic acid)", pp 75–86. Applied Science, London, 1981.

47 Crandon J H *et al:* Ascorbic acid economy in surgical patients. Ann NY Acad Sci *92,* 246–267, 1961.

48 Trope, G E *et al:* Low leucocyte ascorbic acid levels and corneal ulceration. Trans Ophthal Soc UK *99,* 495–496, 1977.

49 Greco, A M *et al:* Relationship between hemorrhagic ocular diseases and vitamin C deficiency: clinical and experimental data. Acta Vitaminol Enzymol *2,* 21–25, 1980.

50 Buzina, R: The impact of marginal malnutrition on health and behaviour. In: Aebi *et al* (eds). "Problems in nutrition research today", pp 57–74. Academic Press, London, 1981.

51 Schorah, C J: Inappropriate vitamin C reserves: their frequency and significance in an urban population. In: Taylor (ed) "Importance of vitamins to human health", pp 61–72. MTP Press, Lancaster, 1979.

52 Schellenberg, B *et al:* The relationship between vitamin status, prematurity and stillbirths. Eur J Clin Invest *13,* 37, 1982.

53 Sexton, M *et al:* Maternal smoking, complications of delivery, and status of the newborn. Fifth World Conference on Smoking and Health, Winnipeg, Canada, July 10–15, 1983, p 160.

54 Yaffe, S J A: A clinical look at the problem of drugs in pregnancy and their effect on the fetus. J Can Med Assoc *112,* 728–733, 1975.

55 Elinder, C G *et al:* Cadmium in kidney cortex, liver, and pancreas from Swedish autopsies. Estimation of biological half time in kidney cortex, considering caloric intake and smoking habits. Arch Environ Health *31,* 292–302, 1976.

56 Creason, J P *et al:* Blood trace metals in military recruits. South Med J *69,* 289–293, 1976.

57 Fox, S M R: Protective effects of ascorbic acid against toxicity of heavy metals. Ann NY Acad Sci *258,* 144–150, 1975.

58 Fox; S M R *et al:* Effects of vitamin C and iron on cadmium metabolism. Ann NY Acad Sci *355,* 249–261, 1980.

D.H. Hornig, PhD, Department of Vitamin and Nutrition Research, F. Hoffmann-La Roche & Co., Ltd., CH-4002 Basle, Switzerland

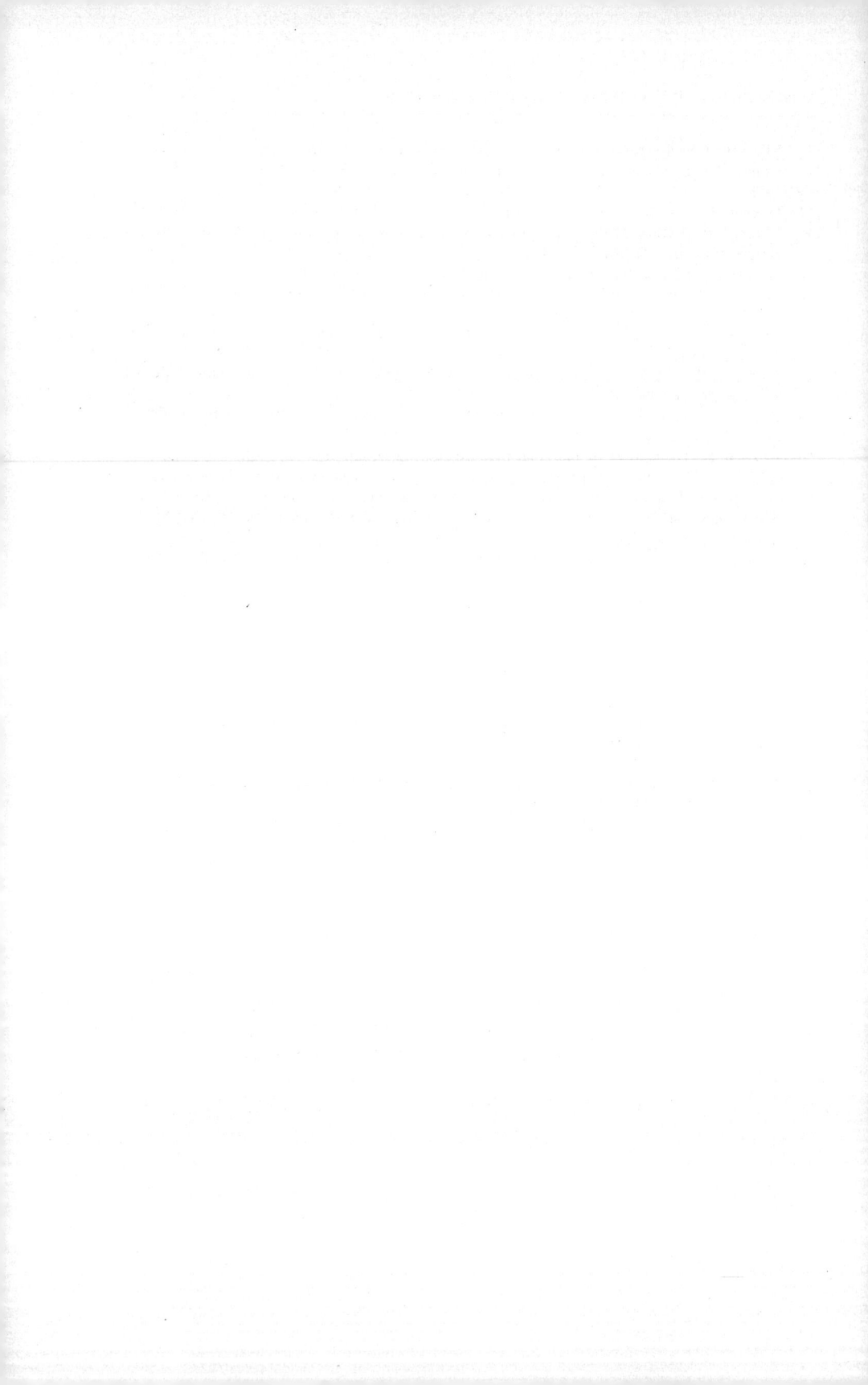

Vitamin C and Physical Working Capacity

R. Buzina and K. Suboticanec

Institute of Public Health, Zagreb, Yugoslavia

Key Words: Adolescents · Physical working capacity · Vitamin C · Riboflavin · Pyridoxine · Iron · Ascorbic acid requirement

Abstract: The results of this study indicate vitamin C to be associated with the aerobic capacity of young adolescents. This association was more pronounced in the subjects having deficient and low plasma vitamin C values. The increase in plasma vitamin C was followed by an increase in $\dot{V}O_2$ max, but only till plasma vitamin C reached the level of 0.8–0.9 mg/dl. No further increase in $\dot{V}O_2$ max was observed when plasma vitamin C rose above that level. On the basis of these data it may be concluded that the optimal aerobic capacity is associated with a daily ascorbic acid intake of 80–100 mg. These results, obtained by use of a functional test, are in good agreement with the results obtained by kinetic studies.

Introduction

A good physical performance is dependent on many factors including physical condition, technical skill, coordination, muscular strength, and optimal nutrition. Chronic undernutrition, or even dieting, as observed during body weight reduction, may have a deteriorating effect on physical performance. In the classical study by Keys *et al* [1] work capacity was substantially reduced by long-term dietary restriction, and a number of other studies indicate that improvement of nutritional status is related to better physical performance and work productivity [2–5].

In one of our previous studies it was found that poor nutritional status defined as low relative body weight (RBW) affected the physical working capacity of otherwise healthy workers [6]. However, the results of food consumption studies indicated that the diet of subjects with lower RBW was inadequate not only with regard to energy but also with regard to some essential nutrients, notably vitamins and minerals. Though it is well known that energy deficient diets are usually deficient in a number of vitamins and minerals, there is very little information, with the exception of iron, as to whether mineral and vitamin deficiencies affect physical working capacity. Since however mild-to-moderate (subclinical) vitamin deficiencies are quite prevalent in some population groups, even in the industrially developed countries [7–9], we decided to study the specific effect on physical working capacity of some more prevalent vitamin deficiencies.

Selection of Subjects

The studies were carried out in adolescent boys aged 13–15 years in a rural district with a high prevalence of subclinical, biochemically defined vitamin malnutrition. The initial nutritional status was assessed on the basis of anthropometric, clinical and biochemical examinations, and physical working capacity was determined by measuring aerobic capacity ($\dot{V}O_2$max). After the baseline study was completed the effect on physical working capacity of the rehabilitation of the three most common vitamin deficiencies, i. e. vitamin C, riboflavin and pyridoxine was studied.

The subjects were therefore divided into two groups, one of which (the experimental group) was treated with tablets containing 70 mg of ascorbic acid, 2 mg of riboflavin and 2 mg of pyridoxine. The tablets were given daily (except Sundays) in the school under teacher's supervision over a period of 3 months. The other group served as control. At the end of the 3-month period all examinations were repeated.

Methods

Nutritional status was assessed on the basis of weight for height (relative body weight), and the following biochemical parameters: serum vitamin A, determined after chromatographic separation from carotenoids by the method of Kahan [10]; plasma vitamin C, by a modification of the fluorometric method by Deutsch and Weeks [11]; thiamine in red cells, by transketolase (ETK) test according to Schouten [12]; riboflavin, by the measurement of activated and non-activated glutathione reductase (EGR) according to Glatzle et al [13]; pyridoxine, by the level of activity of pyridoxal-5-phosphate-dependent glutamic oxalacetic transaminase (EGOT) from hemolysed red blood cells by the method of Scheidt et al [14]; serum iron by a modified method of Bothwell and Mallet [15]; iron-binding capacity by the method of Ramsey [16]; hemoglobin by the use of the cyanomethemoglobin method [17]; and hematocrit by the microhematocrit method. Blood samples were taken from all subjects with the consent of their parents.

Physical working capacity was studied by the bicycle ergometer technique which measures the work load required to elevate the heart rate to above 130 beats/min. Maximal oxygen uptake was predicted from heart rate and work load by the Astrand-Rhyming nomogram [18]. The results are expressed as $\dot{V}O_2$ max (l/min).

Results and Discussion

The results of nutritional status assessment based on RBW data (Table I) show that 85.5 % of the examined subjects had an adequate energy intake, 2.5 % were obese (RBW $>$ 120), and only 12 % were mildly undernourished (RBW $<$ 90).

More significant, however, was the problem of vitamin and iron deficiency.

Tab. I: Relative body weight (weight for height) as percentage of reference median[1] of the examined subjects

80–89		90–109		110–119		≥ 120		Total	
N	%	N	%	N	%	N	%	N	%
28	11.8	181	75.7	24	10.0	6	2.5	239	100.0

[1] NCHS Growth Charts. USDHEW: HRA 76-1120, 25, 3, 1976.

Data summarized in Table II indicate that 33.9 % of the examined subjects were affected by biochemical deficiency of riboflavin, and 30.0 % by vitamin C deficiency. About 17 % of the subjects showed a deficient red cell pyridoxine content, and only 2.7 % had deficient levels of serum vitamin A. With regard to iron nutritional status, the prevalence of anemia diagnosed on the basis of deficient blood hemoglobin values was rather low. Much higher, however, was the prevalence of tissue iron deficiency as diagnosed from low serum iron and transferrin saturation levels, which were found in about 11 to 12 % of subjects, respectively.

Tab. II: Nutritional status of the examined subjects; biochemical evaluation

	Criteria deficiency	n	$\bar{X}$	SD	Subjects with deficient values, %
Vitamin A, µg/dl	< 20.0	226	34.5	8.8	2.7
Vitamin C, mg/dl	< 0.20	230	0.44	0.36	30.0
ETK (α)[1]	> 1.20	231	1.11	0.05	5.2
EGR (α)[1]	> 1.20	239	1.13	0.16	33.9
EGOT (α)[1]	> 2.00	239	1.85	0.18	17.2
Hemoglobin, g/dl	< 12.0	239	14.1	1.00	1.3
Hematocrit, %	< 31.0	237	42.0	2.6	0.0
Serum iron, µg/dl	< 50.0	225	89.9	34.1	10.5
Transferrin saturation, %	< 16.0	212	25.8	9.3	11.8

[1] Reactivation coefficient.

The relation between aerobic capacity and anthropometric and biochemical parameters of nutritional status is presented in Table III.

The $\dot{V}O_2$ max (l/min) was significantly correlated with age and the size of the body as defined by body height and body weight. There was also a small but statistically significant correlation with the blood levels of hemoglobin, hematocrit, vitamin A, vitamin C as well as with the EGR activation coefficient.

Tabl. III: Correlations between $\dot{V}O_2$ max (l/min) and examined anthropometrical and biochemical parameters (Kendall two-sided rank correlation)

		0_2 Consumption			
	$n^{[1]}$	l/min		ml/kg/min	
		$r^{[2]}$	significance	$r^{[2]}$	significance
Age	201	0.496	S	0.031	NS
Body weight	201	0.536	S	−0.101	S
Body height	201	0.504	S	−0.075	NS
RBW	201	0.041	NS	−0.144	S
Hemoglobin	199	0.327	S	0.186	S
Hematocrit	197	0.217	S	0.004	NS
Serum iron	188	0.027	NS	0.271	S
TIBC	176	0.076	NS	0.105	S
Transferrin saturation	176	−0.008	NS	0.028	NS
Vitamin A	188	0.160	S	−0.070	NS
Vitamin C	192	0.107	S	0.034	NS
ETK	191	0.033	NS	−0.024	NS
EGR	199	−0.101	S	−0.179	S
EGOT	199	−0.001	NS	0.023	NS

[1] N = Number of pairs.
[2] Correlation coefficient.

The results of anthropometric and biochemical measurements and aerobic capacity before and after supplementation are summarized in Table IV.

In the experimental group vitamin administration resulted in a significant increase in the mean plasma vitamin C concentration and red cell riboflavin content. The improvement in these two biochemical parameters of vitamin C and riboflavin nutritional status has also been accompanied by a reduction in the prevalence of deficient plasma vitamin C values from 28.8 % to zero, and deficient EGR values from 35.0 to 3.8 %. There was also a slight but statistically non-significant improvement in EGOT activation which was followed by a decrease in deficient EGOT values from 16.3 to 6.3 %. No changes regarding vitamin status were observed in the control group except for an increase in vitamin C content. This increase took place at the very end of the study which terminated at the beginning of June when fresh vegetables and fruits were becoming available and were consumed in greater amounts in the family diet again. This increase in mean plasma vitamin C values had only a slight impact on the prevalence of deficient plasma values which fell from 27.2 to 18.2 %.

The rehabilitation of vitamin deficiencies was accompanied by a statistically significant increase in $\dot{V}O_2$ max, whereas in the control group there was a

Tab. IV: Relationship between vitamin and iron nutritional status and $\dot{V}O_2$ max before (I) and after (II) 3 months of vitamin supplementation in a group of boys aged 12–15 years compared with an unsupplemented group

| | Experimental group (supplemented) n = 80 | | | | | Control group (unsupplemented) n = 66 | | | | |
| | I | | II | | p | I | | II | | p |
	mean	SD	mean	SD		mean	SD	mean	SD	
Age, months	157	21.1	160	21.2	NS	163	22.4	166	22.6	NS
Body height, cm	150.1	8.6	150.6	7.8	NS	154.2	11.3	154.7	11.4	NS
Body weight, kg	38.0	7.6	38.3	8.6	NS	41.3	8.1	41.8	7.9	NS
RBW, %	97.2	9.9	97.1	8.8	NS	97.0	9.0	97.0	8.7	NS
$\dot{V}O_2$ max, l/min	1.84	0.45	2.15	0.52	0.001	2.10	0.56	2.05	0.53	NS
$\dot{V}O_2$ max, ml/kg/min	44.5	8.2	51.6	9.6	0.001	51.4	8.7	48.6	8.5	0.01
Hemoglobin, g/dl	14.0	1.2	14.1	1.1	NS	14.0	0.9	13.8	1.0	NS
Hematocrit, %	42.5	3.0	42.5	3.4	NS	42.2	2.3	41.8	2.5	NS
Serum iron, µg/dl	81.5	25.4	96.2	21.7	0.001	92.2	31.7	71.5	25.8	NS
TIBC, µg/dl	334.4	90.6	284.9	54.1	0.001	329.0	82.1	302.4	75.7	NS
Transferrin saturation, %	25.1	6.7	28.8	5.7	0.001	27.4	10.9	25.1	9.6	NS
Vitamin A, µg/dl	36.3	8.6	35.9	8.9	NS	36.9	9.2	36.6	9.8	NS
Vitamin C, mg/dl	0.42	0.25	1.18	0.28	0.001	0.43	0.36	0.58	0.41	0.05
ETK (α)[1]	1.12	0.05	1.12	0.06	NS	1.12	0.06	1.14	0.06	NS
EGR (α)[1]	1.17	0.16	1.04	0.11	0.001	1.16	0.17	1.17	0.14	NS
EGOT (α)[1]	1.83	0.16	1.81	0.18	NS	1.86	0.19	1.85	0.19	NS

[1] Reactivation coefficient.

slight decrease in $\dot{V}O_2$ max measured in l/min. The correction of ascorbic acid and riboflavin deficiencies was also accompanied by a non-significant increase in blood hemoglobin values and a significant increase in serum iron and transferrin saturation values. At the same time, there was a slight, but non-significant decrease in the parameters of iron nutritional status in the control group.

The presented data suggest that besides an association with the parameters of body size, the $\dot{V}O_2$ max is at least in part associated with vitamin and iron nutritional status. Among the biochemical measurements made, relatively higher correlation with $\dot{V}O_2$ max was observed for hemoglobin and hematocrit, whereas the correlation with the vitamin A, vitamin C and riboflavin status was of a much lower order. However, as hemoglobin, hematocrit and serum iron as well as plasma vitamin A are age-dependent variables [19–22] which, during the growth period, are also positively correlated with body weight and height, we have calculated partial correlations independent of age for those biochemical parameters. The results presented in Table V indicate that hemoglobin, hematocrit, and riboflavin are related to aerobic capacity independently of age.

Tab. V: Partial correlations (independent of age) between $\dot{V}O_2$ max (l/min) and hemoglobin, hematocrit, serum iron, vitamin A and EGR reactivation (α)

Variable	n[1]	r[2]	p
Hemoglobin	199	0.248	<0.001
Hematocrit	199	0.164	<0.01
Serum iron	188	0.082	NS
Vitamin A	188	0.149	<0.05
EGR (α)	199	−0.183	<0.01

[1] Number of pairs.
[2] Partial correlation.

In order to find out which biochemical parameters were associated with the observed increase in aerobic capacity after the supplementation period, we have pooled the data from both the experimental and control group and have divided the subjects to whether their $\dot{V}O_2$ max increased or decreased. The correlation coefficients between the changes in biochemical parameters during the supplementation period and the difference between the second and first $\dot{V}O_2$ max measurement ($\triangle$) are summarized in Table VI.

Tab. VI: The coefficients of correlations between biochemical parameters of nutritional status and increased ($\triangle +$) and decreased ($\triangle -$) areobic capacity ($\dot{V}O_2$ max, l/min)

	Aerobic capacity	
	$\triangle +$	$\triangle -$
Hemoglobin	0.278*	−0.125
Hematocrit	0.113	−0.206
TIBC	−0.106	0.075
Serum iron	0.044	−0.035
Transferrin saturation	0.058	0.005
Vitamin A	0.079	−0.130
Vitamin C	0.226*	0.009
ETK	−0.192	−0.297**
EGR	−0.268*	0.0.44
EGOT	0.043	0.015

* $p < 0.05$.
** $p < 0.01$.

The increase in $\dot{V}O_2$ max (l/min) was positively correlated with the increase in iron nutritional status, the most significant of which was the increase in hemoglobin level ($p < 0.01$). The increase in $\dot{V}O_2$ max was also significantly correlated with the increase in plasma vitamin C and red cell riboflavin content. On the other hand, the decrease in $\dot{V}O_2$ max was associated, though not significantly, with a decrease in hemoglobin, hematocrit, and serum iron values as well as with a decrease in plasma vitamin A values. In subjects with a decreased $\dot{V}O_2$ max, a significant association with the increased red cell thiamin content was observed, as was also the case, though not significantly so, in those with increased $\dot{V}O_2$ max.

However, though the results of this study point to an association between aerobic capacity and vitamin C and riboflavin nutrition, it is not clear from the presented data whether the role of ascorbic acid and riboflavin was a direct one, or rather, whether their effects were exercised through their impact on iron nutrition status which has improved after the improvement of vitamin C and riboflavin nutritional status. Both these vitamins seem to be connected with the absorption and utilization of dietary iron [23–27].

Tab. VII: Means and standard deviations of the physical characteristics, biochemical parameters of nutritional status, and aerobic capacity of the examined subjects before (I) and after (II) vitamin supplementation

	Experimental group (n = 49)			Control group (n = 42)		
	I	II	p	I	II	p
Age, years	12.9 ± 1.1	13.1 ± 1.0		12.4 ± 1.3	12.6 ± 1.4	
RBW, %	96.9 ± 10.0	97.0 ± 10.1	NS	100.7 ± 11.9	100.6 ± 11.4	NS
W/H²	1.7 ± 0.2	1.7 ± 0.2	NS	1.7 ± 0.2	1.7 ± 0.2	NS
Vitamin C, mg/dl	0.33 ± 0.24	1.49 ± 0.25	0.001	0.43 ± 0.34	0.56 ± 0.31	NS
EGR (α)	1.13 ± 0.10	1.01 ± 0.08	0.001	1.10 ± 0.10	0.99 ± 0.05	0.01
EGOT (α)	1.91 ± 0.12	1.73 ± 0.16	0.001	1.81 ± 0.14	1.63 ± 0.13	0.001
Vitamin A, µg/dl	34.1 ± 5.0	33.4 ± 5.3	NS	33.8 ± 6.8	34.6 ± 6.4	NS
Hemoglobin, g/dl	14.2 ± 0.6	14.1 ± 0.9	NS	14.2 ± 0.5	14.3 ± 0.6	NS
Hematocrit, %	40.7 ± 1.4	40.5 ± 2.4	NS	42.0 ± 1.6	41.3 ± 2.3	NS
Transferrin, %	22.3 ± 8.8	20.1 ± 8.2	NS	23.5 ± 51.7	21.0 ± 6.8	NS
$\dot{V}O_2$ max, l/min	2.9 ± 0.3	3.2 ± 0.3	0.01	2.9 ± 0.3	3.0 ± 0.3	NS

In order to find out whether vitamin C deficiency rehabilitation has an independent effect on aerobic capacity, those studies were continued in two populations with comparable and adequate iron nutritional status in which biochemical deficiencies of riboflavin and pyridoxine were corrected by peroral administration of 2.0 mg riboflavin and 2.0 mg pyridoxine over a two-month period. One (experimental) group was simultaneously treated with 70 mg ascorbic acid. The results are summarized in Table VII.

In the control group, riboflavin and pyridoxine supplementation resulted in a statistically significant improvement of average EGR reactivation coefficients (p < 0.01) as well as of EGOT reactivation coefficients (p < 0.001). At the same time, the percentage of subjects with biochemically deficient red cell riboflavin and pyridoxine values was reduced from 12 and 8.5 %, respectively, to zero. With regard to vitamin C nutritional status there was a slight, but statistically non-significant increase in the average plasma vitamin C level toward the end of the study which was associated with a reduction in the proportion of subjects with low vitamin C plasma values (< 0.20 mg/dl) from 30 to 21 %.

In the experimental group, the statistically significant increase in the average riboflavin and pyridoxine red cell content was accompanied by an equally significant increase in vitamin C plasma values (p < 0.001). At the same time the percentage of subjects with deficient plasma vitamin C values was reduced from 52.3 % to zero. During the supplementation period significant changes occurred neither in plasma vitamin A levels nor in the examined biochemical parameters of iron nutritional status.

The supplementation with riboflavin, pyridoxine and ascorbic acid resulted in a small, but statistically significant (p < 0.05) increase in aerobic capacity in the experimental group, whereas the supplementation with riboflavin and pyridoxine alone had no statistically significant impact on aerobic capacity of the control group subjects. As the observed action of vitamin C on aerobic capacity could be clearly dissociated from any effects on iron absorption and utilization, or from an improvement of riboflavin nutritional status, the results of this study indicate that vitamin C may have a small, but independent effect on the aerobic capacity of adolescents.

Tab. VIII: The oxygen intake (l/min) in subjects divided according to the level of vitamin C in plasma

	Group I (n = 32)	Group II (n = 50)	Group III (n = 26)	Group IV (n = 63)
Vitamin C, mg/dl	0.00–0.19	0.20–0.59	0.60–0.99	≥ 1.00
O_2, l/min	2.81 ± 0.22	2.86 ± 0.42	3.13 ± 0.38	3.14 ± 0.31
t	I:II = 0.351	I:III = 3.451	II:III = 2.518	III:IV = 0.556
p	> 0.05	< 0.01	< 0.05	> 0.05

The effect on aerobic capacity of vitamin C supplementation was primarily observed in the subjects with deficient and low plasma vitamin C levels (Table VIII). When vitamin C plasma levels have increased above 1.0 mg/dl, no further increase in aerobic capacity was observed. These data suggest a non-linear relationship between the aerobic capacity and vitamin C plasma levels.

In order to find out the level below which ascorbic acid intake may be inadequate for attaining optimal aerobic capacity, two regression equations, approximating low and high vitamin C plasma concentrations were calculated. The two straight lines crossed at x = 0.86 mg/dl indicating that a further increase of the vitamin C plasma level will have no effect on the improvement of aerobic capacity (Fig. 1).

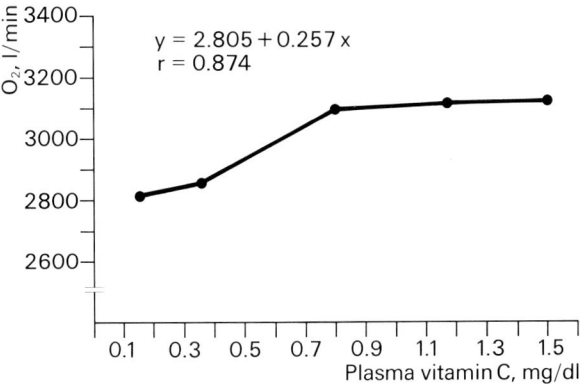

Fig. 1: Correlation of oxygen consumption to plasma vitamin C concentration.

The plasma vitamin C level of 0.86 mg/dl corresponds to an intake of about 80 mg ascorbic acid/day. But, since in most diets a part of dietary ascorbic acid is supplied by foods which are subjected to heat treatment resulting in a 30-60 % loss of ascorbic acid, it seems that the actual amount of dietary ascorbic acid needed for attaining optimal plasma levels may be even higher than 80 mg/day. A similar figure was obtained by KALLNER *et al* [27] who suggested a daily intake of about 100 mg ascorbic acid to be appropriate to cover the daily requirement of this vitamin in at least 95 % of the population, and to maintain a plasma vitamin C concentration of 0.8 to 0.9 mg/dl. Thus, our results, obtained by use of a functional test are in good agreement with the suggested optimal ascorbic acid dietary intake obtained by kinetic studies with (1-¹⁴C)ascorbic acid.

References

1 KEYS, A *et al:* The biology of human starvation. University of Minnesota, Press, Minneapolis, 1950.
2 STEARNS, M: In: LOEWENSTEIN (ed) "Food and nutrition in Africa". WHO/Organization of African Unity. No 6, p 17, 1968.
3 CONSOLAZIO, C F: Nutritional status and work capacity relationship. In: DEBRY and BLEYER (eds) "Alimentation et travail", pp 227-244. Masson, Paris, 1972.
4 DAVIES, C T H: Relationship of maximum aerobic power output to productivity and absenteeism of East African sugar cane workers. Br J Industr Med *30,* 146-154, 1973.

5 Kraut, H: Food intake as a factor of production. In: Debry and Bleyer (eds) "Alimentation et travail", pp 216-225, Masson, Paris, 1972.

6 Buzina, R et al: Nutritional status, working capacity and absenteeism in industrial workers. In: Debry and Bleyer (eds) "Alimentation et travail", pp 141-151. Masson, Paris, 1972.

7 Brubacher, G et al: Transketolase-Aktivität, Thiaminausscheidung und Blutthiamingehalt bei Menschen zur Beurteilung der Vitamin-B_1-Versorgung. Int J Vit Nutr Res 42, 451-456, 1972.

8 Fisher, S et al: Nutritional assessment of senior rural Utahns by biochemical and physical measurements. Am J Clin Nutr 31, 667-672, 1978.

9 Jacob, M et al: Biochemical assessment of the nutritional status of low-income pregnant women of Mexican descent. Am J Clin Nutr 29, 650-656, 1976.

10 Kahan, J: A method for the fluorometric determination of vitamin A. Scand J Clin Lab Invest 18, 679-690, 1966.

11 Deutsch, M J, Weeks, C E: Microfluorometric assay for vitamin C. J Am Org Analyt Chem 48, 1248-1256, 1965.

12 Schouten, M et al: Transketolase in blood. Clin Chim Acta 10, 474-476, 1964.

13 Glatzle, D et al: Method for the detection of a biochemical riboflavin deficiency. Stimulation of $NADPH_2$ dependent glutathione reductase from human erythrocytes by FAD in vitro. Int J Vit Res 40, 166-173, 1970.

14 Scheidt, R A et al: Automated determination of serum glutamic oxalacetic transaminase. Technicon Symposia 1965. Medicaid, New York, 1966.

15 Bothwell, T H, Mallet, B: The determination of iron in plasma or serum. Biochem J 59, 599-602, 1955.

16 Ramsay, W N M: The determination of the total ironbinding capacity of serum. Clin Chim Acta 2, 221-226, 1957.

17 ICNND: Manual for nutrition surveys; 2nd ed. US Government Printing Office, Washington, 1963.

18 Astrand, I: Aerobic work capacity in men and women with special reference to age. Acta Physiol Scand 49, suppl 169, 1960.

19 Wintrobe, M M: Clinical hematology; 8th ed. Lea & Febiger, Philadelphia, 1962.

20 Seltzer, C C et al: Serum iron binding capacity in adolescents. I. Standard values. Am J Clin Nutr 13, 343-353, 1963.

21 Kaspar, H: Die Vitamin A and Carotinkonzentration in Serum. Int J Vit Res 38, 142-148, 1968.

22 Buzina, R et al: Prevention of nutritional deficiency in the community. A study of the effects of medicamentous prophylaxis and nutrition education. Final report. Institute of Public-Health, Zagreb, 1978.

23 Mc Curdy, P R, Dern, R: Effect of ascorbic acid upon iron absorption. Am J Clin Nutr 20, 367, 1967.

24 Sayer, M H et al: Iron absorption from rice meals cooked with fortified salt containing ferrous sulphate and ascorbic acid. Br J Nutr 31, 367-375, 1974.

25 Alfrey, C P, Lane, M: The effect of riboflavin deficiency in erythropoesis. Sem Hematol 7, 49-54, 1970.

26 Sirivech, S et al: NADH-FMN oxydoreductase activity and iron content of organs from riboflavin and iron deficient rats. J Nutr 107, 739-745, 1977.

27 Buzina, R et al: The effects of riboflavin administration on iron metabolism parameters in a school-going population. Int J Vit Nutr Res 49, 136-143, 1979.

Prof. Ratko Buzina, MD, ScD, Head, Nutrition Department, Institute of Public Health of SR Croatia, Rockefellerova 7, Zagreb, Yugoslavia

The Role of Ascorbic Acid in the Bioavailability of Iron from Infant Foods

A. Stekel, M. Olivares, F. Pizarro, M. Amar, P. Chadud, M. Cayazzo, S. Llaguno, V. Vega and E. Hertrampf

Institute of Nutrition and Food Technology (INTA), University of Chile, Santiago, Chile

Key Words: Iron absorption · Ascorbic acid · Milk, infant foods · Food fortification

Abstract: Iron deficiency in infancy continues to be highly prevalent throughout the world. During the initial 4–6 months of life, infants are protected from developing iron deficiency by the iron stores present at birth and the high bioavailability of breastmilk iron. After this initial period, good dietary iron sources are needed to satisfy the high iron demands for growth. Cow's milk, the main source of calories in artificially fed infants, has a very low iron content and this iron is of relatively poor bioavailability. Solid foods, such as cereals, used to supplement the infants' diet have a higher iron content, but the non-heme iron present in these vegetable products is also of low bioavailability. Fortification of milk formulas and infant cereals with iron is recommended and widely used, but the absorption of the inorganic fortification iron is inhibited by dietary factors and is often quite low. Chilean infants from 3 to 15 months of age fed low-fat cow's milk containing 15 mg elemental iron per liter, as ferrous sulphate, were only partially protected from developing iron deficiency. Isotopic absorption studies conducted in our laboratory indicated that iron bioavailability from cow's milk could be increased 2–3 times by the addition of ascorbic acid. The effect of ascorbic acid on absorption was maintained after several months of storage. As a result of these studies, a milk formula containing 15 mg elemental iron and 100 mg ascorbic acid per liter was manufactured. Controlled field trials have shown that, when used after weaning at 3 months of age, this product essentially eradicates iron deficiency anemia during the first year of life in both term and preterm Chilean infants.

Introduction

Infants are highly susceptible to develop iron deficiency. Iron stores present at birth in the form of tissue deposits and a high hemoglobin concentration last for only a few months. When stores are exhausted, the infant depends on dietary sources to meet the high requirements of the mineral and unless the diet is adequately supplemented, there are high chances that it will not meet these requirements [1].

Iron Requirements in Infancy

Iron requirements during infancy are determined by the size of iron stores at birth, the requirements for growth and by the quantity of iron losses. Since most iron is transferred to the fetus during the third trimester of pregnancy, there is a linear relationship between body weight and total body iron, so that newborns have an average of 75 mg iron/kg [2]. The iron nutrition status at birth does not seem to be much influenced by the iron nutrition of the mother [3, 4]; it appears that only very severe iron deficiency in the mother can affect iron stores in the newborn [5].

Knowledge about iron losses in infancy is limited. Using radioisotopic methods, GARBY et al [6] calculated in a small number of infants a mean loss of iron in the feces of 0.03 mg/kg/day. Other authors [7] have estimated total mean daily losses during the first 2 years of life at 0.04 mg/kg.

Requirements for growth can be calculated from estimations of total body iron at various ages. SMITH and RÍOS (7) have made these calculations based on data of iron content of different tissues. Mean daily requirements of absorbed iron for growth determined in this way are 0.25 mg/day in the first semester of life, 0.53 mg/day from 6 months to 1 year, and 0.29 mg/day in the second year of life. Taking into consideration the need to replace losses, requirements of absorbed iron are approximately 0.5 mg/day from 0 to 6 months of age, 0.9 mg/day from 6 months to 1 year, and 0.7–0.8 mg/day from 1 to 8 years [8].

Food Iron Absorption

Recommended intakes of iron to meet requirements must be based on an adequate knowledge of the proportion of the dietary iron that is absorbed. Bioavailability of food iron can vary markedly depending on factors such as the type of iron and the composition of the diet [9]. Heme iron, the iron present in myoglobin and hemoglobin, is well absorbed, and its bioavailability is relatively independent of the composition of the diet. Iron in the diet, however, is mostly present in the form of non-heme, inorganic iron. This is the form of iron present in the main staple foods such as maize, corn and rice, in vegetables and in foods of animal origin such as milk and eggs. It is also the form of iron that is used in food fortification. Non-heme dietary iron is more poorly absorbed than heme iron and is greatly affected by the composition of the diet. Substances such as carbonates, oxalates, phosphates, phytate, bran, vegetable fiber, tea and egg yolk depress non-heme iron absorption. The main enhancers of non-hem food iron absorption are meat and ascorbic acid [10].

Absorption of Iron from Milk

Milk, the main source of calories in the infant diet, has a very low iron content. Both human and cow milk contain less than 1 mg iron/l. For reasons that are not well understood, the iron present in human milk is unusually well absorbed [11], as a result breast fed infants are protected from developing iron deficiency during the first 4–6 months of life [12]. After this age, infants become dependent on other dietary sources to meet their high iron requirements.

Even with an early introduction of solid foods into the diet, many infants develop iron deficiency during the first year of life. For this reason, iron fortification of infant foods has been recommended and is widely used, especially in the more developed countries. Infant formulas and infant cereals are the vehicles most commonly used in iron fortification.

We have studied the influence of various factors on the bioavailability of fortification iron from milk in infants. In these studies, all products were for-

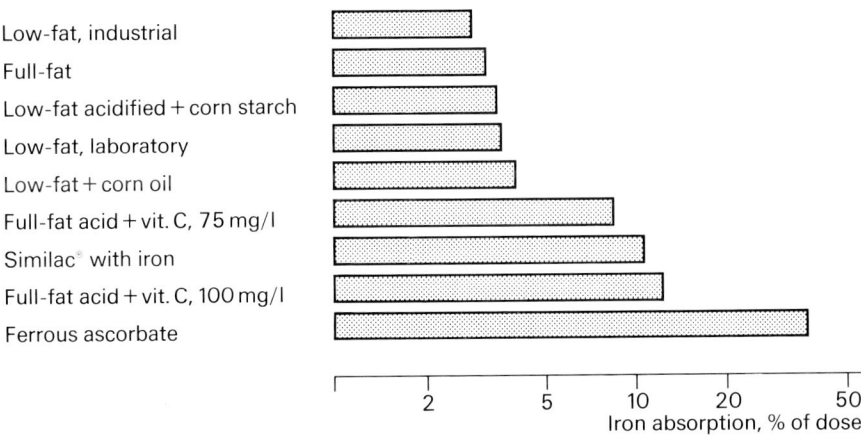

Fig. 1: Absorption of fortification iron from different milk formulas in infants. The length of the bars indicate the geometric mean absorption from each product.

tified with ferrous sulphate in concentrations varying from 10 to 15 mg of elemental iron per liter of formula. Absorption was studied radioisotopically using an extrinsic tag of radioiron. Figure 1 shows that there is a relatively large variation in the mean iron absorption from the different products. Factors such as the amount of fat, the type of carbohydrate and acidification of the milk had little influence on bioavailability. The products with the higher absorption were those containing a significant amount of ascorbic acid.

Effect of Ascorbic Acid on the Absorption of Iron from Milk

The influence of ascorbic acid on the absorption of fortification iron in milk was systematically studied by the use of a double isotope technique. In these studies, infants received on day 1, low-fat cow's milk fortified with 15 mg/l elemental iron as ferrous sulphate. The next day they were given the same product with various amounts of freshly added ascorbic acid, ranging in concentration from 25 to 800 mg/l. Absorption was calculated from the circulating radioactivity on day 15 [13]. Results shown in Figure 2 indicate that with concentrations of 100 mg/l or higher, absorption increased 2 to 3 times over the basal value. The highest effect in our study was found with a concentration of 200 mg/l, representing a molar relationship of ascorbic acid to iron of 4:1. When a milk fortified with 15 mg iron and 100 mg ascorbic acid/100 g powder was industrially produced, the enhancing effect of ascorbic acid was

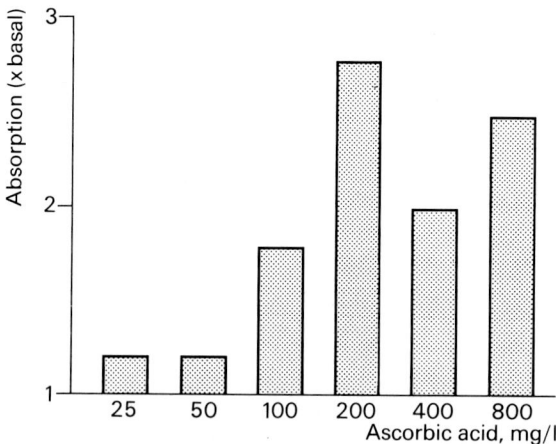

Fig. 2: Effect of ascorbic acid on the absorption of fortification iron in milk. The height of the columns indicate the ratio of iron absorption from milk with different concentrations of ascorbic acid versus milk without ascorbic acid; from STEKEL *et al* [9].

Tab I: Absorption of fortification iron from an acidified milk formula with ascorbic acid

Batch date	Study date	n	Iron absorption, %[1]		
			low-fat milk (A)	acid milk + vitamin C (B)	B / A
7/75	7/75	9	5.5	12.0	2.2
9/75	7/76	17	4.0	10.7	2.7
7/76	7/76	13	4.9	11.3	2.1

[1] Geometric mean values.

maintained 10 months after formula manufacture in products packed in oxygen-tight tin cans (Table I).

An even more marked effect of ascorbic acid on the absorption of iron from infant formulas has been reported by DERMAN et al [14] who found a three fold increase in the absolute amount of iron absorbed with a molar relationship of ascorbic acid to iron of 2:1 and a six fold increase with a molar relationship of 6.3 to 1. These authors also reported a marked effect of ascorbic acid on the absorption of fortification iron from infant cereals.

Field Trials with Iron Fortified Milk

The importance of ascorbic acid on the bioavailability of fortification iron from infant formulas is well demonstrated by the results of field trials we have conducted with various fortified products [1, 15, 16].

Duration of breast feeding in Chile is short. As a means of preventing protein-calorie malnutrition, powdered cow's milk has been distributed to infants for many years under a National Program of Supplementary Feeding (NPSF). Since iron deficiency in Chilean infants is highly prevalent [17] and the program milk reaches a high proportion of the infantile population, fortification of this product with iron seemed a logical way of preventing iron deficiency in the first year of life.

The first field trial with iron fortified milk was conducted with a low-fat (12 %) product fortified with 15 mg of elemental iron per liter, as ferrous sulphate. Geometric mean iron absorption from this milk was 3-4 %. It was thus calculated that infants receiving 750 ml milk/day would absorb an average of 0.4 mg iron, or about half their requirements. At 3 months of age, term infants who had spontaneously discontinued breast milk were randomly assigned to a group receiving fortified milk or a control group receiving the same milk without iron. Solid foods were introduced according to local practice: fruits and eggs at 4 months, vegetables and meat at 5 months, legumes at 6–7 months and regular table food at 9–12 months. At 15 months of age, anemia (hemoglobin concentration below 11 g/dl) existed in 34.6 % of the control infants versus 12.7 % of those receiving fortified milk. A still higher proportion of infants in both groups had biochemical indication of iron deficient erythropoiesis. It was concluded that even though the fortified milk produced a significant improvement of iron nutrition status, not enough iron was absorbed to cover the requirements of all infants.

As a result of the studies indicating the favourable effect of ascorbic acid on absorption, we designed a new milk formula fortified with 15 mg iron and 100 mg ascorbic acid/l. The product was acidified to prevent its use in the house for purposes other than feeding the infant. In a pilot field trial, 280 term infants were given the fortified milk from 3 to 15 months of age. A control group received the unfortified full-fat (26 %) milk being distributed at the time by the NPSF. Solid foods were given as in the previous study. Laboratory studies at 9 and 15 months of age indicated a highly significant difference in iron nutrition status between the two groups (Fig. 3). Anemia at 15 months was present in only 1.6 % of infants receiving the fortified milk versus 27.8 % in the control group. A study conducted in preterm infants confirmed the efficacy of the product in preventing iron deficiency anemia in this highly vulnerable group of infants [18].

The milk fortified with iron and ascorbic acid was then studied in a larger field trial designed to test the product under the regular operating conditions of the NPSF. Starting on August 1, 1978, infants born in a large segment of the city of Santiago received after weaning, the fortified milk instead of the regular unfortified milk powder. Two cohorts of infants, those born in June–July and in August–September, representing the last group of infants receiving unfortified milk and the first group receiving fortified milk, were studied in more detail. At 9 and 15 months of age, samples of approximately 200 infants were randomly selected from each group for laboratory studies, regardless of the age of weaning or the infant's birth weight. At 9 months, 32.5 % of infants receiving unfortified milk were anemic versus 11.8 % of those receiving the fortified product. At 15 months, anemia existed in 29.9 % of the infants born in June–July but only in 5.5 % of those born in August–September (Fig.

Fig. 3: Mean values of hemoglobin (Hgb), transferrin saturation (Sat), free erythrocyte protopor- ▶ phyrin (FEP) and serum ferritin (SF) at 3, 9, and 15 months of age in infants receiving acidified milk fortified with iron and ascorbic acid (○) or unfortified milk (●). Differences significant with p values < .001. From STEKEL *et al* [15].

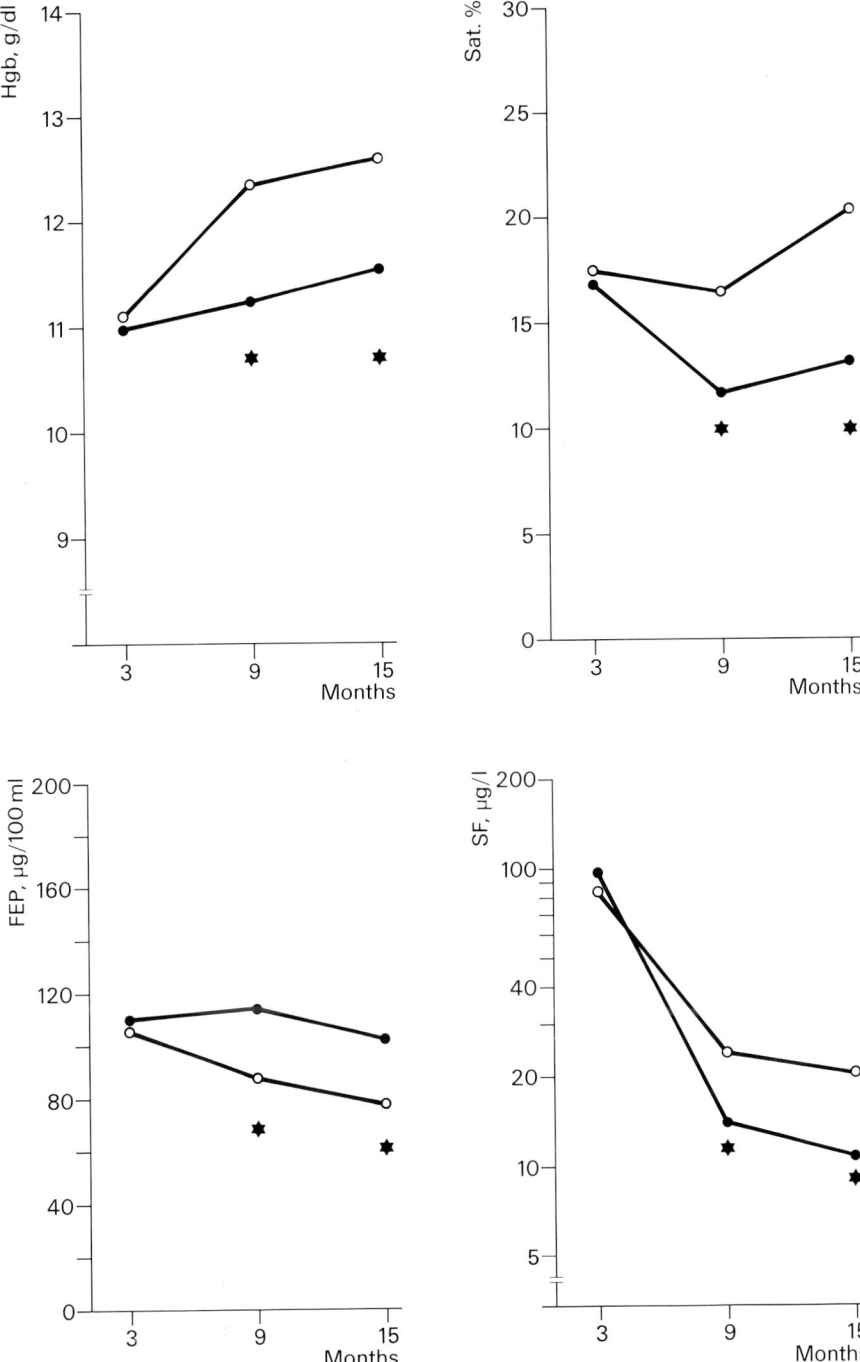

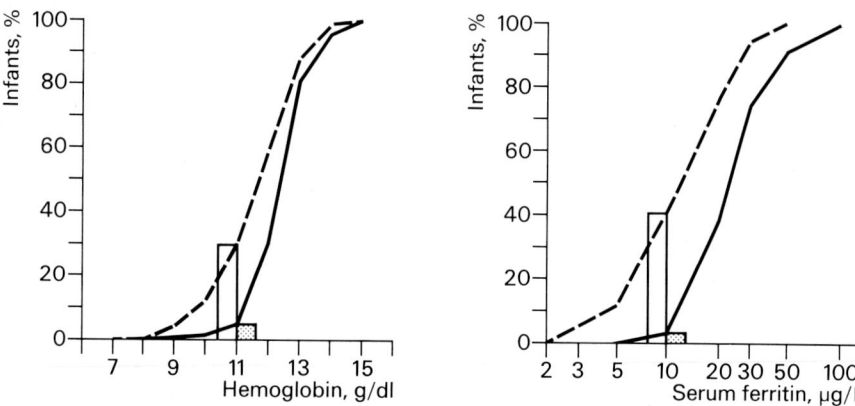

Fig. 4: Regional field trial of acidified milk fortified with iron and ascorbic acid. Cumulative frequency distribution of individual values of hemoglobin and serum ferritin at 15 months of age in infants born on June–July 1978 receiving unfortified milk (- - -) and on August–September 1978 receiving fortified milk (——). The height of the columns indicate the percentage of infants with hemoglobin < 11 g/dl (left) and serum ferritin < 10 μg/l (right) in each of the two groups. From STEKEL [16].

4). A low serum ferritin at this age was present in 41.2 % of infants born before August 1 versus 3.5 % of those born after that date (Fig. 4).

In summary, the studies presented indicate that the simple fortification of milk with seemingly adequate amounts of iron may not be sufficient to prevent iron deficiency in all infants due to the low bioavailability of the iron. Ascorbic acid, a known enhancer of dietary non-heme iron absorption, markedly increases the absorption of iron from milk. A milk formula fortified with iron and ascorbic acid given regularly during the first year of life markedly decreased the prevalence of iron deficiency in Chilean infants.

Acknowledgements: These studies were supported by grants from the Research Corporation, the Departamento de Desarrollo de la Investigación, University of Chile, the United Nations University and the Chilean Ministry of Health.

References

1 DALLMAN P R et al: Iron deficiency in infancy and childhood. Am J Clin Nutr *33*, 86–118, 1980.
2 WIDDOWSON E M, SPRAY C M: Chemical development *in utero.* Arch Dis Child *26:* 205–214, 1951.
3 RIOS E et al: Relationship of maternal and infant iron stores as assessed by determination of plasma ferritin. Pediatrics *55,* 694–699, 1975.

4 Murray M J *et al:* The effect of iron status of Nigerian mothers on that of their infants at birth and 6 months, and on the concentration of Fe in breast milk. Br J Nutr. *39,* 627–630, 1978.

5 Singla P N *et al:* Effect of maternal anaemia on the placenta and the newborn infant. Acta Paediat Scand *67,* 645–648, 1978.

6 Garby L *et al:* Studies on erythro-kinetics in infancy. IV. The long-term behavior of radioiron in circulating foetal and adult haemoglobin, and its faecal excretion. Acta Paediat *53,* 33–41, 1964.

7 Smith N J and Ríos E: Iron metabolism and iron deficiency in infancy and childhood. In: Schulman (ed). Advances in Pediatrics, vol 21, pp 239–280. Year Book Medical Publishers, Chicago, 1974.

8 Stekel A: Iron requirements in infancy and childhood. In: Stekel (ed). Iron nutrition in infancy and childhood, pp 1–10. Raven Press, New York, 1984.

9 Stekel A *et al:* Nutritional significance of interactions between iron and food components. Archos Latinoamer Nutr *33,* 33–41, 1983.

10 Hallberg L: Effect of vitamin C on the bioavailability of iron from food. In: Counsell and Hornig (eds). Vitamin C, pp 49–61. Applied Science, London, 1981.

11 Saarinen U M *et al:* Iron absorption in infants: high bioavailability of breast milk iron as indicated by the extrinsic tag method of iron absorption and by the concentration of serum ferritin. J Pediat *91,* 36–39, 1977.

12 Saarinen U M: Need for iron supplementation in infants on prolonged breast feeding. J Pediat *93,* 177–180, 1978.

13 Stekel A *et al:* Effect of ascorbic acid on the absorption of supplementary iron in milk. Abstr 3–12, 16th Int Congr Hematol, Kyoto, 1976.

14 Derman D P *et al:* Importance of ascorbic acid in the absorption of iron from infant foods. Scand J Haematol *25,* 193–201, 1980.

15 Stekel A *et al:* Prevention of iron deficiency in infants by milk fortification. In: Underwood (ed). Nutrition intervention strategies in national development, pp 315–323. Academic Press, New York, 1983.

16 Stekel A: Prevention of iron deficiency. In: Stekel (ed). Iron nutrition in infancy and childhood, pp 179–184. Raven Press, New York, 1984.

17 Ríos E *et al:* Evaluation of iron status and prevalence of iron deficiency in infants in Chile. In: Underwood (ed). Nutrition intervention strategies in national development, pp 273–283. Academic Press, New York, 1983.

18 Ríos E *et al:* Unpublished observations.

Abraham Stekel, MD, INTA, Casilla 15138, Santiago 11, Chile

The Role of Vitamin C in Improving the Critical Iron Balance Situation in Women

L. HALLBERG

Department of Medicine, University of Göteborg, Sweden

Key Words: Iron absorption · Iron requirements · Iron balance · Vitamin C · Women

Abstract: The more critical iron balance situation in women than in men is due to their additional menstrual iron losses and the iron requirements of pregnancies. The iron requirements in women per unit body weight is probably the same in all populations and has remained unchanged for thousands of years. The prevalence of iron deficiency in female populations is thus mainly determined by the properties of the diet.

In industrialized countries the iron absorption is low due to a low intake of both energy and iron. A contributing factor is sometimes an unsuitable meal composition. In developing countries a main reason for the low iron absorption is the low intake of foods and nutrients stimulating iron absorption such as meat, fish and vitamin C. There is a risk that a further reduction in energy intake in several developing countries due to a rapid technological development will lead to a reduced intake of both energy and essential nutrients as there is usually a marked inertia in changing food habits and meal composition.

The usual measures that are considered in the prevention of iron deficiency are: iron tablet supplementation to certain groups (e.g. pregnant women); iron fortification; food education (use of foods rich in iron or improving iron bioavailability). Recently the addition of small amounts of vitamin C to meals has also been suggested because of the probably important physiological role of vitamin C in iron absorption.

Introduction

The iron balance situation in women is more critical than in men because of their higher iron requirements due to menstrual iron losses and pregnancies and due to their often lower dietary intake of energy and thus also of iron.

The iron requirements of menstruating women is probably the same per unit body weight in all populations. The distribution of the iron losses in a population in Sweden [1] is about the same as in England [2], Canada and even Burma [3]. The basal iron losses due to losses from especially the skin and the gastrointestinal tract are mainly related to body size [4]. The *average* menstrual iron losses in a population is probably also related to the average body size. The mean losses in a 45 kg Burmese woman can thus be expected to be about 20 % lower than in a 55 kg Swedish woman due to the different size of their bodies and uterus. The wide variation in the menstrual iron losses in a population is mainly genetically controlled as we have found in studies on twins [5]. The fact that the average menstrual iron losses per unit bodyweight are probably the same throughout the world and that the variation of the menstrual iron losses are genetically controlled imply that the iron requirements in women have been the same for thousands of years. Differences in the prevalence of iron deficiency between female populations in different parts of the world or in the same population at different times would thus have been determined by differences in iron absorption from the diet. In this presumption differences due to infestation with hookworms or other parasites affecting iron losses will be disregarded.

Iron Absorption from Diet

The absorption of iron from the diet is not only determined by the amount of iron ingested but also by the source of iron and the composition of the main meals. Knowledge about dietary iron absorption has increased very much in the last 10 years and as a basis for the further discussion the main points will be summarized only briefly [for reviews see 6-8].

There are two kinds of iron in the diet with respect to mechanism of absorption - heme iron (derived mainly from hemoglobin and myoglobin in meat) and non-heme iron (derived mainly from cereals, fruits and vegetables). Heme iron is a minor part of the iron intake - it accounts for only 10 - 15 % of the total iron intake in present day diets with a high meat intake. Heme iron is still nutritionally important because of its high bioavailability (about 25 %) in meat containing meals [9]. The intake of heme iron in most developing countries is negligible.

Non-heme iron is thus the main source of dietary iron. The absorption of non-heme iron in a meal is determined by the amount of iron present in the meal and the balance between various factors affecting the absorption of non-heme iron. Research especially in the last decade has greatly increased our knowledge about such factors and how they interact [6-8]. Some factors enhance iron absorption such as meat, fish and ascorbic acid. Meat markedly stimulates the absorption of iron from a meal. This was first shown by LAYRISSE and coworkers in studies on iron absorption from maize [10]. Meat thus has a double effect on iron absorption - it stimulates in some unknown way the absorption of non-heme iron present in other foods and it provides the well-absorbed heme iron in the meat itself. Fish, chicken or mussels have a similar absorption promoting effect on non-heme iron, whereas other protein rich foods such as eggs, or vegetable proteins such as soy protein have no such effects [11-13].

Vitamin C (ascorbic acid) is the other main factor in the diet stimulating non-heme iron absorption. Vitamin C and meat act independently, and the effect of vitamin C seems to be even more marked than that of meat. Already small physiological amounts of vitamin C in the diet such as 25 mg have a marked effect on the absorption of iron [for a review see 14]. This observation suggests that vitamin C has a key physiological role in the absorption of iron from the diet just as it has key roles in several biochemical reactions in the body. This assumption is also supported by the observation that when the native ascorbic acid in a meal is fully or partially destroyed (e.g. by prolonged warming) there is a significant reduction in the absorption of iron [15].

There are also factors in the diet that inhibit the absorption of non-heme iron. Phytates are present in all plant material and are their normal storage form for iron. Cereals are especially rich in phytates, especially in the bran fraction. The addition of phytates or food rich in phytates such as bran, markedly reduces iron absorption. The same is true for tannins (polyphenols). There is a high content of tannins in some vegetables, in tea, and to some extent in coffee [16-18]. Tea taken with a meal has a marked reducing effect on iron absorption. This reduction can be partially counteracted by ascorbic acid.

The addition of other fiber materials such as pectins, ispagula, guar gum etc, has no or only a small effect on iron absorption in man [9].

In addition to the native food iron, meals may contain iron from dirt and dust contaminating the foods or the water used for drinking and cooking. This iron usually originates from the soil. It may be totally unavailable for man. Some types of soil, however, such as iron in clay may be partially available and may thus contribute to the amount of iron absorbed [19,20].

In summary, a good iron absorption can be expected from a diet with a high content of meat, fish or ascorbic acid. The absorption of iron from fully vegetarian diets depends mainly on its content of ascorbic acid.

Iron Balance in Earlier Days

The fact that the iron losses in women probably have been the same for a very long time, the fact that today iron deficiency is very common in almost all developing countries and is the only deficiency disorder of importance in industrialized countries makes it important to assess the changes in the properties of the diet, with respect to iron nutrition, that have occurred in the course of time.

Early man was probably living as a nomad in constant search for food, mainly consisting of fruits, berries, vegetables, insects and small animals. Later and for at least about half a million years small groups of men were living in caves. They probably also spent much time hunting, fishing and gathering various plants, nuts, insects etc. Analyses of findings in these caves indicate that iron nutrition must have been quite good in our hunting - gathering ancestors - the intake of animal protein (meat, fish etc) was probably high, and it is also probable that the intake of ascorbic acid was high [21-24].

Just before what has been called the agricultural revolution, which started to occur about 8 -10000 years ago, there are findings indicating a domestication of animals, for example sheep, which was used as food, and there also seems to have been some cultivation of plants.

The domestication and cultivation of wheat in the Middle East, the cultivation of maize in the American continents and rice especially in Southeast Asia was the basis for the agricultural revolution. Archeological findings indicate that over the last 10000 years an earlier ratio animal/plant food of 70/30 was successively reversed to 30/70. In late prehistoric time the proportion of plant material in the food increased to about 85 %. The agricultural revolution was the basis of the enormous population growth, in turn leading to a further shortage in animal protein in most developing countries where the diet today has become mainly vegetarian.

Industrialization starting less than 200 years ago had a marked influence on nutrition first in Europe and later on in other parts of the world. Over a period of 100-200 years machines have little by little taken over the heavy work. This increased mechanization was also utilized in farming; more food was produced, but gradually man needed less energy (less food) to do the work.

Iron Balance Today in Industrialized and Developing Countries

The trends outlined for both developing and industrialized countries have continued.

In *industrialized countries* the decrease in energy expenditure has continued with increased mechanization and automation. Machines have taken over the main part of the more energy-demanding elements in different jobs. Transportation of the human body is made easier by elevators, escalators, cars, busses, trains etc. The housework is also facilitated by various appliances. Less time is spent standing or walking and more time sitting at work, in cars, and at home reading or looking at TV etc.

Several dietary surveys during the last century have shown a constant relationship between intake of energy and iron [25]. The reduced energy expenditure thus means that the intake of iron has been proportionally reduced.

Another new trend related to nutrition is the increased proportion of meals and snacks consumed outside the home - in restaurants, canteens etc. We have thus been more and more dependent on the quality of food prepared by the food industry, as various food items or whole meals.

In *developing countries* there are marked differences between countries. Usually, however, the diet is monotonous, mainly vegetarian with staple foods such as wheat, rice, maize, cassava or millets. In some countries beans, potatoes etc contribute much to energy consumption. The intake of fish and meat is low, sometimes negligible. The intake of vitamin C is also often low considering the requirements of ascorbic acid for iron absorption (even if it seldom reaches the scorbutic levels). The content of food components such as phytates and tannins inhibiting food iron absorption is often high.

The intake of energy in Western women with a sedentary lifestyle is often only around 1 500 kcal/day. In women in developing countries the energy consumption is usually reported to be higher, often about 2 400–2 500 kcal/day.

In several developing countries there is a rapid technological development -an industrialization with introduction of effective transportation systems, of machines taking over more and more of the heavy part of manual work. This change will probably take place more rapidly in developing countries than it did in the Western world during its industrial development as an advanced technology is already at hand and has only to be transplanted to the previously more slowly developing country. It should be noted that a close relationship between intake of iron and energy has also been observed in developing countries, and an extensive study was recently reported from India [SRIKANTIA, personal communication]. There is thus an imminent risk that the expected reduced requirements for energy, due to the technological development, is not accompanied by corresponding adjustments in the composition of the diet. In Western countries we have seen a reduction in energy intake in women to about one half in the last few generations without any significant adjustment in meal composition which means that the intake of iron has also been reduced. This is the main factor explaining the fairly recent critical iron balance situation in industrialized countries. There is a risk that something similar will occur in developing countries - the difference being, however, that the change will probably occur much faster, not over generations but perhaps within a generation. It is likely that the conservatism in the choice of meal composition seen in the Western countries will be valid also in developing countries and that the ongoing industrialization in developing countries thus carries the risk of the development of nutritional deficiencies which must be carefully considered especially taking into account the present poor diet in many developing countries which is often borderline for several nutrients.

In *summary* - both in industrialized, Western-type countries, and in developing countries iron requirements have remained the same, but the dietary supply of iron has successively become impaired. In Western-type countries the intake of iron has gone down, due mainly to the reduction in energy intake with no adequate adjustment in meal composition. In most developing countries the intake of iron is often higher but the content of factors in the diet stimulating the iron absorption such as meat, fish and vitamin C is often low.

Strategies to Improve Iron Balance

Several measures may be taken to prevent iron deficiency in women. In most countries it is possible and advisable to use not one but several methods at the same time [26].

1) *Iron supplementation* is useful to certain groups, especially pregnant women and sometimes schoolchildren. It is effective provided adequate doses of good iron preparations are given, the subjects are well motivated and a good delivery system is available. In populations with severe hookworm infestation it is probably the only effective method besides antiparasitic treatment to combat iron deficiency.

2) *Iron fortification* can be used in some countries. It is often difficult, however, to find a suitable vehicle, which reaches the target groups in a population. It may also be difficult to find suitable iron compounds which are well absorbed and do not interfere with other components in the diet.

3) *Improvement of the bioavailability of dietary iron.* By *food education* it is at least theoretically possible to change the meal composition or the technique for meal preparation in order 1) to reduce the content of inhibitors of non-heme iron absorption (e.g. phytates and tannins) or 2) to increase the content of foods enhancing iron absorption. An increased intake of foods

such as fish and meat is usually not economically possible in any country. An increased intake of foods rich in ascorbic acid (e.g. various fruits, cabbage, green leafy vegetables etc.) may be feasible in certain populations. Another main alternative to improve the bioavailability of the iron already present in the diet would be the *addition of ascorbic acid* to the meals. It would certainly be very effective provided suitable techniques are developed at reasonable costs.

Considerations about the Rationale of Adding Ascorbic Acid to Meals
A Summary

1) The native ascorbic acid in the diet has probably an important *physiological* role in iron absorption. A reduction of the content of native ascorbic acid, for example, by prolonged warming reduces the absorption of non-heme iron from the diet [13].

2) The effect on iron absorption is the same of synthetic ascorbic acid and native ascorbic acid in foods [12].

3) Even small amounts of ascorbic acid added to a meal stimulate markedly non-heme iron absorption from meals. In studies on a simple maize meal [27] and on a semisynthetic meal [28] a marked continuous increase in iron absorption was seen with increasing doses of ascorbic acid. When other types of meals were studied a marked absorption increase was seen with small doses of ascorbic acid just as in the previously mentioned studies. However, with increasing doses of ascorbic acid the absorption increase was much less marked. This was valid both for a continental breakfast, for a simple Southeast Asian type of rice meal and it seems to be true also for a hamburger meal (Figs. 1 and 2). This means that for most diets an almost optimal absorption promoting effect is obtained already with 25–50 mg ascorbic acid per meal. It also means that the risk of developing an iron overload by the addition of ascorbic acid to meals seems to be negligible based on the preliminary results so far available.

4) A comparison of various methods to increase the iron absorption from meals clearly shows that ascorbic acid is a very potent stimulator of iron absorption [for a review see 12]. In one study on a Latin-American type of meal composed of rice, maize and black beans we compared the effect of various measures to improve iron absorption [29] (Fig. 3). 50 mg of ascorbic acid in pure form or as cauliflower (65 mg) markedly increased the absorption of non-heme iron, actually to about the same degree as 75 g of meat or 6 mg of iron as ferrous sulphate. As little as 25–50 mg ascorbic acid added to a meal

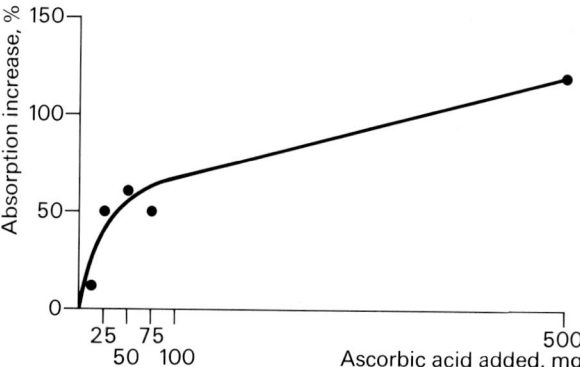

Fig. 1: The effect of ascorbic acid on iron absorption from a continental breakfast [30]. The absorption increase (%) is plotted against the amount of ascorbic acid added.

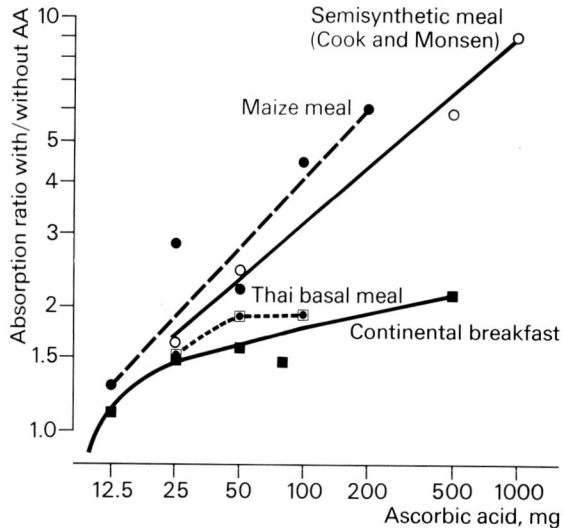

Fig. 2: The effect of ascorbic acid on iron absorption from different meals – a semisynthetic meal [28], a maize meal [27], a breakfast meal [30] and a simple Southeast Asian meal of rice, vegetables and a curry. The log mean ratio of iron absorption with to without ascorbic acid is plotted against the log amount of ascorbic acid added.

Fig. 3: Comparison of various methods to increase non-heme iron absorption from a simple▶ Latin-American type of meal composed of maize, rice and black beans [29]. Expressed in amount (top) and percentage (bottom).

Meal	Non-heme iron content, mg	Non-heme iron absorption, mg

Meal	Non-heme iron content, mg	Non-heme iron absorption, %

thus improves iron absorption significantly. To achieve the same effect by iron fortification the addition of very large quantities of fortification iron would be needed.

Conclusions

Considering the probably high intake of ascorbic acid in early man and its probably physiological role in the absorption of iron from diet and considering the present often low content of ascorbic acid in meals in both industrialized and developing countries, an addition in some form of ascorbic acid to meals will be a rational solution to improve iron nutrition. We still don't know, however, how best to do it. It is a technological challenge for food industry to find effective and economically feasible solutions to increase or normalize the vitamin C content of the diet – up to the probably more physiological levels of our predators. It seems to be the most effective way to improve iron nutrition in both developing and industrialized countries.

References

1 HALLBERG, L et al: Menstrual blood loss – a population study. Variation at different ages and attempts to define normality. Acta Obstet Gynec Scand 45, 320–351, 1966.
2 COLE, S K et al: Sources of variation in menstrual blood loss. J Obstet Gynec Br Commonwlth 78, 933–939, 1971.
3 AUNG-THAN-BATU et al: Iron balance in young Burmese women. Union Burma J Life Sci 4, 327–333, 1971.
4 GREEN, R et al: Body iron excretion in man. A collaborative study. Am J Med 45, 336–353, 1968.
5 RYBO, G, HALLBERG, L: Influence of heredity and environment on normal menstrual blood loss. Acta Obstet Gynec Scand 45, 57–78, 1966.
6 HALLBERG, L: Bioavailability of dietary iron in man. Am Rev Nutr 1, 123–147, 1981.
7 HALLBERG, L: Iron. In: OLSSON (ed) "Present knowledge in nutrition", Vth ed. Nutrition Foundation, Washington, 1983.
8 BOTHWELL, T H, CHARLTON, R W: Iron deficiency in women. Rep Inter Nutr Anemia Consult Group (INACG). Libr Congr Cat no 81-83358, 1981.
9 HALLBERG, L et al: Dietary heme iron absorption. A discussion of possible mechanisms for the absorption – promoting effect of meat and for the regulation of iron absorption. Scand J Gastroenterol 14, 769–779, 1979.
10 LAYRISSE, M et al: The effect of interaction of various foods on iron absorption. Am J Clin Nutr 21, 1175–1183, 1968.
11 International Nutritional Anemia Consultative Group (INACG). The effects of cereals and legumes on iron availability. Report June 1982. Libr Congr Cat no 82-60413, 1982.
12 HALLBERG, L, ROSSANDER, L: Effects of soy protein on nonheme iron absorption in man. Am J Clin Nutr 36, 514–520, 1982.

13 COOK, J D *et al:* The inhibitory effect of soy products on non-heme iron absorption in man. Am J Clin Nutr *34,* 2622–2629, 1981.

14 HALLBERG, L: Effect of vitamin C on the bioavailability of iron from food. In: COUNSELL and HORNIG (eds) "Vitamin C (ascorbic acid)", pp 49–61. Applied Science, London, 1981.

15 HALLBERG, L *et al:* Deleterious effects of prolonged warming of meals on ascorbic acid content and iron absorption. Am J Clin Nutr *36,* 846–850, 1982.

16 DISLER, P B *et al:* The effect of tea on iron absorption. Gut *16,* 193–200, 1975.

17 HALLBERG, L, ROSSANDER, L: Effect of different drinks on the absorption of non-heme iron from composite meals. Hum Nutr Appl Nutr *36A,* 116–123, 1982.

18 MORCK, T A *et al:* Inhibition of food iron absorption by coffee. Am J Clin Nutr *37,* 416–420, 1983.

19 HALLBERG, L, BJÖRN-RASMUSSEN, E: Measurement of iron absorption from meals contaminated with iron. Am J Clin Nutr *34,* 2808–2815, 1981.

20 HALLBERG, L *et al:* Iron absorption from some Asian meals containing contamination iron. Am J Clin Nutr *37,* 272–277, 1983.

21 NEWMAN, M T: Nutritional adaption in man. In: BAMON (ed) "Physiological anthropology". Oxford University Press, New York, 1975.

22 BRAIDWOOD, R J: From cave to village. Sci Am, October 1952.

23 RENFREW, J M: Palaeoethnobotany: The prehistoric food plants of the Near East and Europe. Colombia University Press, New York, 1973.

24 STRAUS, L G *et al:* Ice-age subsistence in Northern Spain. Sci Am June 1980, pp 120–129.

25 BLIX, G: A study on the relation between total calories and single nutrients in Swedish food. Acta Soc Med Upsal *70,* 117–129, 1965.

26 WHO Technical Report Ser 580, 1975. Control of Nutritional anemia with special reference to iron deficiency. Report of an IAEA/USAID/WHO Joint meeting.

27 BJÖRN-RASMUSSEN, E, HALLBERG, L: Iron absorption from maize. Effect of ascorbic acid on iron absorption from maize supplemented with ferrous sulphate. Nutr Metabol *16,* 94–100, 1974.

28 COOK, J D, MONSEN, E R: Vitamin C, the common cold and iron absorption. Am J Clin Nutr *30,* 235–241, 1977.

29 HALLBERG, L, ROSSANDER, L: Improvement of iron nutrition in developing countries. Comparison of adding meat, soy protein, ascorbic acid, citric acid and ferrous sulphate on iron absorption from a simple Latin-American type of meal. Am J Clin Nutr (in press).

30 ROSSANDER, L *et al:* Absorption of iron from breakfast meals. Am J Clin Nutr *32,* 2484–2489, 1979.

Prof. Leif Hallberg, MD, Department of Medicine II, University of Göteborg, Sahlgrenska Sjukhuset, S-41345 Göteborg, Sweden

Analgesic and Anti-Inflammatory Properties of Vitamins

A. Hanck and H. Weiser

Unit of Social and Preventive Medicine, University of Basle, Switzerland, Pharma Clinical Research Department, and Central Research Units, F. Hoffmann-La Roche & Co., Ltd., Basle, Switzerland

Key Words: Vitamins · Anti-inflammatory · Analgesic properties · Rat paw test · Prophylactic, therapeutic use · Carrageenan, kaolin · Hyaluronidase · Phylloquinone, analogs · Cyanocobalamin · Vitamin C · Acetylsalicylate · Phenylbutazone

Abstract: Pain and inflammation connected with vitamin deficiencies have been known since ancient times. Many vitamin deficiency diseases such as beriberi, scurvy, and pellagra are associated with unspecific pain. Peripheral or central neurological changes and inflammation of the skin and mucosae are a feature. Pain and inflammation resulting from vitamin deficiencies can be easily treated by administration of the appropriate vitamin. Outside this context, however, vitamins possess analgesic and anti-inflammatory properties which correspond to those of conventional analgesics and anti-inflammatory agents, but without their side effects, which, particularly in long-term use, can become very troublesome. Vitamins appear to be suitable for use alone as mild analgesics, or in combination with conventional analgesic and anti-inflammatory agents. Of particular interest are the analgesic and anti-inflammatory properties of the vitamins of the B-complex, used either alone or combined. Vitamin B_{12} and its combination with vitamin B_1 and vitamin B_6 produced significant, dose-dependent pain relief and inhibition of inflammation, comparable to the action of phenylbutazone, a standard treatment. A significant anti-inflammatory and analgesic effect was also demonstrated with vitamin K and some of its metabolites, and with vitamin C. The combination of vitamin C with sodium acetylsalicylate was more effective than sodium acetylsalicylate alone. The mechanism of action of the individual vitamins appears to differ.

Introduction

Pain is probably the oldest and best-known symptom to be recorded in the history of the art of healing. Today it remains one of the most important reasons for consulting a physician. Pain is an important alarm signal, and can be described as a "guardian" of health. However, this interpretation has its limitations, as many life-threatening illnesses often cause no pain in their initial stages.

Pain and inflammation associated with vitamin deficiency diseases have been known since olden times. In the case of beriberi, for example, pain of indeterminate origin is reported, and neuritis features among the various manifestations of this disease.

Electron microscopic examination of the peripheral nervous system, e. g. peroneal nerve, sciatic nerve, spinal root, in animal experiments shows definite pathological abnormalities characterized by a marked axonal degeneration. Myelin sheath breakdown appears as a secondary phenomenon. Thick myelinated nerve fibers are more involved than thin myelinated ones [7]. This axonal degeneration is also seen in man. Neuropathy predominantly affects motor neurons. TAKAHASHI [41] reported that the conduction velocity in posterior tibial nerves was reduced from 80–120 m/sec to 38–43 m/sec.

In scurvy, in addition to the conspicuous symptom of extensive bleeding areas, we also find extremely painful swelling around the joints.

A clinical sign of vitamin B_{12} deficiency is the painful HUNTER's glossitis but the main neuropathological lesions in vitamin B_{12} deficiency affect the thickly myelinated axons of the spinal cord, the brain and peripheral nerves. The pronounced demyelination is perhaps secondary to axonal degeneration.

A feature of pellagra is the painful inflammation of skin and mucosae, while an early sign of vitamin A deficiency is increased light sensitivity. The recommendation to treat this condition with vitamin A is probably one of the oldest prescriptions in the world, being recorded in the Eber papyrus, which 3500 years ago recommended raw liver to treat nightblindness, which includes bright light sensitivity. As we now know, raw liver is a good source of vitamins, and contains a large amount of vitamin A.

Pain and inflammation originating from vitamin deficiencies can be appropriately and effectively treated with specific vitamins. However, outside this context, vitamins also possess analgesic and anti-inflammatory properties corresponding to those of traditional analgesics and anti-inflammatories, but are devoid of the known side effects of these compounds which, especially in long-term use, can be very troublesome. Known side effects of weak analgesics are: formation of methaemoglobin, anaemia, interstitial nephritis, bone-marrow depression and formation of carcinogenic products. The use of strong analgesics such as opiates always involves the risk of dependence.

Pain is felt as a psychological experience. It can, however, be influenced by pharmacological means at two somatic levels: peripheral and central. Appropriate combinations of analgesics may exert a stronger effect due to a simultaneous action at both levels.

In the periphery, the sensitivity of pain receptors can be dampened to the point where their stimulation by pain stimuli is either reduced or completely blocked. Centrally, the transmission of impulses from the hypothalamus to the sensitive cerebral cortex can be suppressed, and the perception of painful stimuli either weakened or abolished. These properties are found in, for example, the opiates, but neuroleptics also impair the registration of pain.

Weak analgesics are suitable for the relief of slight or moderate pain; severe pain usually requires treatment with opiates. However, weaker analgesics have the advantage over opiates that they do not lead to dependence or habituation on chronic use. Their margin of safety is greater than that of the opiates.

Vitamins could be used as mild analgesics or in combination with conventional analgesics and anti-inflammatory agents. The analgesic and anti-inflammatory properties of the B vitamins, alone or combined, are of particular interest.

High doses of vitamin B_1 have been reported to produce ganglionic blockade and to suppress the transmission of neural stimuli to skeletal muscles [9, 14]. This effect has been demonstrated in man using 10 to 30 g vitamin B_1 intravenously, but has not led to a general use in anaesthesia [13, 30, 31]. SMALL [38] reported on successful relief of pain by thiamin injections in combination with infiltration of autonomic ganglia in patients suffering from severe neuritis. An interesting interaction between thiamin and morphine in the central nervous system has been reported by MISRA et al [33]. Morphine significantly increased the amount of thiamin in the cortical hemisphere by 21 %, in the cerebellum by 44 %, and in the brain stem by 29 %.

In animal experiments [27], vitamin B_6 and several of its derivatives have shown a central analgesic effect which is, however, weaker than morphine · HCl. The most potent central analgesic effect was demonstrated for 4-pyridoxic acid, a metabolite of pyridoxine, pyridoxine-4'-disulfide · 2HCl, pyridoxal-5'-phosphate, and pyridoxamine-5'-disulfide · 4HCl. The experiments showed no correlation between the specific activity of vitamin B_6 and the cerebral analgesic action of the vitamin B_6 derivatives examined.

Vitamin B_6 works by acting on the tryptophan metabolism. Pyridoxal-5'-phosphate acts as a co-enzyme of 5-hydroxytryptophan-decarboxylase in transforming 5-hydroxytryptophan into serotonin. Serotonin exists in relatively high concentrations in the central nervous system (hypothalamus). Here, it exerts a transmitter function and appears to possess both a psychostimulant effect and a sedative effect. In the presence of vitamin B_6 deficiency, the serotonin concentration in the brain is decreased. This relationship with serotonin might also explain the slight central depressant effect of vitamin B_6.

Several investigators have reported on the effect of high doses of vitamin B_{12} on pain.

To treat vitamin B_{12} deficiency states, an initial daily dose of 1 000 µg vitamin B_{12} is injected intramuscularly. This is later reduced to 1 000 µg monthly, depending on the etiology. For the treatment of vertebral pain and sensory disturbances, HIEBER [24] administered 5 000 µg daily either i.m. or i.v. to 400 patients for 6 to 16 days. The analgesic action of the vitamin was very good or good in about 50 % of the cases, absent in 10 patients and satisfactory in the rest. DETTORI et al [15] treated two groups of patients with 10 000 µg vitamin B_{12} daily for two weeks, one group suffering from degenerative neuropathy, the other group with similar pain from malignancies. Marked and prompt relief of pain was recorded in 80 % of patients of the first group, but less dramatic benefit in the others. There was disappearance of pain in 27 % and improvement in 33 %. However, no central activity of the compound could be demonstrated by HOLM et al [25] in cats, following 2 000 µg/kg i.m. This prompted us to investigate the analgesic effect of vitamin B_{12} and other vitamins and vitamin combinations in rats.

Material and Methods

Male, specific pathogen-free albino rats, weighing 65–70 g, were kept under standardized optimal hygienic conditions and were fed on NAFAG 850 ad libitum.

All vitamins used, vitamin B_{12}, vitamin K, vitamin C, their combinations and derivatives were of highest purity and pharmaceutical quality.

0.1 ml of either kaolin 10 %, or calcium carrageenan 1 %, or 125–250 USP-U of hyaluronidase, all in sterile sodium chloride solution, were injected into the paw of the right hind leg to induce inflammation. The anti-inflammatory activity of drugs, administered either orally or parenterally, was evaluated by standard planimetric and plethysmometric methods.

Analgesic activity was evaluated by determining the pain threshold with an analgesiometer Type No 7200, Ugo Basile, I-21025 Comerio-Varese. The pain threshold was registered as the difference in pressure perception (in grams) between injected and non-injected paw. The determinations were carried out always 4 hours after induction of edema. Oral test drugs were administered by stomach tube No 10. To test prophylactic activity, drugs were administered 0.5 hours before initiation of inflammation. To test therapeutic activity, drugs were administered 2 hours after initiation of inflammation. In all trials the test drugs were administered only once, with the exception of one trial. All test drugs were compared with a known analgesic or anti-inflammatory agent, and with placebo. To determine dose levels at which the vitamins were effective an ascending dose schedule was used. Route and dosage are always stated in the tables of results.

Results

Vitamin B_{12} showed in three independent trials a dose-dependent analgesic effect: 5–10 μg/kg given orally was comparable to 20 mg oral phenyl-butazone. The results are summarized in Table I, and a dose effect relation-ship is given in Figure 1.

Tab. I: Anti-inflammatory and analgesic effect of orally administered cyanocobalamin (0.1 % SD powder); "therapeutic test": 2 hours after paw injection (trial R 11/80; N = 10 rats per group). Parameter: 4 hours after local carrageenan injection (0.1 ml, 1 % sol)

	Control	Cyanocobalamin/kg body-weight			Phenylbutazone (20 mg)
		2.5 μg	5.0 μg	10.0 μg	
Anti-inflammatory effect					
Mean increase of dor/plan					
paw diameter, mm	1.74	1.59*	1.20***	1.14***	0.86***
SEM[1]	0.05	0.05	0.09	0.06	0.06
Inhibition, %		8.6	31.0	34.0	50.6
Analgesic effect					
Mean improvement of					
pain tolerance, g	33.0	22.00*	13.00***	13.00***	14.00***
SEM[1]	3.35	2.00	3.00	2.13	2.21
Inhibition, %		33.3	60.6	60.6	57.6

[1]   Difference between injected and non-injected paw.
  * = Significant (p < 0.05) in comparison with untreated controls.
*** = Significant (P < 0.01) in comparison with untreated controls.

The anti-inflammatory effect of vitamin B_{12} was also significant, but less pronounced than that of 20 mg phenylbutazone. The combination of vita-mins B_1, B_6, B_{12} combined in Cobenexol Fuerte showed an excellent effect, dose-dependent and comparable to phenylbutazone in both the therapeu-tic anti-inflammatory and in the analgesic test. Tables II and III show the results of independent trials, in which Cobenexol Fuerte was administered orally, and intravenously. Figure 2 shows the dose-effect relation of Cobene-xol Fuerte.

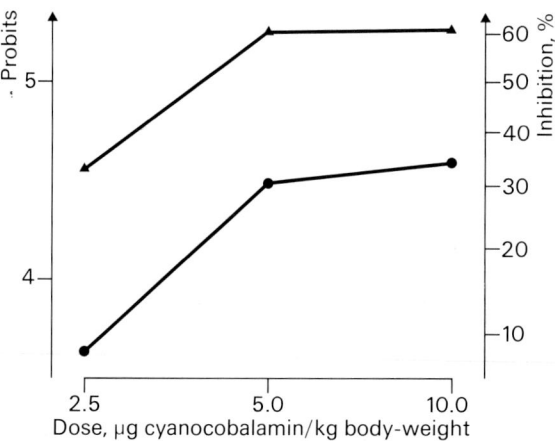

Fig. 1: Dose efficacy response of orally administered cyanocobalamin (vitamin B_{12}). Irritation by 0.1 ml carrageen 1 %; single oral dose of vitamin B_{12}. Therapeutic assay: 2 hours after paw injection (trial R 11/82; N = 10 rats per group). ▲ = Anti-inflammatory effect; ● = analgesic effect.

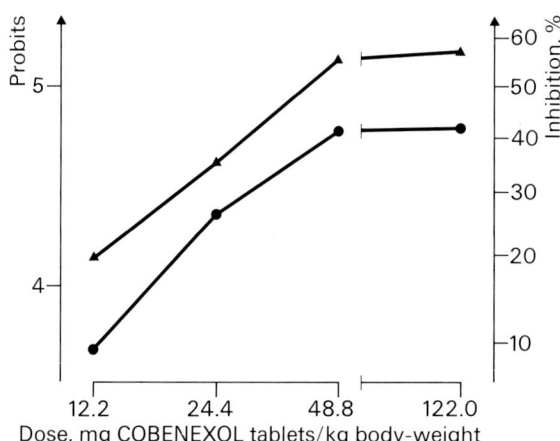

Fig. 2: Dose efficacy response of orally administered Cobenexol Fuerte (CF). Irritation by 0.1 ml carrageen 1 %; single oral dose of CF. Therapeutic assay: 2 hours after paw injection (trial R 26 + R 50/80; N = 10 rats per group). ▲ Anti-inflammatory effect; ● = analgesic effect.

The anti-inflammatory and analgesic activity of vitamin K_1 is demonstrated in Table IV showing a significant inhibition of inflammation and pain by 4 mg/kg body-weight orally. The influence of the vehicle, waterdispersible or oily, on the efficacy of vitamin K_1 could be demonstrated by the higher inhibiting effects of the oily solutions.

Tab. II: Anti-inflammatory and analgesic effect of orally administered Cobenexol Fuerte (tablets[1]); "therapeutic test": 2 hours after paw injection (trial R 50/80; N = 10 rats per group). Parameter: 4 hours after local carrageenan injection (0.1 ml, 1 % sol)

	Control	Cobenexol Fuerte/kg body-weight			Phenylbutazone (20 mg)
		5 mg B_1, 5 mg B_6, 0.06 mg B_{12} (12.2 mg tablet)	10 mg B_1, 10 mg B_6, 0.12 mg B_{12} (24.4 mg tablet)	20 mg B_1, 20 mg B_6, 0.24 mg B_{12} (48.8 mg tablet)	
Anti-inflammatory effect					
Mean increase of dor/plan					
paw diameter, mm	1.79	1.64[ns]	1.33***	1.06***	0.90***
SEM[2]	0.05	0.02	0.06	0.03	0.09
Inhibition, %		8.4	25.7	40.8	49.7
Analgesic effect					
Mean improvement of					
pain tolerance, g	36.00	28.00[ns]	23.00***	16.00***	14.00***
SEM[2]	3.7.	3.27	2.13	1.63	1.63
Inhibition, %		22.2	36.1	55.6	61.1

[1] Tablet 610 mg (components): thiamin · HCl 250 mg, pyridoxine · HCl 250 mg, cyanocobalamin 3 mg.

[2] Difference between injected and non-injected paw.

ns = Not significant, in comparison with untreated controls.

*** = Significant (p < 0.01)

Tab. III: Anti-inflammatory and analgesic effect of i.v. Cobenexol Fuerte (tablets[1]); "therapeutic test": 2 hours after paw injection (trial R 48/80; N = 10 rats per group). Parameter: 4 hours after local carrageenan injection (0.1 ml, 1 % sol)

	Control	Cobenexol Fuerte/kg body-weight			Phenylbutazone (20 mg, oral route)
		5 mg B_1, 5 mg B_6, 0.06 mg B_{12} (12.2 mg tablet)	10 mg B_1, 10 mg B_6, 0.12 mg B_{12} (24.4 mg tablet)	20 mg B_1, 20 mg B_6, 0.24 mg B_{12} (48.8 mg tablet)	
Anti-inflammatory effect					
Mean increase of dor/plan					
paw diameter, mm	1.77	1.61[ns]	1.19***	1.06***	0.94***
SEM[2]	0.06	0.04	0.05	0.03	0.05
Inhibition, %		9.0	32.8	40.1	46.9
Analgesic effect					
Mean improvement of					
pain tolerance, g	35.00	30.00[ns]	19.00***	16.00***	15.00***
SEM[2]	4.01	3.33	2.77	2.21	1.67
Inhibition, %		14.3	45.7	54.3	57.1

[1] Tablet compositios as in Table II; dissolved in saline solution.

[2] Difference between injected and non-injected paw.

ns = Not significant, in comparison with untreated controls.

*** = Significant (p < 0.01)

Tab. IV: Anti-inflammatory and analgesic effect of orally administered phylloquinone in arachis oil; "therapeutic test": 2 hours after paw injection (trial R 22/81; N = 10 rats per group). Parameter: 4 hours after local carrageenan injection (0.1 ml, 1 % sol)

	Control	Phylloquinone (Sic)/kg body-weight		Phenylbutazone (30 mg)
		2 mg	4 mg	
Anti-inflammatory effect				
Mean increase of dor/plan				
paw diameter, mm	2.01	1.52***	1.22***	0.93***
SEM[1]	0.06	0.07	0.05	0.07
Inhibition, %		24.4	39.3	53.7
Analgesic effect				
Mean improvement of				
pain tolerance, g	46.00	28.00***	23.00***	19.00***
SEM[1]	2.21	2.49	3.00	1.79
Inhibition, %		39.1	50.00	58.7

[1] Difference between injected and non-injected paw.
*** = Significant (p < 0.01) in comparison with untreated controls.

Tab. V: Anti-inflammatory and analgesic effect of water-dispersible phylloquinone preparations in dependence of intramuscular administration. "Therapeutic test": 2 hours after paw injection (CARR-oedema); N = 10 rats/group. Paramters: increase in paw diameter (mm ± SEM); impairment of pain tolerance (g ± SEM); Inhibition (%) in comparison with untreated controls

Trial	Control		Vitamin K_1 (prep. SIC), 2 mg/kg body-weight		Phenylbutazone (oral), 20 mg/kg body-weight	
	antiphlogistic, mm	analgesic, g	antiphlogistic, mm	analgesic, g	antiphlogistic, mm	analgesic, g
R 33/80						
Inhibition	2.06 ± 0.05	40.0 ± 3.33	1.29 ± 0.08	26.0 ± 2.66	1.02 ± 0.04	27.0 ± 3.35
vs. controls, %			37.4	35.0	50.5	32.5
R 34/80						
Inhibition	2.07 ± 0.06	40.0 ± 3.33	1.30 ± 0.10	25.0 ± 2.24	1.01 ± 0.05	23.0 ± 3.00
vs. controls, %			37.2	37.5	51.2	42.5
R 35/80						
Inhibition	1.86 ± 0.08	42.0 ± 2.00	1.02 ± 0.10	23.0 ± 3.00	1.03 ± 0.07	26.0 ± 2.67
vs. controls, %			45.2	45.2	44.6	38.1
R 37/80						
Inhibition	1.86 ± 0.04	42.0 ± 2.00	1.01 ± 0.04	23.0 ± 3.00	0.91 ± 0.04	21.6 ± 2.33
vs. controls, %			45.7	45.2	51.1	50.0
Mean inhibition, %			41.37	40.73	49.35	40.78

The probability of finding an analgesic or anti-inflammatory efficacy of test drugs was higher in the group with carrageenan-induced irritation of the paw. Tables V and VI show the reproducibility of our animal model in measuring anti-inflammatory and analgesic effects of vitamin K_1 given intramuscularly or intravenously.

Tab. VI: Anti-inflammatory and analgesic effect of water dispersible phylloquinone preparations in dependance of intravenous administration; "therapeutic test": 2 hours after paw injection (CARR-oedema; 0.1 ml, 1 % sol). Paramters: increase in paw diameter (mm ± SEM); impairment of pain tolerance (g ± SEM); Inhibition (%) in comparison with untreated controls

Trial	Control		Vitamin K_1 (prep. SIC), 2 mg/kg body-weight		Phenylbutazone (oral), 20 mg/kg body-weight	
	antiphlogistic, mm	analgesic, g	antiphlogistic, mm	analgesic, g	antiphlogistic, mm	analgesic, g
R 38/80 Inhibition vs. controls, %	2.06 ± 0.05	41.0 ± 3.14	1.52 ± 0.06 26.2	29.0 ± 2.77 29.3	1.05 ± 0.03 49.0	28.0 ± 2.91 31.7
R 41/80 Inhibition vs. controls, %	2.04 ± 0.06	40.0 ± 2.54	1.70 ± 0.05 16.7	29.0 ± 2.57 27.5	1.08 ± 0.03 47.1	26.0 ± 2.11 35.0
R 43/80 Inhibition vs. controls, %	2.00 ± 0.05	39.0 ± 2.11	1.68 ± 0.04 16.0	29.0 ± 2.15 25.6	1.07 ± 0.02 46.5	25.0 ± 2.09 35.9
R 44/80 Inhibition vs. controls, %	2.09 ± 0.07	45.0 ± 2.45	1.73 ± 0.08 17.2	37.0 ± 2.60 17.8	1.10 ± 0.05 47.4	30.0 ± 2.05 33.3
Mean inhibition, %			19.03	25.05	47.50	33.98

Two analogs of vitamin K_1, displaying basically the same ring structure as vitamin K but with a short side chain ending with a carboxy group, and its ethyl ester derivative also demonstrated marked pharmacological effects but no antihemorrhagic properties [43].

A metabolite of vitamin K_1, the 2,3-epoxide was less active as an anti-inflammatory agent than vitamin K_1 and had no analgesic effect.

The anti-inflammatory and analgesic effect of oral vitamin C was examined in the following trials. There was a dose-dependent significant reduction of pain and inflammation by therapeutic administration of vitamin C. The prophylactic efficacy of vitamin C is shown in Tables VII and VIII. To achieve an

Tab. VII: Anti-inflammatory and analgesic effect of vitamin C; «prophylactic test»: 0.5 hour before paw injection (trial R 6 / 81; N = 10 rats per group). Parameter: 4 hours after local carrageenan injection (0.1 ml, 1 % sol)

	Control	Vitamin C (oral)/kg body-weight			Phenylbutazone (oral), 20 mg
		62.5 mg	125 mg	250 mg	
Anti-inflammatory effect					
Mean increase of dor/plan					
paw diameter, mm	2.05	1.97^{ns}	1.61^{***}	1.28^{***}	0.88^{***}
SEM[1]	0.06	0.04	0.07	0.06	0.06
Inhibition, %		3.9	21.5	37.6	57.1
Analgesic effect					
Mean improvement of					
pain tolerance, g	38.00	36.00^{ns}	35.00^{ns}	31.00^{ns}	21.00^{***}
SEM[1]	2.01	1.51	3.00	3.32	2.44
Inhibition, %		5.3	7.9	18.4	44.7

[1] Difference between injected and non-injected paw.
ns = Not significant, in comparison with untreated controls.
*** = Significant (p < 0.01).

Tab. VIII: Anti-inflammatory and analgesic effect of vitamin C; «prophylactic test»: 0.5 hour before paw injection (trial R 4 / 81; N = 10 rats per group). Parameter: 4 hours after local carrageenan injection (0.1 ml, 1 % sol)

	Control	Vitamin C (oral)/kg body-weight			Phenylbutazone (oral), 20 mg
		250 mg	500 mg	1000 mg	
Anti-inflammatory effect					
Mean increase of dor/plan					
paw diameter, mm	2.04	1.30^{***}	1.04^{***}	1.04^{***}	0.85^{***}
SEM[1]	0.05	0.04	0.07	0.07	0.06
Inhibition, %		36.3	49.0	49.0	58.3
Analgesic effect					
Mean improvement of					
pain tolerance, g	37.00	30.00^{ns}	17.00^{***}	15.00^{***}	20.00^{***}
SEM[1]	2.13	1.49	2.13	3.42	2.11
Inhibition, %		18.9	54.0	59.5	46.0

[1] Difference between injected and non-injected paw.
ns = Not significant, in comparison with untreated controls.
*** = Significant (p < 0.01).

analgesic effect, higher doses of vitamin C are necessary than for its anti-inflammatory effect.

Table IX shows the anti-inflammatory effect of an oral daily intake of vitamin C during eight consecutive days after 15 to 60 min of irritation with hyaluronidase. Non-parametric statistical analysis showed the anti-inflammatory effect to be highly significant. The dose-effect relation of vitamin C as an anti-inflammatory agent is given in Figure 3 and that of its analgesic in Figure 4.

Tab. IX: Anti-inflammatory effect[1], of orally administered vitamin C during consecutive days; "prophylactic test": 15, 30 and 60 minutes after local paw injection of hyaluronidase (125 USP units/0.05 ml NaCl-sol.) on day 9, difference between injected and non-injected paw (mm ± SEM)

Time after irritation	Control	Vitamin C		Phenylbutazone (oral), 2 mg/kg
		250 mg	500 mg	
15 min	1.94 ± 0.13	1.72 ± 0.18	1.09 ± 0.16	1.40 ± 0.11
vs. controls, %		11.0	43.9	27.7
30 min	2.10 ± 0.12	1.69 ± 0.14	1.27 ± 0.15	1.26 ± 0.10
vs. controls, %		19.6	39.3	39.9
60 min	1.49 ± 0.06	1.26 ± 0.16	0.94 ± 0.11	0.87 ± 0.10
vs. controls, %		14.3	37.0	41.2

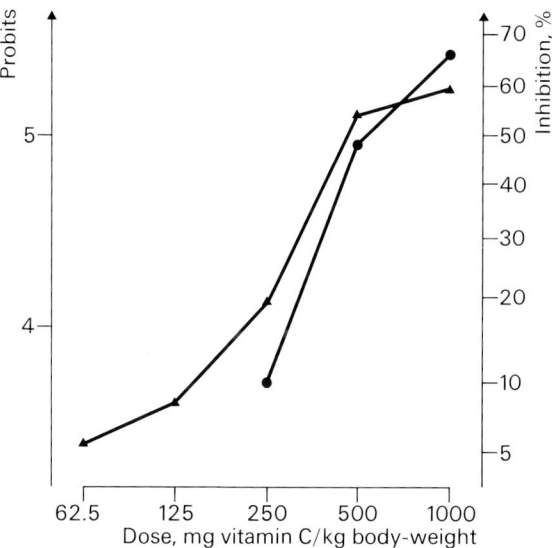

Fig. 3: Analgesic dose efficacy response of orally administered vitamin C. Irritation by 0.1 ml carrageenan 1%; single oral dose of vitamin C (trial R 4 + R 6/81; N = 10 rats per group). ▲ = Prophylactic assay: 0.5 hour before paw injection: ● = therapeutic assay: 2 hours after paw injection.

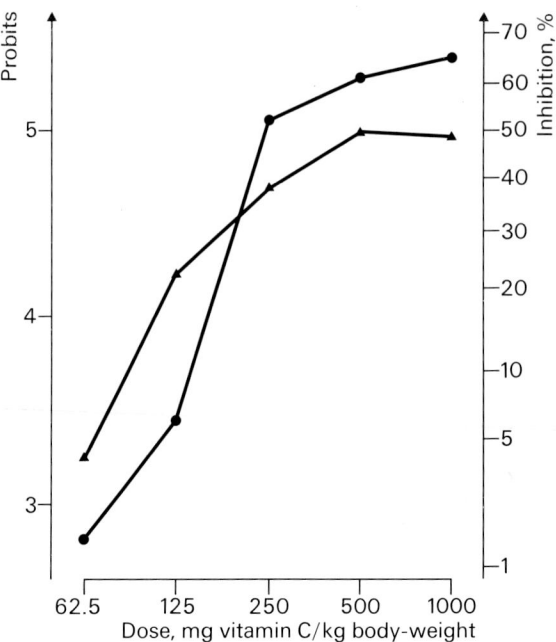

Fig. 4: Anti-inflammatory dose efficacy response of oral vitamin C. Irritation by 0.1 ml carrageenan 1 %: single oral dose of vitamin C (trial R 4 + R 6/81; N = 10 rats per group.) ▲ = Prophylactic assay: 0.5 hour before paw injection; ● = therapeutic assay: 2 hours after paw injection.

Tab. X: Anti-inflammatory and analgesic effect of orally administered sodium acetylsalicylate (AcSal) or/and vitamin C (C); "therapeutic test": 2 hours after paw injection (trial R 23/82; N = 10 rats per group). Parameter: 4 hours after local carrageenan injection (0.1 ml; 1 % sol)

	Control	AcSal or/and vitamin C/kg body-weight		
		100 mg AcSal	100 mg C	100 mg AcSal + 100 mg C
Anti-inflammatory effect				
Mean increase of dor/plan				
paw diameter, mm	1.86	1.23***	1.46*	1.02***
SEM[1]	0.08	0.09	0.05	0.10
Inhibition, %		33.9	21.5	45.2
Analgesic effect				
Mean improvement of				
pain tolerance, g	35.00	14.00***	22.00**	13.00**
SEM[1]	2.69	2.67	2.49	2.60
Inhibition, %		60.0	37.1	62.9

[1] Difference between injected and non-injected paw.

   * =Significant (p < 0.05) in comparison with untreated controls.

  ** =Significant (p < 0.02).

*** =Significant (p < 0.01).

Tables X and XI show the dose-response of vitamin C and sodium acetylsalicylate in our therapeutic test after carrageenan irritation. Two different dose levels of acetylsalicylate and vitamin C were given alone or in combination, and resulted in a significant anti-inflammatory and analgesic effect. However, the most effective was the combination of acetylsalicylate with vitamin C.

Tab. XI: Anti-inflammatory and analgesic effect of orally administered sodium acetylsalicylate (AcSal) or/and vitamin C (C); "therapeutic test": 2 hours after paw injection (trial R 23/82; N = 10 rats per group). Parameter: 4 hours after local carrageenan injection (0.1 ml; 1 % sol)

	Control	AcSal or/and vitamin C/kg body-weight		
		500 mg AcSal	500 mg C	500 mg AcSal + 500 mg C
Anti-inflammatory effect				
Mean increase of dor/plan				
paw diameter, mm	1.82	0.87***	1.22***	0.64***
SEM[1]	0.06	0.07	0.08	0.06
Inhibition, %		52.2	33.0	64.8
Analgesic effect				
Mean improvement of				
pain tolerance, g	30.00	9.00***	17.00**	7.00**
SEM[1]	2.98	4.07	3.00	2.13
Inhibition, %		70.0	43.3	76.7

[1] Difference between injected and non-injected paw.
*** =Significant (p < 0.01) in comparison with untreated controls.

Discussion

Our results show that several vitamins, some of their metabolites and their combinations, administered in appropriate doses, are capable of significantly reducing pain and inflammation in test animals under standardized conditions. These results have been reproducible within narrow limits over several years. The vitamins studied bring about a reduction of pain and inflammation by about 50%, which is comparable to other commonly used anti-inflammatory agents or analgesics. To discover rather weak anti-inflammatory or analgesic activities a suitable model, that is, induction of a mild inflammation or pain, and the use of an appropriate and bioavailable form are both essential. Our new data are in agreement with earlier findings by ourselves [20] and others [17], and back the reports on anti-inflammatory and analgesic actions of vitamins and their combinations in man. To demonstrate these actions of vitamins it is essential to administer the correct dose according to body-weight. In contrast to clinical investigations of anti-inflammatory and analgesic drug activities in man, animal tests are not affected by a placebo effect. A number of clinical investigations have also demonstrated analgesic and anti-inflammatory activities of vitamins.

Vitamin C administered in high doses of 10 g/day to severely ill cancer patients in a double-blind controlled study showed a significant reduction of pain [12]. This result is in agreement with our own observations. In some cases of breast cancer, patients suffering from pain, and no longer responding to usual analgesics, became pain-free when the analgesic was administered together with 10–25 g vitamin C i.v.

BASU et al [4,5] reported a significant relief of bone pain in PAGET's disease by 3 g vitamin C per day given orally. Pain relief by high doses of vitamin C has been reported in various conditions: GREENWOOD [18] reported a significant reduction of pain from the lumbar disk. KURZ and EYRING [28] administered high doses of vitamin C successfully in osteogenesis imperfecta. CAMERON and CAMPBELL [10] reported significant reduction of pain from bone metastases. GUPTE and SAVANT [19] studied the effect of vitamin C on post-suxamethonium pains following procedures such as oesophagoscopy, bronchoscopy and direct laryngoscopy. Their results show a reduction in muscle pains significant at the 1 % level when tested by the chisquare test. Further, the severity of pain was greater in the control group than in the group given vitamin C.

The basis of the analgesic action of vitamin C is not clear but there may be central and peripheral foci of action.

Vitamin C has been shown to be released from nervous tissue by depolarising stimuli [32]. It may modulate dopaminergic mechanisms by inhibiting dopamine binding to striatal membranes and can antagonise dopamine mediated behaviours [22]. With respect to peripheral effects, it is of interest that vitamin C blocks the activation of phospholipase by catecholamines. The action of myocardial phospholipase A, or its surfactant product, lysophosphatidylcholine, on plasma membrane associated phospholipids has been suggested as the cause of the pain in angina pectoris [34].

Phospholipase A also catalyses the release of fatty acids for the formation of prostaglandins. In prostaglandin synthesis, endoperoxides occur as intermediate products in a process mediated by a dioxygenase. The formation of these endoperoxides is inhibited by reduction agents such as vitamin C and vitamin E [29]. This process provides a simple biomolecular basis to explain the reduction of pain and inflammation obtained with these two vitamins. Analgesics, antipyretics and antiphlogistics such as acetylsalicylic acid, indomethacin and phenacetin are known to act by inhibiting prostaglandin synthesis at the dioxygenase level.

The inhibitory action of vitamin C has been established in tissue homogenates and in intact tissue. Stimulation of prostaglandin biosynthesis by vitamin C has also been reported: whilst 15 mM vitamin C inhibited the formation of prostaglandins in endothelial and epithelial cells, production of prostaglandins from arachidonic acid was stimulated in smooth muscle cells and fibroblasts 20- to 50- fold, respectively [35].

DOLBEARE and MARTLAGE [16] have also reported on some anti-inflammatory properties of vitamins in comparison with aspirin and phenylbutazone (Table XII).

Tab. XII: Anti-inflammatory effects of vitamin C, aspirin and phenylbutazone in different animal models; according to DOLBEARE and MARTLAGE [16]

Animal model	Inhibition of inflammation, %		
	vitamin C (50 mg/kg)	aspirin (100 mg/kg)	phenylbutazone (50 mg/kg)
UV Erythema	0	80 ± 1.5	90 ± 1.3
Carageenan	12 ± 1.1	29 ± 2.5	49 ± 0.6
Adjuvant arthritis			
7 days	21 ± 0.1	12 ± 2	33 ± 0.1
14 days	25 ± 0.2	0	43 ± 0.1

The anti-inflammatory efficacy of vitamin C was also demonstrated in two groups of guinea pigs in which osteoarthritis was induced by severance of the anterior cruciate ligament, transaction of the major portion of the medial collateral ligament and removal of the anterior portion of the medial meniscus [36, 37].

One group received 2.4 mg vitamin C/animal/day, the other 150 mg vitamin C/day. After about 21 weeks a significant difference in the cartilage surface of the studied joints was visible. The joints of the guinea pigs with low vitamin C intake showed osteophyte formation in medial and lateral compartments, extensive surface fibrillation, flattening and widening of joint structures. Guinea pigs on high vitamin C intake showed only slight surface fibrillation and osteophyte formation in the medial compartment. Significant differences were found in the activities of crucial cartilage enzymes of the joints studied. In supplemented animals vitamin C markedly inhibited activity of alkaline phosphatase and increased the net synthesis of sulfated proteoglycans. Low dietary levels of vitamin C promoted the development of surgically induced osteoarthritis. In vitro vitamin E also inhibited the activities of lysosomal enzymes, in particular arysulfatase A and acid phosphatase. The inhibition resulted from a direct interaction between these enzymes and vitamin E. Vitamin C and vitamin E appear to stabilize sulfated proteoglycans, essential structures of the cartilage and thus to inhibit inflammation. Treatment of osteoarthritis with effective amounts of these vitamins, either alone or together with other therapeutic means, is suggested as a means of retarding the erosion of the cartilage, giving less pain to the patients and postponing surgical intervention, e.g. hip replacement, for years.

As already mentioned, vitamin E too shows an analgesic effect, most probably via inhibition of prostaglandin synthesis. Clinical reports on pain relief include leg cramps that responded to 300 IU vitamin E/day [2], other idiopathic cramps, pain in the neck and the lower part of the back [11], and post-herpes zoster neuralgia [3].

HIEBER [23] has obtained surprisingly good results in the intra-articular treatment with panthenol of arthrotic and prearthrotic irritation in the knee and hip joint.

Lately another B-vitamin, vitamin B_6 has become popular in treatment of a special pain situation, the premenstrual syndrome (PMS). PMS comprises a group of affective and somatic symptoms occurring seven to ten days premenstrually with marked improvement at menses. The patients complain of headache, depression of mood, breast tenderness, irritability, lethargy, oedema and impaired coordination. After a first paper dating back to the early 1940's [8], in which a lack of the B-complex vitamins was brought into context with PMS, successful treatment of about 300 women with vitamin B_6, suffering from PMS was not reported until the 1970's. In different clinical trials (open, double-blind and cross-over) partial improvement up to complete recovery was seen with an average intake of 100 mg vitamin B_6 daily [1,6,21,26,39,40,42].

Vitamin B_6 plays an essential role in tryptophan metabolism. As shown previously serotonin formation from tryptophan is directly dependent on vitamin B_6. Besides this, vitamin B_6 also plays a role in the biosynthesis of dopamine, another very important transmitter substance.

Many of the results with vitamin B_6 are encouraging, as it would appear to be an effective and well-tolerated form of treatment.

The examples given demonstrate that vitamins, administered in amounts far above the normal doses show analgesic and anti-inflammatory properties that are unrelated to a vitamin deficiency or their intrinsic vitamin nature. These activities derive from their chemical nature as oxidants or antioxidants, for example changing the activity of certain enzymes involved in pain perception. Unlike the usual analgesics and anti-inflammatories, vitamins are well tolerated and especially pose no difficulties on long-term use. There is no danger of addiction.

In some of the clinical situations described, the application of vitamins alone or in combination appears to be of particular interest and should encourage further clinical investigation.

References

1 ABRAHAM, G E, HARGROVE, J T: Effect of vitamin B_6 on premenstrual symptomatology in women with premenstrual tension syndromes: double blind crossover study. Infertility *3*, 155–165, 1980.

2 AYRES, S, MIHAN, R: Leg cramps and vitamin E. J Am Med Assoc *219*, 216–217, 1972.

3 AYRES, S, MIHAN, R. Post-herpes zoster neuralgia: response to vitamin E therapy. Arch Dermatol *108*, 855–856, 1973.

4 BASU, T K et al: Effect of ascorbic acid on urinary hydroxyproline and calcium excretion in patients with Paget's disease. Scand J Rheumatol *4*, suppl 8, p 29, 1975.

5 BASU, T K et al: Ascorbic acid therapy for the relief of bone pain in Paget's disease. Acta Vitaminol Enzymol (Milano) *32*, 45–49, 1978.

6 BAUMBLATT, M J, WINSTON, F: Pyridoxine and the pill. Lancet *i*, 832–833, 1970.

7 BISCHOFF, A et al: Neurophysiological and electron-microscopic studies in experimental thiamine-deficient polyneuropathy. In: CHAVEZ et al (ed). Nutrition, vol, 2, pp 254–259. Karger, Basel, 1975.

8 BISKIND, M S, BISKIND, G R: Effect of vitamin B-complex deficiency on inactivation of estrone in the liver. Endocrinology *31*, 109, 1942.

9 BOISSIER, J-R et al: Action de la thiamine sur les potentiels des nerfs moteurs de la queue de rat provoqués par stimulations electriques et mécaniques. Thérapie *21*, 159–165, 1966.

10 CAMERON, E, CAMPBELL, A: The orthomolecular treatment of cancer. II. Clinical trial of high-dose ascorbic acid supplements in advanced human cancer. Chem Biol Interact *9*, 285–315, 1974.

11 CATHCART, R F et al: Leg cramps and vitamin E. J Am Med Assoc *219*, 216–217, 1972.

12 CREAGAN, E T et al: Failure of high-dose vitamin C (ascorbic acid) therapy to benefit patients with advanced cancer. New Engl J Med *301*, 687–690, 1979.

13 DAY, J B: Clinical trials in the premenstrual syndrome. Current Med Res Opinion *6*, suppl 5, pp 40–45, 1979.

14 DE CASTRO J.: Synaptanalgésie a base de fortes doses de thiamine. Méd Hyg (Genève) *23*, 1012–1013, 1965.

15 DETTORI, A G, PONARI, O: Effetto antalgico della cobamamide in corso di neuropatie periferiche di diversa etiopatogenesi. Minerva Med *64*, 1077–1082, 1973.

16 DOLBEARE, F A, MARTLAGE, K A: Some anti-inflammatory properties of ascorbic acid. Proc Soc exp Biol (NY) *139*, 540–543, 1972.

17 EICHBAUM, F W et al: Anti-inflammatory effect of warfarin and vitamin K. Naunyn-Schmiedeberg's Arch Pharmacol *307*, 185–190, 1979.

18 GREENWOOD, Jr: Optimum vitamin C intake as a factor in the preservation of disc integrity. Med Ann DC *33*, 274, 1964.

19 GUPTE, S R, SAVANT, N S: Post suxamethonium pains and vitamin C. Anaesthesia *26*, 436–440, 1971.

20 HANCK, A, WEISER, H: Physiological and pharmacological effects of vitamin K. Int J Vit Nutr Res, suppl 24, pp 155–170, 1983.

21 HARGROVE, J, ABRAHAM, G E: Effect of vitamin B_6 on infertility in women with the premenstrual tension syndrome. Fert Sterility *30*, 736, 1978.

22 HEIKKILA, R E et al: Differential inhibitory effects of ascorbic acid on the binding of
    dopamine agonists and antagonists to neostriatal membrane preparations: correlations with
    behavioral effects. Res Commun Chem Pathol Pharmacol 34, 409–421, 1981.
23 HIEBER, F: Erfahrungen mit intraartikulären Injektionen von Pantothensäure bei ar-
    throtischen und präarthrotischen Reizzuständen der Knie- und Hüftgelenke. Therapiewoche
    29, 978, 1967.
24 HIEBER, H. Die Behandlung vertebragener Schmerzen und Sensibilitätsstörungen mit
    hochdosiertem Hydroxocobalamin. Med Monatsschr 28, 545–548, 1974.
25 HOLM, E et al: Neurophysiologische Befunde nach hochdosierter Applikation von
    Hydroxocobalamin-Base bei Katzen. Arneimittel-Forsch 24, 1289–1290, 1974.
26 KERR, G D: The management of the premenstrual syndrome. Current Med Res Opinion 4,
    suppl 4, pp 29–34, 1977.
27 KRAFT, H G et al: Zur Pharmakologie des Vitamins B$_6$ und seiner Derivate. Arzneim Forsch
    11, 922–929, 1961.
28 KURZ, D, EYRING, E J: Effect of vitamin C on osteogenesis imperfecta. Pediatrics 54, 56–61,
    1974.
29 LANDS, W E M et al: In: BERGSTRÖM (ed) "Advances in biosciences", pp 15 ff. Pergamon
    Press, Oxford, 1973.
30 LENOT, G: Note sur l'aneurine, anesthésique général. Ann Anesthésiol franc 7, suppl 1, pp
    173–175, 1966.
31 MAZZONI, P, VALENTI, F: Un nuovo anestetico generale per via endovenosa – la tiamina. Ac-
    ta anaesth (Padova) 15, 815–828, 1964.
32 MILBY, K H et al: In vitro and in vivo depolarization coupled efflux of ascorbic acid in rat
    brain preparation. Brain Res Bull 7, 237–242, 1981.
33 MISRA, A L et al: Differential effects of opiates on the incorporation of (^{14}C) thiamine in the
    central nervous system of the rat. Experientia 33, 372–374, 1977.
34 OSTER, K A et al: Pharmacodynamics of angina pectoris palliation by nitroglycerin. J Clin
    Pharmac 14, 398–399, 1974.
35 POLGAR, P, TAYLOR, L: Stimulation of prostaglandin synthesis by ascorbic acid via hydrogen
    peroxide formation. Prostaglandins 19, 693, 1980.
36 SCHWARTZ, E R: The modulation of osteoarthritic development by vitamins C and E. Int J
    Vit Nutr Res, suppl 26, pp 141–146, 1984.
37 SCHWARTZ, E R: Vitamin C: effect on arylsulfatase activities and sulfated proteoglycan
    metabolism in cultures derived from human articular cartilage. Int J Vit Nutr Res, suppl 19,
    pp 113–125, 1979.
38 SMALL, F B: Relief of pain by infiltration of autonomic ganglia with steroids. Can Med Assoc
    J 118, 375, 1978.
39 SNIDER, B L, DIETEMAN, D F: Pyridoxine therapy for premenstrual acne flare. Arch Der-
    matol 110, 130–131, 1974.
40 STOKES, J MENDELS, J: Pyridoxine and premenstrual tension. Lancet i, 1177–1178, 1972.
41 TAKAHASKI, K, NAKAMURA, H: Axonal degeneration in beriberi neuropathy. Arch Neurol
    33, 836–841, 1976.
42 TAYLOR, R W, JAMES, C E: The clinician's view of patients with premenstrual syndrome.
    Current Med Res Opinion 6, suppl 5, pp 46–51, 1979.
43 WEISER, H, KORMANN, A W: Biopotency of vitamin K. I. Antihemorrhagic properties of
    structural analogs of phylloquinone as determined by curative prothrombin time tests. Int J
    Vit Nutr Res 53, 143–155, 1983.

*A. Hanck, MD, PhD, Unit of Social and Preventive Medicine, University of Basle, St. Alban-
vorstadt 19, CH-4000 Basle, and Pharma Clinical Research Department, F. Hoffmann-La
Roche & Co., Ltd, CH-4002 Basle, Switzerland*

Vitamin Requirements in Human Pregnancy

G.A. Hauser

Lucerne, Switzerland

Key Words: Pregnancy · Vitamin requirements · Prophylaxis · Iron-multivitamin-mineral preparations · Risk factors

Abstract: Today, prophylactic administration of iron and all vitamins is now practised on a large scale, especially in the industrialized countries. All recent studies on vitamin levels in the blood of pregnant women reveal a high incidence of vitamin deficiency. Studies on individual vitamins reveal that on average 20–30 % of pregnant women suffer from a deficiency. Without prophylaxis about three-quarters of pregnant women would show a deficiency of at least one vitamin. Prophylactic treatment of pregnant women with all necessary vitamins and minerals, especially iron and folic acid in adequate amounts, is therefore indicated. For this purpose we have had excellent results with the iron-multivitamin-mineral preparation Elevit ® Pronatal.

During pregnancy, vitamin requirements are increased by those of the conceptus (fetus, amniotic fluid and placenta) and the uterus, which is then five times larger in size. Above all, an important role is played here by the blood volume, the plasma volume rising by about 50 %. When iron supplements are taken, the erythrocyte volume is increased by over 25 %, when they are not taken, by only 20 % [1]. When vitamins are not administered, on average the plasma vitamin B_{12} level during pregnancy falls to 80 % of the normal, the vitamin C level to 60 %, the folic acid, vitamin B_6 and biotin levels to 50 % of the normal [2]. The additional amounts required during pregnancy are not known for all vitamins, biotin being a case in point.

The general rule of thumb [3] laying down a vitamin requirement in pregnancy twice that of the non-pregnant woman is much too simple. This alleged rule is inaccurate as well as incorrect (Table I).

A key role in the vitamin requirement of the fetus is played by the placenta. For many vitamins the fetal blood level is in equilibrium with the maternal level, for others, a higher level has been observed in the fetal than in the maternal blood. This is due to the ability of the placenta to act as a selective filter and pump vitamins out of the maternal into the fetal circulation as soon as the placental concentration has sunk to a critical level [4].

Tab. I: Daily requirements of vitamins in young adult women, and supplementary daily vitamin requirements in pregnancy and lactation [2, 3]

Vitamin	Daily requirement	Supplementary daily requirement
A	800 RE	200 RE (1000 IU), during lactation 400 RE; one authority (4) recommends a supplement of 3000 IU
D	300 IU	200 IU
E	8 mg	One-fifth, during lactation a supplement of 3 mg
C	60 mg	20 mg, during lactation a supplement of 40 mg
K	100 µg	2–5 mg
B_1	1.1 mg	0.4 mg
B_2	1.3 mg	0.3 mg
B_{12}	3 µg	1 µg
B_6	2 mg	0.6 mg (2); other authorities recommend up to 8 mg (6) with an additional 0.5 mg during lactation
Folic acid	400 µg	400 µg (5, 6)
Nicotinamide	14 mg	2 mg; during lactation 5 mg

[1] 1000 µg retinol equivalents (RE) correspond to 3333 IU retinol or 5000 IU vitamin A from the diet.

Malnutrition aside, among the factors affecting the availability of vitamins one must take into account the socioeconomic context and social class. Especially in developing countries seasonal differences also play a role, as is the case in Gambia and Senegal in particular for vitamin A, a deficiency of which can cause serious damage to both mother and child [5-7]. Seasonal variations of vitamin blood levels can however also be measured in industrialized regions [8].

Only very few studies are concerned with more than one vitamin. As Smithells [9] reported, even in the United Kingdom – that is to say, in an advanced and highly industrialized country – there is a deficiency of vitamin B_1, riboflavin and retinol in the diet of pregnant women. This investigator found that two-thirds of women in early pregnancy suffered from a dietary deficiency of calories, iron and vitamin D in comparison with non-pregnant women. In more than one-third of cases there was a demonstrable deficiency also of vitamins B_1, B_2 and A.

The studies of Dostalova [10] merit particular attention. They involved assays of nine vitamins in the blood of pregnant women in the Basle (Switzerland) region. Deficiencies of one or more vitamins were recorded in 78 % of the subjects. Deficiencies of a single vitamin occurred with the following frequencies: vitamin B_1 36 %, vitamin B_{12} 31 %, pyridoxine 29 %, vitamin C 27 %, folic acid 24 %, biotin 5 %. Women who become pregnant within three months of ceasing to take ovulation inhibitors run an increased risk of deficiency in vitamins B_1 and B_6 and folic acid. A deficiency of vitamins B_6, B_{12} and B_1 has been reported in women with pregnancy toxemia [11].

General vitamin prophylaxis, although only rarely recommended in the textbooks, is practised world-wide, mainly in combination with iron and folic acid [12, 13]. Among 17 different studies carried out in the United Kingdom, Germany and Scandinavia on the subject of combined vitamin-iron prophylaxis and reviewed by HEMMINEKI and STARFIELD [14], there is only a single study in which cases of pregnancy toxemia (pre-eclampsia) occurred. Whether periconceptional multivitamin treatment would in fact reduce the incidence of neural tube deformities – as SMITHELLS *et al* [15] claim – remains to be confirmed.

Results of Trials With a New Iron-Multivitamin-Mineral Preparation (Elevit ®)

The iron-multivitamin-mineral preparation Elevit®, containing iron, folic acid and electrolytes was given prophylactically to 121 pregnant women at the rate of one tablet per day.[1] The effect of this preparation on the hemoglobin level of the mother has been evaluated in 95 cases to date. In 27 of the subjects the hemoglobin level rose by an average of 0.67 g %, in 5 it remained unchanged. In the remainder of the women the level fell by an average of 1.33 g %.

In a control group of 100 pregnant women not given vitamins and minerals prophylactically, a rise in the hemoglobin level was recorded in only 12 cases, and it remained unchanged in only 3 cases. This result means that the frequency of a rise in the hemoglobin level was over twice as great in the Elevit® group.

As a rule, the maternal hemoglobin level declines during the course of pregnancy. In the above-mentioned control group we found a fall in the hemoglobin level in 85 % of patients (on an average by 1.4 g %), while in 74 % (63 patients) the value fell below 12 g %. Under Elevit®, the fall in the hemoglobin level was less, a result confirming the favourable prophylactic effect of a multivitamin-mineral preparation. In anemic patients given Elevit®, we were able to record a rise in the hemoglobin level in as many as 44 % of cases.

---

[1] Elevit® contains 6000 IU vitamin A, 500 IU vitamin D, 10 mg vitamin E (α-TE), 1.6 mg vitamin B_1, 1.8 mg vitamin B_2, 2.6 mg vitamin B_6, 4.0 µg vitamin B_{12}, 10 mg calcium pantothenate, 100 mg vitamin C, 0.8 mg folic acid, 0.2 mg biotin, 125 mg calcium, 125 mg phosphorus, 100 mg magnesium, 60 mg iron, 1 mg copper, 1 mg manganese, 7.5 mg zinc.

Particular attention was paid to the tolerance shown by patients to the preparation Elevit®. Among a total of 110 evaluated cases we found side effects in 5.4 % (6 patients) (Table II), whereby in two cases the symptoms were not true side effects: one patient described the tablets as being too large, while another reported having diarrhea. Compared with other iron preparations used in similar groups of pregnant patients (Table III), this iron-polyvitamin-mineral preparation is generally very well tolerated. During pregnancy, women tend in any case to experience nausea. All drugs are less well tolerated than when they are taken outside pregnancy. When it is borne in mind moreover that Elevit® contains – in addition to the iron mainly responsible for the side effects – all vitamins including folic acid together with the essential minerals and metals, it can be regarded as a particularly well tolerated preparation.

Tab. II: Side effects of Elevit® when administered in pregnancy

Side effect	Cases (N = 6, i.e. 5.4 %)	Connection with ingestion of the preparation	
		established	not established
Nausea, vomiting	1	—	+
Nausea, eructation	1	—	+
Nausea, vertigo	1	—	+
Nausea	1	—	+
Diarrhea	1	—	+
Capsules too large	1	+	—

Tab. III: Frequency of side effects of preparations containing iron when given during pregnancy, as determined in comparable patient populations

Iron salt (IS)	IS dosage unit, mg	Fe^{++} content, mg	No. of patients, N	Side effects, %
Ferrous gluconate	200	22	71	20.4
Ferrous sulphate	200	50	71	15.3
Ferrous succinate	120	37	155	4.0
Ferrous sulphate with 80 mg gastrointestinal mucoprotease and 350 µg folic acid	270	80	250	1.6
Ferrous fumarate[1]	187	60	110	5.3[2]

[1] Elevit® Pronatal.
[2] Established connection with ingestion of the preparation only 0.9 %.

Discussion

For many years, prophylaxis with iron alone was the mainstay of care of the pregnant woman. Today, this is usually combined with folic acid administration, and in this form has become widely accepted practice, as has general prophylaxis with vitamins and/or minerals.

In the literature, the subject of vitamin deficiency in pregnancy was formerly discussed mainly in connection with the developing countries. More recently, however, there have been increasingly frequent reports of vitamin deficiency states among pregnant women in the advanced and highly industrialized countries. These reports – unfortunately relating mostly to individual vitamins – have aroused wide interest and reveal that some 20–30 % of pregnant women in the population as a whole suffer from some particular isolated deficiency condition. Even in Switzerland, three-quarters of pregnant women have a demonstrable deficiency of at least one vitamin. The problem is therefore an extremely important one calling for action. In the light of our most recent knowledge, general polyvitamin prophylaxis during pregnancy, combined with iron and folic acid in particular as well as with other minerals, is urgently necessary. This applies also to the advanced, highly industrialized countries, particularly where women in the less affluent classes are concerned.

References

1 PITKIN, R M: Assessment of nutritional status of mother, fetus and newborn. Am J Clin Nutr 34, 660, 1981.
2 HYTTEN, F E: Maternal nutrition during pregnancy and lactation. In: AEBI et al (ed) "Maternal nutrition during pregnancy and lactation", p 34. Huber, Bern, 1980.
3 NICHOLS, B L, NICHOLS, V N: Nutrition in pregnancy and lactation. Review in clinical nutrition. Nutr Abstr Rev 53, 259–273, 1983.
4 BAKER, H et al: Role of placenta in maternal-fetal vitamin transfer in humans. Am J Obstet Gynecol 141, 791, 1981.
5 SARMA, V: Maternal vitamin A deficiency and fetal microcephaly and anophthalmia. Obstet Gynecol 13, 299–301, 1959.
6 LAMBDA, P A, SOOD, N N: Congenital microphthalmus and colobomata in maternal vitamin A deficiency. J Pediat Ophthalmol 5, 115, 1968.
7 GEBRE-MEDHIN, M: Maternal nutrition during pregnancy and lactation. In: AEBI et al (ed) "Maternal nutrition during pregnancy and lactation", p 100. Huber, Bern, 1980.
8 BATES, C J: Vitamin A in pregnancy and lactation. Proc Nutr Soc 42, 65–79, 1983.
9 SMITHELLS, R W: Maternal nutrition during pregnancy and lactation. In: AEBI et al (ed) "Maternal nutrition during pregnancy and lactation", p 123. Huber, Bern, 1980.
10 DOSTALOVA, L: Correlation of the vitamin states between mother and newborn during delivery. Dev Pharmacol Ther 4, suppl 1, pp 45–57, 1982.

11 Lu, J Y *et al:* Intake of vitamins and minerals by pregnant women with selected clinical symptoms. J Am Diet Ass *78,* 477–482, 1981.
12. KULLANDER, S, KALLEN, B: A prospective study of drugs and pregnancy. 4. Miscellaneous drugs. Acta Obstet Gynecol Scand *55,* 287–295, 1976.
13. PALUMBO, G, MESSANA, C: Vitamins in pregnancy. Submitted for publication.
14. HEMMINEKI, E, STARFIELD, B: Routine administration of iron and vitamins during pregnancy. Review of controlled clinical trials. Brit J Obstet Gynecol *85,* 404–410, 1978.
15. SMITHELLS, R W *et al:* Apparent prevention of neural tube defects by periconceptional vitamin supplementation. Arch Dis Child *56,* 911–918, 1981.

G.A. Hauser, MD, Allenwindenstrasse 7, CH-6004 Luzern (Switzerland)

Vitamin B$_6$ and the Premenstrual Syndrome (PMS)

A.D.G. GUNN

University Health Service, Reading, Berkshire, UK

Key Words: Premenstrual syndrome · Incidence-treatment survey · Pyridoxine · Vitamin B$_6$

Abstract: The premenstrual syndrome undoubtedly exists as a recurring physical, psychological and physiologically disturbing entity. Its recognition by the consulting physician depends on the taking of an accurate and specific history, and its identification depends on the symptoms and signs exhibited by the patient fitting a precise pattern. There are no simple or inexpensive biochemical tests, therefore, its diagnosis is frequently disputed. Its cause is not simple either, the complications of the hypothalamic influence on hormonal secretions, the suggested metabolic pathways of biochemical breakdown and the assumed requirement of enzyme-catalysts are all involved in the syndrome's development. The treatment necessary may vary on a spectrum from simple consolation and dietary advice to diuretics, short or prolonged hormonal interference or supplementation, to psychotropic or antidepressant intervention. Trials of therapy with vitamin B$_6$ (pyridoxine) have been undertaken in several centres in recent years and new research suggests that this substance with, in particular the advantages of no teratogenic, accumulative, or foreseeable unwanted side effect in normal dosage, has particular benefits. The rationale for such treatment is explained in this survey of the current therapy for the premenstrual syndrome. Preliminary information of a new double-blind trial in the UK is reported.

Introduction

There is nothing pleasant about menstruation. At best it is a physiological inconvenience, at worst it contributes to chronic ill health through menorrhagia, dysmenorrhoea or premenstrual tension and its concomitant syndrome of allied disorders and distress [1]. It may be felt by contemporary physicians and gynecologists that female patients consult in ever-increasing numbers about this latter disorder associated with their menstrual cycle – but, this is no new phenomenon, nor one confined to the modern woman of the developed world.

It was not until 1931, however, that Robert Frank defined "a large number of women who are handicapped by premenstrual disturbances of a manifold nature" [2]. He went on with accuracy and precision to describe the handicap as: "a condition of indescribably tension, and a desire to find relief by foolish actions difficult to restrain. Often severe headaches and palpable edema, especially of the face, hands and feet, were accompanied by oliguria and an increase in weight. All symptoms were rapidly relieved at the onset of the menstrual flow, but, recurred at varying times as the end of the cycle drew near. The condition of the patients became worse if the onset of flow was delayed". The description was classic and the occurrence was explained in terms of faulty ovarian function. At the same time, however, Karen Horney, the psychoanalyst, published "Die Prämenstruellen Verstimmungen" [3] and she explained the symptomatology as the "manifestation of repressed sexual desire and power".

The controversy about cause and effect has remained with us for nearly fifty years, constantly influencing attitudes, treatment and exploration, and only in the last decade have some of the physiological and psychological knots of the premenstrual syndrome (PMS) been unravelled.

Incidence

Where a syndrome is precisely defined and its biochemical parameters agreed then its incidence can be accurately assessed. With the premenstrual syndrome difficulties in agreement with regard to its definition, lead to the greatest of variations reported in the literature. It has been reported as affecting as high a proportion of the female population, between the ages of 15 and 50, as 73% (in nursing students in the USA) [4], and as low as 10–15% (in self-selected clinic attenders in the UK) [5]. Estimates have been made that it affects between 40–50% of sophisticated women seen in any gynecological practice [6] and between 20% of woman in rural villages of the developing world [7]. What is intriguing is that recent papers are emphasising its frequent development in women who have had their first baby (and suffered post-natal depression) [8] in those who have had tubal ligation and sterilisation operations [9, 10] – a rising number – , and in those who suffer involuntary infertility [11]. The association of seeking help for the complaint, with other added stress in life is clear. In university students, there is nothing seasonal – one must assume – about menstrual problems, yet consultations about the premenstrual syndrome occur with the greatest frequency during the summer months (in the UK) – the time of impending examinations [12, 13].

Others have noted this clear correlation of "psychological ill health" leading to a greater frequency of complaints [14], as well as complaints that the normally tolerated syndrome becomes unbearable, at times when other aspects of life become unduly stressful. Thus, the extra straw on the camel's back leads to the break in toleration. In consequence, the diverse range in reported incidence of premenstrual syndrome must reflect not only the normal diagnostic dilemmas of any doctor but also the tolerance of the female population being cared for.

There are social changes also that are important in their influence on the reporting of any medical complaint. Literacy and the influence of the media is rising everywhere in the world and many clinics report the attendance of women who only sought treatment for PMS when they read in the press about its availability [8]. Female equality and "liberation", educational changes and improvement, a voluntary delay in the onset of childbearing, the growing use of the oral contraceptive – all in their way lead to increasing numbers of women who, quite rightly, will not tolerate their monthly inconvenience. A recurrent and cyclical syndrome is a cross fewer women wish to bear.

Symptomatology

The list of associated symptoms with the syndrome of PMS is almost endless (Table I). One author [5] lists 54 common complaints from "a change in sleep patterns" to "stimulus overload" and with such other confusing contrasts as "constipation or diarrhea". FRANK's original description has only been little improved with the test of time. What is clear is that for the syndrome to be present it must: 1) be cyclical – with relief occurring in at least the 7 days of the postmenstruum; 2) involve manifestations of an electrolyte disorder – reflected by weight gain, edema, or feelings of bloatedness; 3) involve behavioural changes or mood swings – recognised by the woman herself or others, as being associated with the physical manifestations; 4) in general affect women of reproductive age – although it may rarely occur just before menarche and in some women perimenopausally.

The danger of assuming PMS to be the cause of symptomatology when other disorders are present (e.g. endometriosis and prolactin-secreting tumours [10], as well as of assuming that any simple endocrine parameter is responsible [16] have been reported. There are "diagnostic pointers" (Table II) that are of value in identifying the syndrome, which are by no means exclusive – but, in the long run the completion by the patient of a questionnaire gives the best selection – for it is a disorder with many and varied manifesta-

Tab. I: Women reporting with major symptoms of PMS, before treatment; according to Taylor and James [8]

Symptom	% of total
Depression	55
Irritability/bad temper	40
Tension	12
Increased liability to accident	6
Migraine and other headaches	22
Abdominal distension	22
Breast discomfort	20
Edema	12
Purpura	1
Loss of libido	40
Increase in libido	8
Epilepsy	1

Tab. II: "Diagnostic pointers" in the histories of 100 consecutive patients with PMS; according to Norris [9]

Painless menstruation
Onset after puberty, oral contraceptive use, pregnancy, episode of amenorrhea or tubal ligation
Increased severity after oral contraceptive use, pregnancy, episode of amenorrhea, tubal ligation or hysterectomy
Craving for sweet or salty food in premenstrual phase
Increased sex drive in premenstrual phase
Side effects with oral contraceptive use
Weight fluctuations in adult life exceeding 28 pounds
Alcohol intolerance in premenstrual phase
Postpartum depression
Threatened abortion or miscarriage in first trimester
Pre-eclampsia or toxemia of pregnancy

tions [12]. The questionnaire designed by Moos [17] offers a standard interpretive tool that can be modified to suit the needs of any therapeutic trial, and a diary card can be kept by the patient to rate any deviations in experience as each menstrual cycle passes by.

Because there is no simple, inexpensive biochemical test that can be applied, the diagnosis of PMS is always, in truth, "assumed" or "agreed" by the patient and the physician, after extensive and probably repeated consultations. Proof that the disorder is the cause of the patient's complaint is only obtained in the absence of any other pathological or psychological disorder that might be responsible for some of the manifestations. PMS is thus almost unique in medical practice in having this characteristic – whereas for most physical disorders the diagnosis has been classically defined as being obtained from the history (60 %) and from the examination (40 %) – in PMS it is probably derived solely from the history.

Physiological Changes Involved

Since PMS is a psychoneuroendocrine dysfunction, the physiological processes involved are virtually those of the whole body. In 1973 high premenstrual levels of circulating estrogen and low levels of progestogen were held to be responsible for women suffering from the anxiety symptoms associated with PMS [18]. In 1978 low estrogen levels and high progestogen levels were said to be the cause of the depressive symptoms that other women experienced [19]. Clearly an imbalance between these two groups of hormones is involved – but then the menstrual cycle is by definition a physiological process brought about by normal changes in hormonal relationships. One might ask philosophically whether a women is "designed" to menstruate – or to ovulate? In terms of evolution truly the latter, and menstruation thus marks the body's failure to achieve its objective – physiologically and psychologically.

There is little doubt therefore that unless women are to be constantly pregnant, or lactating throughout their reproductive lives, they will be physiologically exposed to a cyclical imbalance between estrogens and progestogens – thus PMS must originate in an excessive imbalance.

Estrogens are secreted mainly by the ovary (although some are derived from adrenal and ovarian androgens) and are bound to plasma proteins. The liver conjugates estrogens to make them water soluble and inactive (thus excreted via the kidney). Is any excess thus due to secretion, failure to conjugate, or failure to excrete?

Estrogens influence a woman's mood and this may be brought about by the oxidation effect on neurobiochemical amines – notably serotonin and dopamine. Serotonin excess is said to lead to nervous tension, palpitations, inability to concentrate [15], and dopamine induces relaxation. Again a balance between the two is held to be necessary. Estrogens can suppress certain monoamine oxidases and increase others – their full effect on neurochemistry is still to be precisely defined.

Inescapable from any attempt at simplicity in this however, is the recognition of the hypothalamic role in achieving "biological feedback" with regard to balancing hormonal secretion. When in 1971 it was demonstrated anatomically that there were direct access vascular channels between the

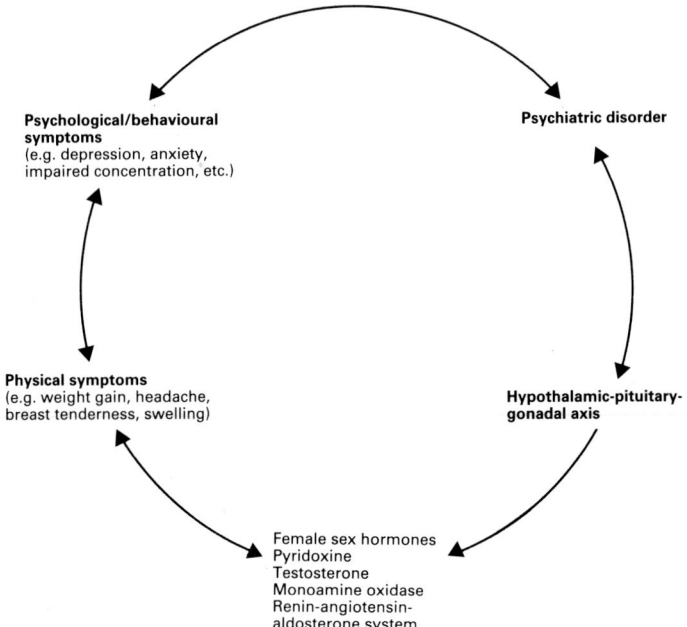

Fig. 1: Circular interactions underlying PMS; according to Clare [14].

hypothalamus of the brain and the pituitary gland below – the influence of psyche over soma and the "nervous" control of hormonal secretion became more clearly appreciated.

Thus estrogen excess may initiate a progestogen response and not be alone responsible for the manifestation of PMS (Fig. 1). Undoubtedly there is a domino effect since elevated prolactin levels have also been determined in some women with PMS [20] – though not in most. Tissue sensitivity may be enhanced to certain hormonal levels as a result of the domino effect, since clearly no one hormone can be responsible. Thus salt and water retention occur premenstrually (hence the bloatedness and edema) as a result of complex estrogenic and aldosterone alterations. Similarly stress in the woman may release β-endorphins [16] which inhibit dopamine, and increase prolactin release – so within the cycle, other cyclical effects are interdependent.

Interdependent also for many of these changes occurring within the woman's body is the role of vitamin B$_6$ (pyridoxine), as shown in Figure 2. When it is deficient there is a decreased liver conjugation of estrogens and thus a decreased renal clearance and excretion rate [11]. As the co-factor, pyridoxal phosphate, it corrects hypothalamic levels of 5-hydroxytryptamine and dopamine, thus influencing pituitary, ovarian and neural activity [14]. If

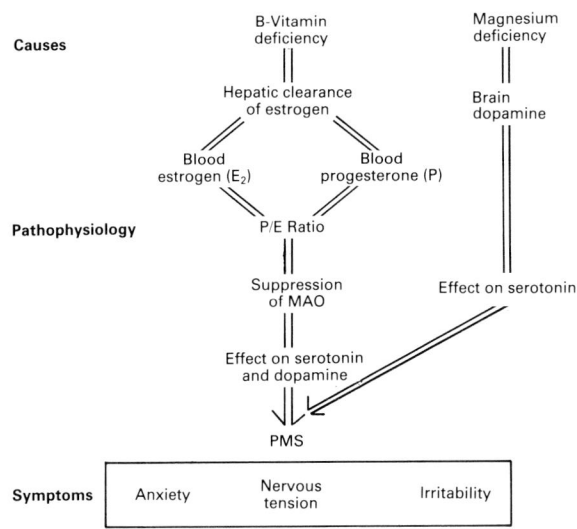

Fig. 2: Postulated pathophysiology of PMS; according to ABRAHAM [32].

deficient there is a diminished biosynthesis of serotonin from dietary tryptophan. Pyridoxine is a co-factor for the conversion of linoleic acid to DGLA [21] – but where it acts in the chain is uncertain, and it may also act to lower prolactin levels, as well as those of estrogen. Pyridoxine certainly relieves the depressive symptoms experienced by users of estrogenic oral contraceptives, though the mechanism is difficult to describe [22]. Its activity by phosphorylation is however said to require sufficient magnesium in the diet [11].

Treatment

It is essential always to remember as a practising physician that it is the patient who is to be treated – not the syndrome, tempting though it might be to the biochemist to do otherwise, and with PMS a constantly recurring finding has been the placebo effect of almost every form of treatment offered. Not surprisingly perhaps after a woman has experienced "many years of discomfort due to enforced lack of attention" [23] – the "placebo" effect of a physician's interest, the reaching of a mutually agreed diagnosis, and the achievement of a sympathetic interest is more than remarkably therapeutic. In one trial 40 % of those allocated to hormonal treatment for their PMS experienced benefit with the placebo [23]. There is a clear "counselling and psychotherapeutic effect" from being entered in a trial if it offers the sufferer hope of relief.

The most frequently tested form of treatment for PMS in the past has been hormonal – but in a new era where there is natural concern about hormonal interference in the cycles of women who might become pregnant, this form of treatment has its limitations. (It also has its cost – an estimate of annual treatment for 25% of the sufferers in the UK would be a cost of £30 million per year [24].) It is also counterproductive for the secondarily infertile women anxious to conceive, and inappropriate for the "pill taker" for despite their use of hormones they may still suffer some of the PMS manifestations.

Diuretics have been employed [12], but have limited benefits in only relieving one manifestation of PMS and again may be inappropriate for the woman who wishes to conceive. The use of lithium has also been assessed [25], but it is by no means appropriate for large numbers of women with PMS.

The use of pyridoxine, therefore, has much to offer – a physiological rationale, safety from unwanted side effects, freedom from teratogenic danger and mounting evidence of its effectiveness.

The Evidence for Vitamin B₆

In 1973 Adams et al [22] showed that in some women who were using oral contraceptives and experiencing depression, there was a disturbance of tryptophan metabolism with an associated tendency to pyridoxine deficiency. This confirmed the work of others who had found vitamin B₆ to be of benefit to both oral contraceptive users and sufferers from PMS.

In 1977 Kerr [26] reported the benefits of pyridoxine (in dosages of 40–100 mg daily) in a trial involving 70 women (mean age 34 years) where pre-entry hormonal tests had shown no abnormality with regard to progesterone or prolactin. There was a 45% "cure rate" for the majority of symptoms and most notably 80% of those with premenstrual headache were considerably improved (Table III). It was remarkable that the women studied were those "who had been treated unsuccessfully in the past".

In 1979 Taylor [8] surveyed the experience of the clinic at St. Thomas' Hospital, London, where in the previous five years nearly 2000 women suffering from PMS had been treated. Treatment with pyridoxine was employed in those women in whom hormonal therapy had not been effective or not desired. Of especial note was the benefit experienced when breast discomfort and breast nodularity were part of the woman's PMS.

This led to the conclusion that vitamin B₆ is best tried *first* when breast discomfort is a major problem.

Tab. III. Women cured or markedly improved on pyridoxine treatment; according to Kerr [26]

Symptom	Women with symptom (N = 70), %	Favourable response, % of those with symptom
Depression (mood)	71	60
Irritability	81	56
Lethargy	27	53
Lack of co-ordination	21	27
Breast tenderness	33	52
Edema and bloatedness	46	59
Headache	23	81

Day [23], from the same clinic, reported on pyridoxine (100 mg) used in a long-acting form and taken only for the post-ovulatory part of the cycle, and found overall improvement in 63 % of the patients.

Taylor [5] summarised their experience stating that "both physical and mental symptoms were improved in more than half of the patients, including those suffering from breast discomfort (Table IV)".

Tab. IV. Proportion of patients cured or greatly improved on pyridoxine treatment (dose of 40 mg twice daily, from day 12 to 26 of menstrual cycle); according to Taylor [5]

Symptom	Proportion cured or greatly improved, % of those with symptom
Depression	60
Irritability/bad temper	56
Abdominal distension	50
Headaches	40
Tension	55
Edema	59
Breast discomfort	50
Purpura	0
Overall	55

In 1980 reporting from California, Abraham et al [11] described a placebo-vitamin B$_6$ double-blind crossover trial in which the dosage was 500 mg daily. There were 25 women involved and a significant and favourable response was found in 21 – with, in particular, the observation that premenstrual weight gain in three patients was markedly decreased. Further they recommended that in view of a high conception rate in PMS patients treated with vitamin B$_6$, who otherwise had unexplained infertility, all infertile women should be similarly evaluated.

In 1982 Colin [27] – also using a 500 mg sustained release preparation of vitamin B$_6$ – found especial benefit (60 %) for women with breast discomfort and Brush [28] reported that because vitamin B$_6$ is a nonprescription medicine, many thousands of women are now taking pyridoxine on their own initiative. Based on the experience at St. Thomas's, he considered it essential that pyridoxine be taken three days before any symptoms (of PMS) would normally be expected and continued until the second day of the next cycle. If the cycle is very irregular vitamin B$_6$ should be taken continually. The dosage involved was 40 mg twice daily working up to 75 mg twice daily and 100 mg twice daily in very severe cases.

A recent extensive review of PMS describes the rationale, benefits and place of pyridoxine in the treatment of this syndrome [16, 29].

Goei and Abraham [6] noted significant difference in dietary habits between normal women and PMS patients. PMS patients consume more refined sugar, refined carbohydrates and dietary products, whereas normal women consume more B vitamins, iron, zinc, and manganese. With a special nutritional supplement containing vitamin B$_6$ and other vitamins and minerals they found a significant improvement in their PMS patients.

Shangold [30] stated that of women with PMS, many benefit from pyridoxine beginning with 50 mg/day and increasing to 200 mg/day if symptoms persist.

Norris [9] recommended an educational program of stress-reduction, regular exercise and improved nutrition for the woman with mild to moderate PMS.

Budoff [31] advised careful initial conservative treatment for PMS patients. She emphasised further that healthy young women must not be exposed chronically to drugs with major side-effects, that may adversely affect their health or mental well being.

Horrobin [21] described how pyridoxine is an essential requirement for the conversion of essential fatty acids and any defective formation of prostaglandins may aggravate some features of PMS.

Labrun [15] proposed a common etiology for PMS involving abnormal fluctuations in brain levels of serotonin, aminobutyric acid (GABA) and interrelated neuroendocrine processes where vitamin B$_6$ was involved.

Abraham [32] stated clearly that administration of vitamin B$_6$ at doses of 200/800 mg a day, reduces blood estrogen, increases progesterone and results in improved symptoms under double-blind conditions.

The evidence thus, for the place of vitamin B$_6$ in the treatment of PMS is rapidly accumulating. In consequence, earlier this year in the UK a multicentre trial involving 1000 women – that was designed to be controlled, randomised and double-blind with dosages of placebo versus pyridoxine (Benadon® by Roche) over three cycles (average 100 mg daily) was started.

Patients admitted to the trial were those suffering from at least one of the following ten symptoms in a cyclical and premenstrual occurrence: tension, irritability, depression, violent tendencies, lethargy, lack of co-ordination, breast tenderness, edema and bloatedness, headache, acne.

The results are currently being analysed, but, this will be the largest single trial conducted under specifically testing conditions of the place of pyridoxine in the treatment of premenstrual tension. On the evidence already available the results will be encouraging and physicians can look forward to a constant improvement in the care of their patients with PMS by the use of safe, non-hormonal, nutritional vitamin therapy.

References

1   LEADER: Br Med J *1*, 212, 1979.
2   FRANK, R T: The hormonal causes of premenstrual tension. Arch Neurol Psych *26*, 1053–1057, 1931.
3. HORNEY, K: Die prämenstruellen Verstimmungen (1931). In: KELMAN (ed) "Feminine psychology", pp 99–106. Norton, New York, 1967.
4   LAMB, W M *et al:* Premenstrual tension, EEG, hormonal and psychiatric evaluation. Am J Psych *109*, 840–848, 1953.
5   TAYLOR, R W: Premenstrual syndrome a successful protocol for all. Mod Med (GB) *25*, 49–53, 1980.
6   GOEI, G S, ABRAHAM, G E: Effect of nutritional supplement Optivite on symptoms of premenstrual tension. J Reprod Med *28*, 527–531, 1983.
7   BUDOFF, P W: No more menstrual cramps and other good news. Putman, New York, 1980.
8   TAYLOR, R W, James, G E: The clinician's view of patients with premenstrual syndrome. Curr Med Res Opinion. *6*, 46–51, 1979.
9   NORRIS, R V: Progesterone for premenstrual tension. J Reprod Med *28*, 509–516, 1983.
10 HARGROVE, J T, ABRAHAM, G E: The ubiquitousness of premenstrual tension in gynaecologic practice. J Reprod Med *28*, 435–437, 1983.
11 ABRAHAM, G E, HARGROVE, J T: Effects of vitamin B$_6$ on premenstrual symptomatology. Infertility *3*, 155–165, 1980.
12 GUNN, A D G: The premenstrual syndrome and its management at a University Health Centre. Br J Sex Med *3*, 21–22, 1975.
13 LONGRICK, A F, GUNN, A D G: A comparison of naproxen sodium and dextropropoxyphene in the treatment of primary dysmenorrhoea in university students. Br J Clin Pract *36*, 181–184, 1982.
14 CLARE, A W: Psychiatric and social aspects of premenstrual complaint. Monographs in Psychology Medicine, vol 4. Cambridge University Press, Cambridge, 1983.
15 LABUNN, A H: Hypothalamic, pineal and pituitary factors in the premenstrual syndrome. J Reprod Med *28*, 438–443, 1983.
16 LONDON, R S *et al:* Education and treatment of breast symptoms in patients with premenstrual syndrome. J Reprod Med *28*, 503–508, 1983.
17 MOOS, R H: The development of a menstrual distress questionnaire. Psychosom Med *30*, 853, 1968.
18 BACKSTROM, T, CARSTENSEN H: Oestrogen and progesterone in relation to menstrual tension. J Steroid Biochem *5*, 257, 1974.

19 ABRAHAM, G E *et al:* Hormonal and behavioural changes during the menstrual cycle. Sendogia *3,* 33, 1978.
20 HORROBIN, D F: In: Prolactin: physiology and clinical significance. MTP Press, Lancaster, 1973.
21 HORROBIN, D F: The role of essential fatty acids and prostaglandins in the premenstrual syndrome. J Reprod Med *28,* 465–468, 1983.
22 ADAMS, P W *et al:* Effects of pyridoxine hydrochloride (B_6) on depression associated with oral contraception. Lancet *1,* 897, 1973.
23 DAY, J B: Clinical trials in the premenstrual syndrome. Curr Med Res Opinion *6,* 40–45, 1979.
24 MARTIN, M: Is PMS a social problem? Pulse, Nov. *29,* 35, 1980.
25 SINGER, K *et al:* A controlled evaluation of lithium in the premenstrual tension syndrome. Br J Psych *124,* 50, 1974.
26 KERR, G D: The management of the premenstrual syndrome. Curr Med Res Opinion *4,* 29–34, 1977.
27 COLIN, C: Etudes contrôlées de l'administration orale de progestagènes, d'un antioestrogène et de vitamin B_6 dans le traitement des mastodynies. Rev Méd Brux *3,* 605–609, 1982.
28 BRUSH, M: The pill, pyridoxine, and PMS symptoms. Mims Mag *1,* 18–24, 1982.
29 CHAKMAKJIAN, Z H: A critical assessment of therapy for the premenstrual tension syndrome. J Reprod Med *28,* 532–538, 1983.
30 SHANGOLD, M M: Drug therapy for the premenstrual syndrome. J Reprod Med *28,* 525–526, 1983.
31 BUDOFF, P W: The use of prostaglandin inhibitors for the premenstrual syndrome. J Reprod Med *28,* 469–478, 1983.
32 ABRAHAM, G E: Nutritional factors in the aetiology of the premenstrual tension syndromes. J Reprod Med *28,* 446–464, 1983.

Dr. A.D.G. Gunn, MD, Director, University Health Centre, Northcourt Avenue, Reading, Berkshire RG2 7HE, United Kingdom

Aspects of Vitamin A Metabolism in Sensory Epithelia (Inner Ear, Olfactory Bulbus, Pineal Gland)

H.K. Biesalski

Institute of Physiological Chemistry II, University of Mainz, Mainz, West Germany

Key Words: Inner ear · Olfactory bulbus · Pineal gland · Vitamin A derivatives · Photosensitivity · HPLC

Abstract: Vinnikov has postulated that ciliated cells contain vitamin A which is essential to their function. To test this hypothesis vitamin A derivatives were determined in different structures of the inner ear, the olfactory bulbus and, as a model for a rudimentary sense organ in vertebrates, the pineal gland.

By means of special HPLC methods we were able to detect different retinyl esters and retinal with high selectivity and sensitivity. In sensory epithelia we found retinyl palmitate and stearate in different ratios as well as uptake of orally administered ^{14}C-retinyl acetate, which was present as retinyl palmitate, showing the ability of sensory tissues to esterify exogenous vitamin A.

In the rat pineal gland 11-cis and all-trans retinal, retinylesters, as well as rhodopsin-like protein were detected. Differences in the isometric configuration during light and dark adaptation of the retinyl esters were demonstrated. All the vitamin A derivatives are well known to play a role in the visual process in the retina. Whereas the retinyl esters and the rhodopsin-like protein were demonstrable in pineal glands exclusively processed in the dark, 11-cis and all-trans retinal were detectable only in light-exposed pineal glands.

Introduction

In 1965, Vinnikov [1] speculated that, like other ciliated cells, sensory cells contain vitamin A which is essential to their function. He pointed out that the origin of structural and functional evolution of all the receptor cells in sense organs of vertebrates and apparently in most invertebrates, may be traced to modified cells or flagellae (Fig. 1).

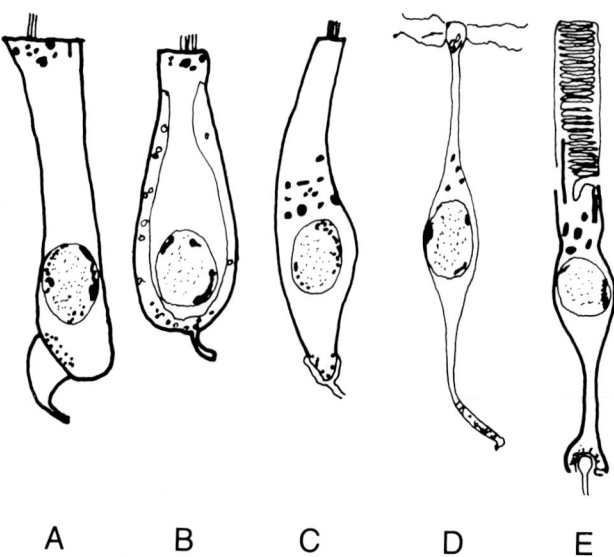

Fig. 1: Mammalian sensory receptor cells. A = Hair cell; B = vestibular hair cell; C = gustatory cell; D = olfactory cell; E = rods and cones.

Until now the involvement and functional significance of vitamin A has been demonstrated in the photochemistry of vision, in the rhodopsin cycle.

Since Wald's [2] fundamental research on the role of vitamin A in the vision process, it has been demonstrated that vitamin A has functional significance in light perception. In vitamin A deficiency, besides many other alterations, nightblindness is an early sign and, at a later stage, xerophthalmia occurs. Only few aspects of vitamin A deficiency affecting other sensory epithelia such as the inner ear, and olfactory and gustatory epithelia are known. From the literature there are some indications that in deficiency, smell and taste decrease [3, 4] and from experimental results it may be assumed that the inner ear is affected by an increased susceptibility to noise and ototoxic drugs [5-9]. Hearing loss has been observed in humans [10, 11] and animal experiments [14, 15] in vitamin A deficiency.

However, these results have to be verified because the authors did not clearly demonstrate whether they found sensorineural or conductive hearing loss due to middle ear infections.

Morphological observations of the inner ear have yielded contradictory results. Exostosis of the internal auditory channel sufficient to touch the eighth cranial nerve and a periostal deposit in relation to the otic capsule [13-15], slight differences of the cuticular membrane [16], as well as other distinct but not significant alterations of the inner ear epithelia were found [17, 18]. However, there is no agreement on a morphological finding typical of vitamin A deficiency.

Clinical observations concerning the protective action of vitamin A against the ototoxic side effects of aminoglycoside antibiotics [19], and noise [20], have yet to be confirmed by experimental results.

Vitamin A depletion in addition to the classically described symptoms is accompanied by a gradual loss of normal taste preferences in rats [21]. The tongue shows increased keratinization of the lingual papillae including the pore area of the taste buds and adjacent epithelial and glandular tissues [22].

Furthermore, the gustatory epithelium is affected during vitamin A deficiency resulting in metaplasia of the epithelium of the nasal mucosa followed by a gradual loss of the sense of smell [4].

In addition to their typical sensory epithelia, vertebrates have retained a sensory organ of invertebrates which has, however, lost its original function: the pineal gland. In lampreys, fishes, amphibians and reptiles, the pineal com-

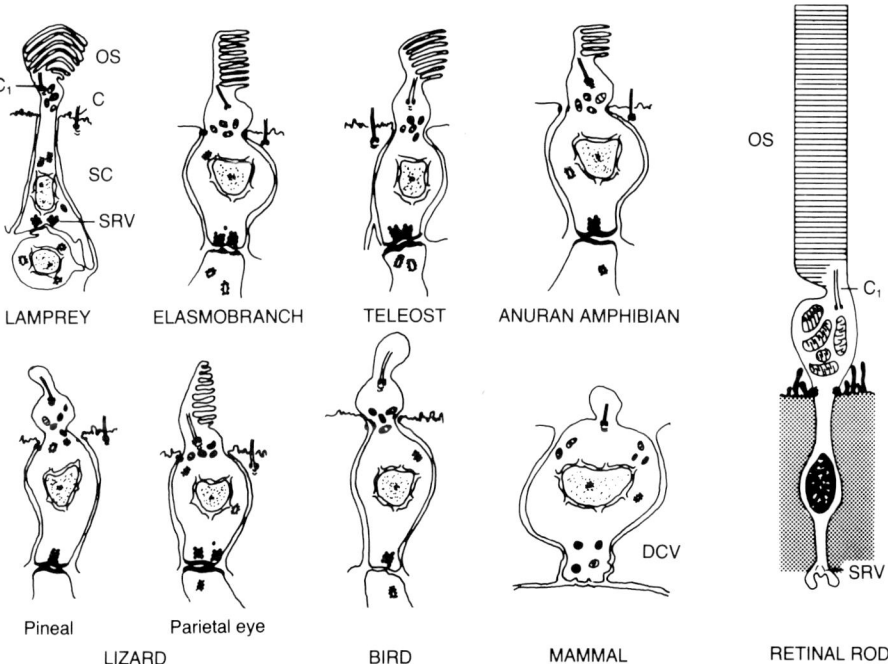

Fig. 2: Morphologic changes of pineal photoreceptor cells in different animals. OS = Outer segment; C = cilium; C_1 = centriole; SC = supporting cell; SRV = synaptic ribbon and vesicles; DCV = dense-cored vesicles.

plex, due to the presence of cone-like structures, is directly photosensitive, and afferent nervous connections from the pineal complex to the brain are prominent [23]. During evolution, pineal photoreceptors in vertebrates lost their outer segments and remained as cone-like structures (Fig. 2).

Rhodopsin-like and opsin-like substances have been demonstrated by means of immunohistochemistry in pineal photoreceptor cells of teleosts, anurans, chelonian reptiles, and birds [24–26]. The presence of photopigments in anurans has been demonstrated also by microspectrophotometric analysis. Whereas the frontal organ contains a photolabile substance with an absorption maximum between 560 nm and 580 nm, in the pineal organ proper a rhodopsin-like pigment 502_1 has been found [27–29]. In the avian pineal gland photoreceptor cells are not consistently present and show clear signs of rudimentation, the majority of pineal cells being the pinealocytes [23, 30, 31].

In good agreement with these ultrastructural findings is the observation that opsin immunoreactivity in birds varies from species to species [26].

Interestingly, there is clear evidence that, in some avian species, organ-cultured pineal glands are directly photosensitive, as demonstrated biochemically [32–37], and that the action spectrum of photosensitivity of the isolated chicken pineal gland resembles the absorption spectrum of rhodopsin [38].

In view of these findings it was decided to study biochemically whether there are any indications that vitamin A and related substances are present in the mammalian pineal gland, despite the fact that in this order the adult pineal gland does not contain photoreceptor cells, is not directly light-sensitive [23, 39], and shows no immunoreactivity for opsin [26].

Methods

Chemicals and equipment

All chemicals used were p.a. quality and purchased from Merck (Darmstadt, FRG). Chromatography was carried out with a Perkin Elmer HPLC-pump (Serie 1), Perkin Elmer Fluorescence detector 650 – 10 S and a Perkin Elmer UV detector LC 85 with Auto control. Columns and special performances of chromatography are given in Table I. Furthermore, for special experiments, we used a Beckman UV detector 165 with on-line scanning of the detected peaks.

Standards

As external standards we used retinol (protected in sealed ampoules) (25 mg, crystalline, Sigma Munich) all-trans retinyl palmitate (1g, crystalline, Sigma Munich) all-trans retinal (1g, crystalline, Sigma Munich). 9-cis-, 13-cis retinyl palmitate, 11-cis retinyl stearate and 11-cis retinal (all crystalline) were a kind gift from Hoffmann-La Roche (Basle).

Tab. I: Chromatographic conditions for determination of different vitamin A derivatives in biological samples.

Derivatives	Column[1]	Flow, ml/min	Mobile phase	t_r, min
I				
Total ester fraction	Spherisorb	3.0	N-Hexane:Isopropanol	4.0
Retinol	Silica 3μ		94:6	
II				
Total ester fraction	Spherisorb	1.5	N-Hexane:Dioxane	9.0
Retinal (all trans-,	Silica 3μ		94:6	
9-cis-,11-cis-,13-cis-)			(dried)	
III				
Ester separation	RP – 18	1.5	Acetonitrile:Water	14.0
Stearate	Hypersil		90:10	
Oleate	3 μ			
Palmitate				
IV				
Ester separation	Spherisorb	1.0	N-Hexane:Diisopropylether	11.0
9-,11-,13-cis, all trans	Silica 3 μ		98:2	
Stearate			(dried)	
Oleate				
Palmitate				

[1] All columns: Ø = 4.6 mm; length = 250 mm.

Standards were dissolved in isopropanol as stock solution. This stock solution is stable at –20 °C for at least four weeks. To check the concentration an aliquot of the stock solution was diluted with isopropanol and its absorbance at typical wavelength was measured against isopropanol in a 1-cm cuvette. Purity was checked by measuring derivative spectra and calculating the ratio of minima (UV/VIS spectrophotometric detector 550, Perkin Elmer). Standard solutions were prepared carefully (avoidance of air, moisture and light) by appropriate dilutions of the stock solution in n-hexane. These standard solutions were reasonably stable in a brown teflon screw cap sample bottle for a whole working day.

The sample concentration was calculated on the basis of the volumes of sample and n-hexane, and the response factor of the linear standard curve.

Qualitative analysis

Identification of different vitamin A derivatives in unknown composition in biological samples is a major problem. Comparison of retention times or adding equivalent standards to unknown samples does not ensure sufficiently precise results. Especially in separation of retinyl esters and their isomeric configurations it may happen that esters such as retinyl palmitate, retinyl stearate and retinyl oleate which are at present the most interesting retinyl esters in biological samples are not clearly separated in an isocratic straight phase HPLC system. Furthermore the absorption spectra of these retinyl esters are very similar so that a mixture of retinyl palmitate and retinyl stearate does not show significant differences in comparison with pure standards in small quantities. To ensure the specificity of our qualitative analysis we separate biological samples according to the conditions in Table I as shown in Figure 3.

When the ester composition is clarified, separation of different isomeric configurations can start, probably again followed by identification of different isomeric structures.

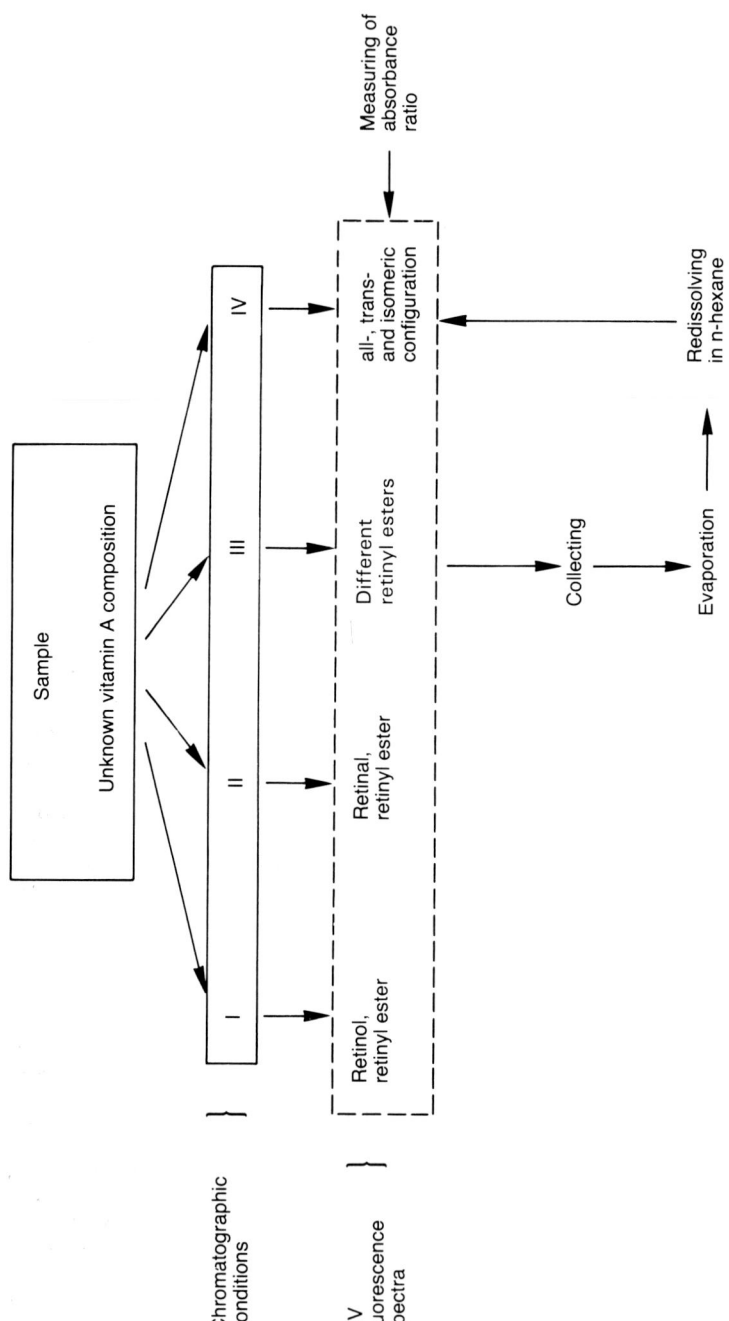

Fig. 3: Procedure followed for determination of unknown vitamin A composition in biological samples (for conditions, see Table I).

To test the purity of separated peaks it may be helpful to calculate them by measuring the absorbance ratio at different wavelengths (255, 305, 328, 380 nm for retinyl esters) in distinct points of the respective peak.

As in quantitative analysis it must be taken into account, that vitamin A is readily oxidized when exposed to air, and all-trans vitamin A isomerizes in solution upon exposure to light. For these reasons, samples must be handled under nitrogen and dim red light.

Sensitivity

To ensure high sensitivity and reproducibility, as well as to avoid alteration of vitamin A derivatives, we used a closed thermostatically controlled recycling system (Fig. 4).

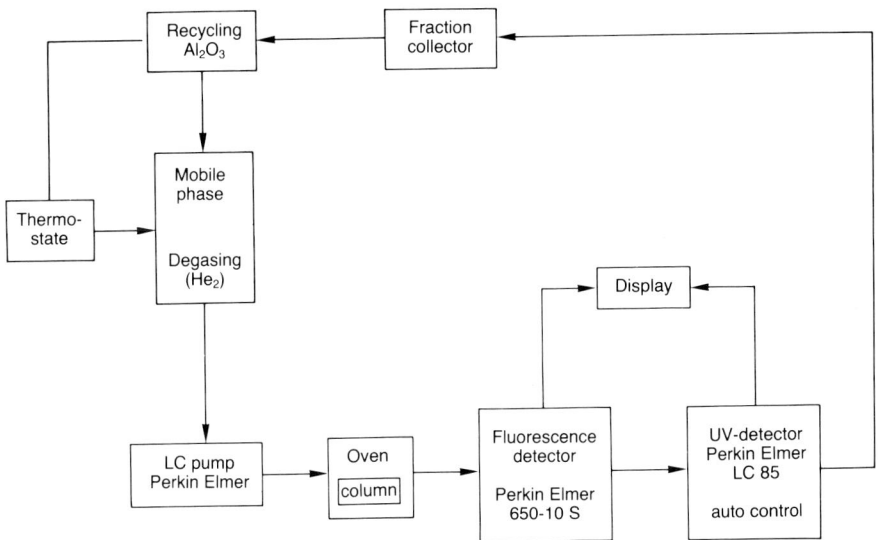

Fig. 4: HPLC recycling system.

Solvents were carefully degassed with helium (dried over sulfuric acid) and stored in brown glass bottles over sodium. After separation the different peaks were collected by a time- and concentration-dependent fraction collector (GILSON) and the mobile phase recycled over a thermostatized Al_2O_3-column back in the solvent sore. Thus we were able to detect 1 ng/ml extraction volume of different retinyl esters and aldehydes with a noise signal ratio of 5:1.

Constant solvent temperature and composition, as well as column equilibration under constant conditions for longer periods, are necessary to ensure sufficient separation and high sensitivity.

Animals

Determinations of vitamin A derivatives in sensory tissues were carried out in normally fed or vitamin A-deficient male guinea pigs. Pineal gland studies were done with normally fed or vitamin A-deficient male Sprague Dawley rats. Rats were chosen because they are the vertebrates in which most pineal gland experiments have been carried out, and the metabolism of different compounds (e.g. melatonin) is better understood in these animals.

Tissue handling and extraction procedure

48 normally nourished and 62 vitamin A-deficient guinea pigs were used. In all animals the Preyer reflex as a parameter for normal hearing function could be triggered easily. After weighing the animals were deeply anaesthetized and decapitated. Thereafter the tissues were removed and quick frozen immediately. The quick freezing was carried out in a mixture of propane:propylene (9:1) as intermediate in liquid nitrogen to avoid hindering heat conduction through nitrogen steam formation. Subsequently the tissues were dried for 48 h at –55 °C in a vacuum of 0.3×10^{-3} torr. Inner ear tissues were specially prepared. The bony cochlea was removed so that the membranous structures remained in situ and could be separated from each other easily. The tissue pieces were transferred into a dessicator until weighing to avoid adulteration of the weight due to absorption of humidity.

The tissue work up and vitamin A determination followed immediately after weighing on a Mettler analysis balance. The sensory epithelia were homogenized in a micro tissue grinder in 100 µl n-hexane. After freeze-drying, further protein denaturation was not necessary and extraction was possible in pure n-hexane. After centrifugation (10 min, 5000 rpm) the organic phase was pipetted off and analyzed.

Other organs such as liver, kidney and lung were first homogenized in a mortar and then aliquots of the organ powder were further homogenized in n-hexane using an Ultra Turrax.

Uptake of ^{14}C-retinyl acetate in sensory epithelia

Determinations were carried out in 36 vitamin A-deficient guinea pigs. Vitamin A-deficient guinea pigs were chosen because the vitamin A stores in sensory tissues are fully depleted so that no endogenous vitamin A is detectable. After oral administration of ^{14}C-14,15-retinyl acetate (5.1 µCi / animal in 250 µl olive oil), the animals were housed in metabolic cages for different time periods. Excretions and exhaled CO_2 (over 10 % KOH) were monitored separately. At predetermined intervals (2,4,6,8 and 12 h) the animals were sacrificed under light ether anaesthesia, and the different organs dissected and weighed.

Liquid samples (perilymph, serum, urine, bile) were counted immediately in a liquid scintillation counter (Packard 460 CD). The other organs were dried and oxidized (Packard sample oxidizer 30). Liver and the remaining tissues (skin, muscle, bone etc.) were homogenized and aliquots measured. The gastrointestinal tract was purified with chloroform:methanol (1:1) and aliquots measured. To ensure that the activity in different epithelia is due to vitamin A, a chemical identification was carried out by HPLC. The tissues were prepared as described above and chromatographically separated. The peaks were collected and the activity was measured in a liquid scintillation counter.

Determination of light-dependent behaviour of vitamin A derivatives in the pineal gland

The animals used were 24 vitamin A-deficient and 32 normally nourished male Sprague Dawley rats. Before the experiment, the animals had been kept for at least two weeks under LD 12:12 (lights on 7.00 h – 19.00 h, fluorescent bulbs Osram L 65410, «white universal»), five per cage under routine laboratory conditions (300 lux, 24 ± 2 °C room temperature, 50 % relative humidity, water ad libitum and special vitamin A-free or vitamin A-supplemented diet). The procedure of experiment is given in Figure 5. Determination of vitamin A derivatives was carried out as described above (Tables I, II).

Determination of the isomeric configuration of retinyl ester during light- and dark-adaptation

Retinyl esters and their isomeric configurations were measured as given in Table I (III, IV) in 60 light-adapted (48 h) and 60 dark-adapted (48 h) male Sprague Dawley rats. After decapitation all handling of samples and extraction procedures were carried out under dim red light to avoid further changes in vitro.

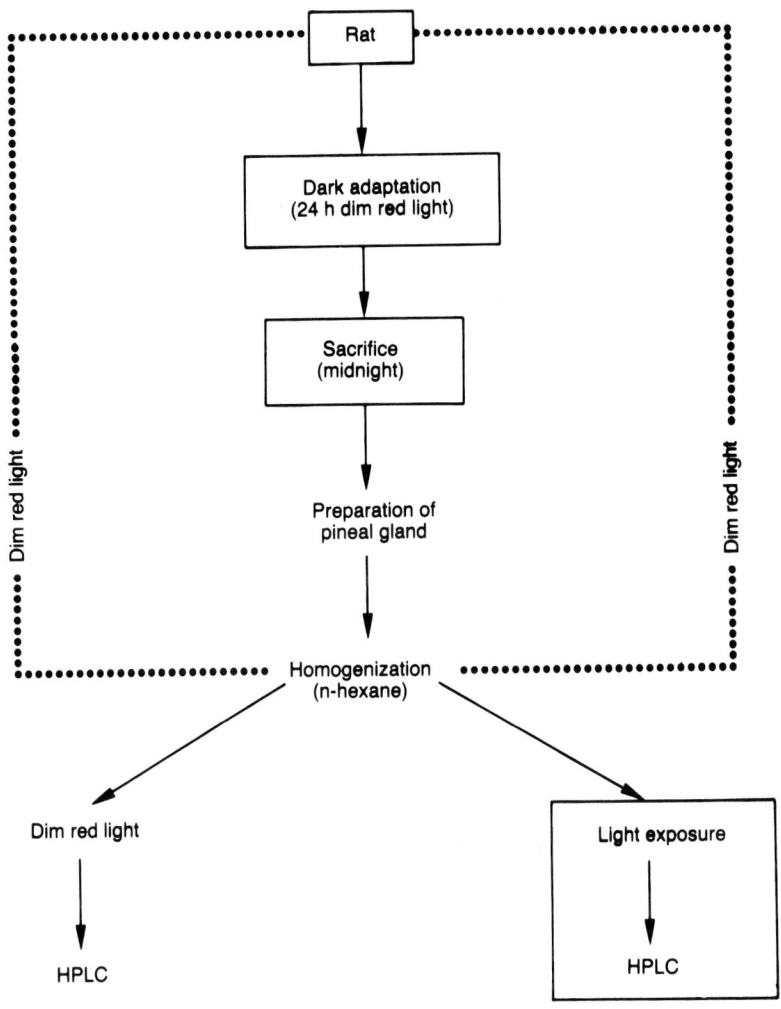

Fig. 5: Experimental procedure for determination of light-dependent behavior of vitamin A derivatives in the pineal gland.

Results

In sensory epithelia of normally nourished guinea pigs we detected all-trans retinyl palmitate and all-trans retinyl stearate in different ratios. In the sensory tissues of vitamin A-deficient guinea pigs, no vitamin A derivatives were detectable. In the rat pineal gland and in both normal and deficient animals, only all-trans palmitate was found (Fig. 6) in equivalent amounts. Compared with other organs the concentrations in sensory tissues of the guinea pig are very high, except in the liver (345 ± 85 µg retinyl ester/g dry weight), the main storage organ (Fig. 7). Similar high values were found only in the testicles pointing to the often observed dependence of spermatogenesis on vitamin A.

Figure 8 shows the time-dependent distribution of the orally administered ^{14}C-retinyl acetate in vitamin A-deficient guinea pigs after distinct time periods. During the first five hours we found decreasing amounts of retinyl palmitate in serum as a sign of excessive vitamin A feeding. After this time no further retinyl palmitate could be detected in serum. The tissue levels of ^{14}C-vitamin A remained constant after 6 hours and were identified as retinyl palmitate (Fig. 9).

No significant uptake of exogenously administered vitamin A could be detected in the pineal gland. Whereas during deficiency the tissue stores of in-

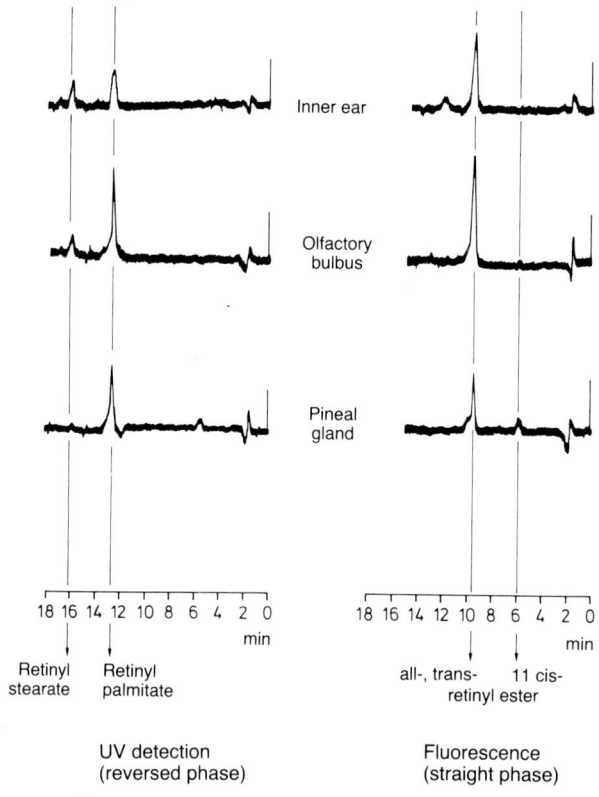

Fig. 6: Retinyl ester composition in sensory tissues.

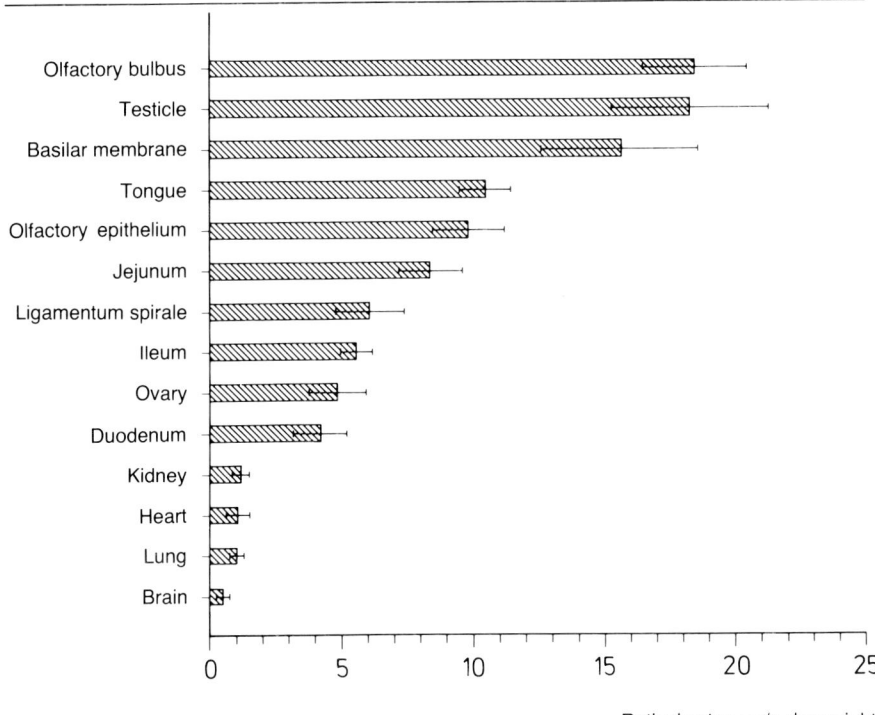

Fig. 7: Total amount of retinyl esters in different tissues of the guinea pig.

ner ear and olfactory bulbus are totally depleted, the pineal gland shows no alteration of retinyl ester content. Thus we assume that the pineal gland needs no further supplementation of this vitamin. The determination of vitamin A in the rat pineal gland (115 µg/g dry weight) shows retinyl esters when exposed to either dim red light or to polychromatic bright light for 45 min (Figs. 10, 11). In contrast – under the same chromatographic conditions – all-trans retinal and 11-cis retinal were demonstrable only after 45 min. exposure of the homogenate to polychromatic bright light (Fig. 11).

Identical results were obtained in animals killed at noon and at midnight, provided that the glands had been processed identically, i.e. without exposure of the homogenate to daylight or to artificial room light at night. During longer lasting dark adaptation (48 h) mainly 11-cis retinyl esters were detected in the rat pineal gland whereas during light adaptation (48 h) only all-trans retinyl esters (in both cases retinyl palmitate) were detectable (Fig. 12).

On-line scanning of the peaks clearly demonstrates the UV spectrum of vitamin A compared with external standards. External standards were handled under the same conditions as pineal glands after dissection to ensure that

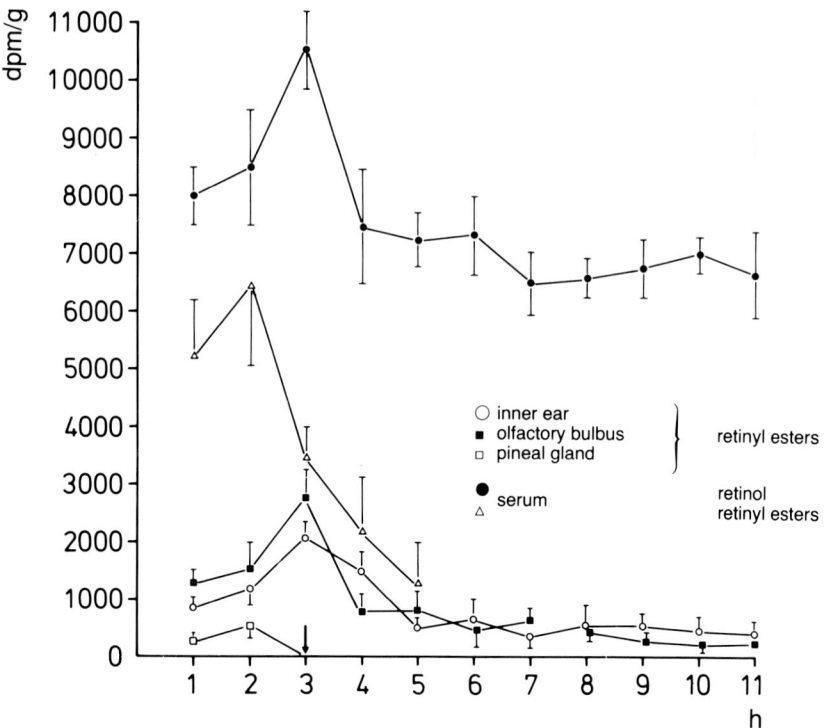

Fig. 8: Time-dependent distribution of orally administered ¹⁴C-retinyl acetate in sensory tissues and serum of vitamin A-deficient guinea pig.

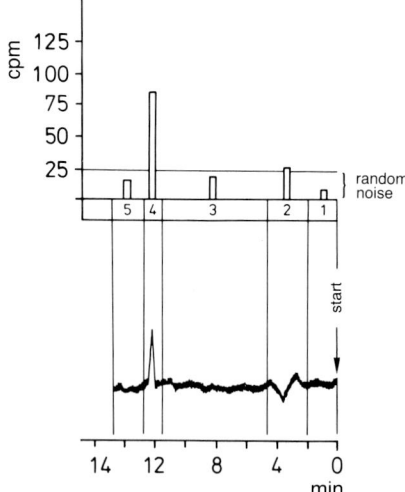

Fig. 9: Identification of radioactivity in the inner ear after 8 hours by HPLC. Main activity is related to all-trans retinyl palmitate.

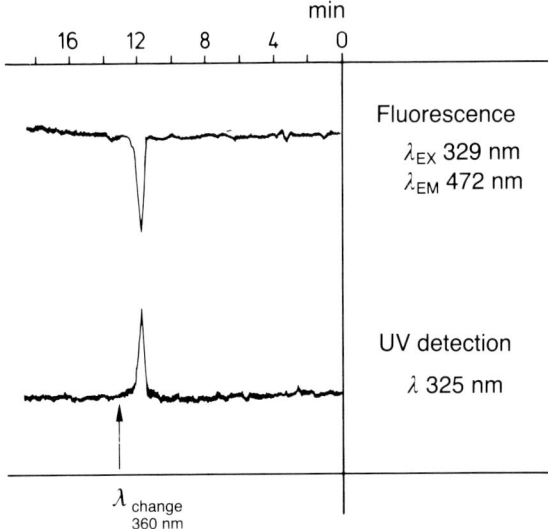

Fig. 10: Retinyl esters (all-trans retinyl palmitate) in dark-adapted rat pineal gland homogenates.

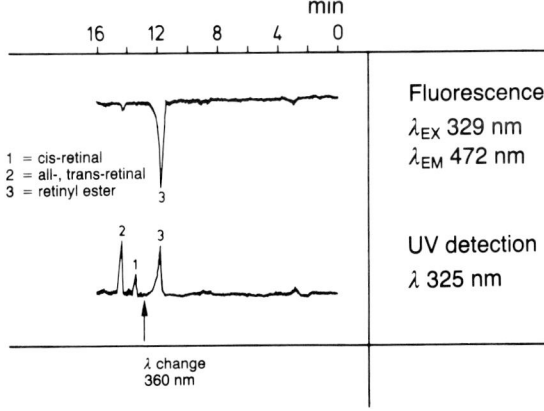

Fig. 11: Retinyl esters and retinal (all-trans, 11-cis) in light-exposed rat pineal gland homogenates.

no changes occurred in pineal gland homogenates in vitro. No alterations of the isometric configuration was observed during extraction and determination.

Discussion

The presence of the retinyl esters in the inner ear (mainly in the basilar membrane) and in the olfactory bulbus of the guinea pig is important. These are the storage forms of the vitamin, whereas the vitamin A alcohol – the

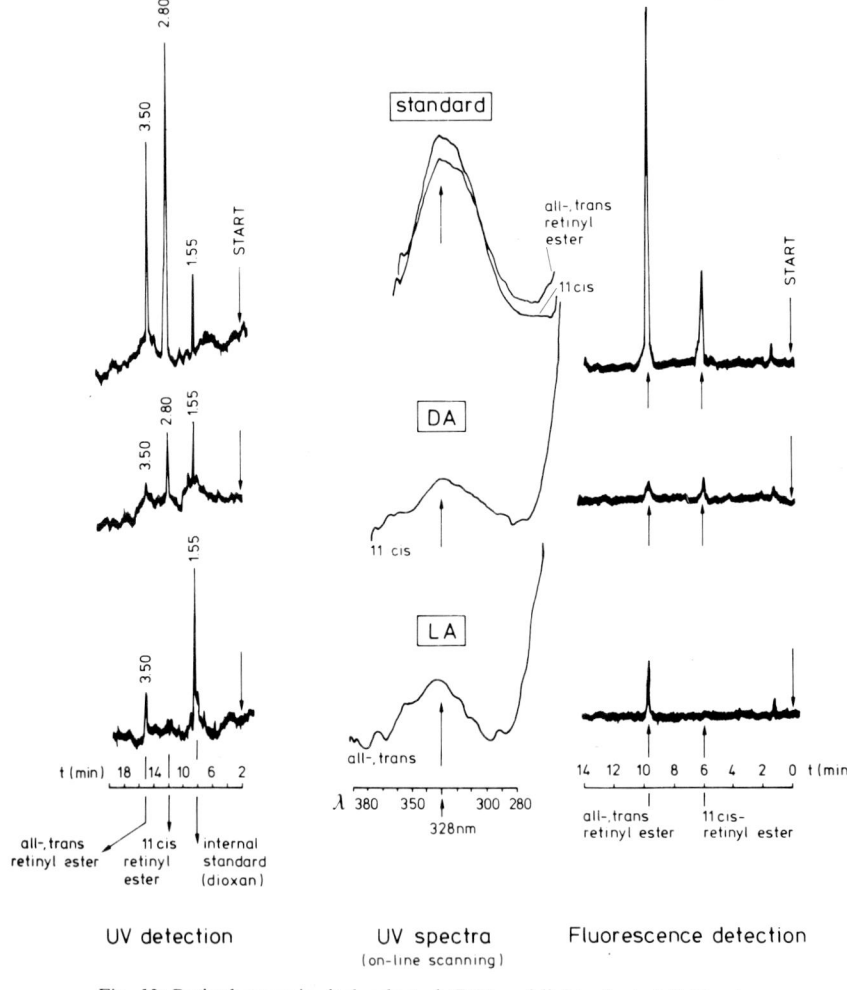

Fig. 12: Retinyl esters in dark-adapted (DA) and light-adapted (LA) rats.

retinol – is the transport form and can be detected only in small amounts in the stria vascularis. One can suppose that the inner ear and olfactory bulbus are capable of storing vitamin A in the form of its esters in a way similar to that of the eye [41–43].

As in the retina, we found retinyl palmitate and stearate in different ratios. In the inner ear the stearate: palmitate ratio ranged from 1:3.5 to 1:1.5. In the retina, other investigators found a stearate: palmitate ratio of 1:4.8 [44] to 1:4.3 [45] whereas the retinyl esters consist almost exclusively of the palmitate. In the retinas of light-adapted rats, a stearate: palmitate ratio of 1:1.3 was detected (44). The question arises as to whether this ratio has any significance or is due to distinct distribution of the different esters in the epithelia. With regard to the inner ear epithelia, it must be determined whether different esters have different locations in the basilar membrane because direct light-dependent alteration of ester composition might be excluded. However, another compound shows cyclic light changes in the inner ear: melatonin. We measured melatonin and melatonin-forming enzymes in the inner ear [46], and showed that melatonin synthesis is low during the day but increases five-fold during the night (maximum at 02.00 h). Thus the possibility arises that inner ear ester composition follows an unknown rhythm which has yet to be identified. An interesting aspect of this melatonin metabolism in the inner ear is that the retina also shows a circadian rhythm of melatonin and, like the inner ear, is capable of synthesizing melatonin, which until now has been known only for the pineal gland and harderian gland.

The uptake of exogenously administered ^{14}C-retinyl acetate, and esterification in the inner ear and olfactory bulbus of the transport form retinol indicate that the sensory tissues need vitamin A for either epithelial integrity or perceptive function.

However, since many tissues can esterify exogenous retinol (liver, intestinal mucosa, sertoli cells, pigmented retinal epithelium), the esterification of exogenous retinol by sensory tissues such as the inner ear and olfactory bulbus may not necessarily imply any functional significance of vitamin A.

Pineal gland

All the substances demonstrated in this study are known to be present in the retina where they play an integral role in light perception. All the visual pigments known at present follow the same principle. The photosensitive pigments of rods are known as rhodopsin, a combination of the protein opsin and a prosthetic group, 11-cis retinal. The pigment of the cones is iodopsin, a combination of retinal and protein, very similar to opsin, called photopsin.

Under the influence of light, rhodopsin is split into all-trans retinal and opsin, which is the appropriate stimulus for hyperpolarization of the photoreceptor cell membrane. By means of an isomerase, all-trans retinal is converted to 11-cis retinal which during dark adaptation together with opsin reforms rhodopsin.

The demonstration of vitamin A derivatives in the rat pineal gland is somewhat surprising. In lower vertebrates the functionally important cells of the pineal gland are cone-like photoreceptors [23]. In mammals, the fully differentiated pinealocytes lack outer segments, though early in development in rats [47–49] and in adult moles [50] structures vaguely resembling rudimentary outer segments have been detected. In one exceptional case, in the pinealocyte of an adult hamster, cone-like lamellar discs of outer segments were found [51]. In rat pinealocytes, the mitochondria are not evenly distributed throughout the cytoplasm, but form aggregations resembling the elipsoids of photoreceptor cells [23, 52].

There is ample biochemical evidence that the mammalian pineal gland is indirectly light-sensitive [23]. Pineal melatonin formation is low during photophase and high during scotophase. In sympathetically denervated pineal glands, the nocturnal increase of melatonin formation is no longer demonstrable, and exposure of animals to continuous illumination depresses the melatonin-forming activity of the pineal gland.

In adult mammals clear evidence has been obtained that the pineal gland does not respond directly to light. However there are some indications that direct light sensitivity of pineal gland exists in the newborn [53, 54] which is apparently lost during postnatal development.

In this context it is interesting to note that according to the results of the present study the components of a (functioning) rhodopsin cycle as well as different alterations during light and dark adaptation are demonstrable in pineal glands of adult rats. Especially important is the observation that all-trans and 11-cis retinal were not detectable in pineal glands dissected and processed under dim red light but only in light exposed glands. The fact that both 11-cis and all-trans retinal occur after light exposure seems strange but according to Bok [55] a pool of 11-cis vitamin A should be readily available during dark adaptation close to the site of synthesis. This should consist mainly of the 11-cis retinyl esters but the possibility must be considered that, in pineal glands, even 11-cis retinal is detectable during the process of combination with the presumed opsin.

The differences in the isomeric configurations of retinyl esters during light-

and dark-adaptation are in good agreement with the findings of BRIDGES [56] who showed that during dark adaptation in the frog retina the all-trans retinyl ester is partly isomerized to 11-cis ester.

The retinyl esters are the precursors of 11-cis retinal used for visual pigment regeneration during dark adaptation. In the pigmented epithelium of frogs about 99 % of the vitamin A is esterified and up to 55 % is in the form of the 11-cis isomer [57].

Whereas vitamin A in the retina of light-adapted rats consists of all-trans retinyl palmitate and all-trans retinyl stearate, in the dark-adapted albino rat eye the esters were not detectable [58, 59].

The question arises as to whether in vitro isomerization took place in our experiments. Although extraction of tissues in organic solvents was carried out under dim red light, isomerization of vitamin A compounds especially retinal might have been possible. The amount of this isomerization was determined for the retinal [60], for free 11-cis isomers of retinol and retinyl esters. The percent isomerization of 11-cis to all-trans ranged from 25.4 % for retinal to 8.7 % for retinol and 7.7 % for retinyl esters.

In light-adapted pineal glands we did not find any 11-cis isomer, and in dark-adapted pineal glands a small amount of all-trans retinyl ester might have been due to changes in vitro. No isomerization from all-trans to 11-cis retinyl ester was detected during handling with external standards. Thus it may be assumed that in the pineal gland an isomerase is acting on alltrans retinyl ester which might be involved by indirect light exposure. To test whether direct light exposure can split retinal or can involve isomerization of retinyl esters in the pineal gland, a pilot experiment was carried out in which intact rats and rats with shaved heads were exposed to natural daylight of 12 000–16 000 lux (between 11.00 h and 12.00 h). This experiment showed that apparently high light intensities are insufficient to demonstrate vitamin A derivatives in the pineal gland in situ. No isomerization takes place in these light-adapted rats.

Thus another way of inducing isomerase activity of retinyl ester must be sought. Whether there is any nervous or biochemical control which influences isomeric configuration during light- and dark-cycle is still a matter of speculation.

The functional significance of the present findings remains unclear. Vitamin A derivatives may be involved in the metabolic regulation of melatonin formation. The circadian rhythm of melatonin formation in the retina [61] suggests a fundamental similarity in their underlying organization. One may speculate that the rhythmic features of melatonin in retina, inner ear and pineal gland represent fundamental aspects of receptor metabolism. The question arises as to whether vitamin A metabolism in sensory epithelia is involved in circadian melatonin rhythm or itself involves this rhythmic pattern.

Conclusions

Different vitamin A derivatives could be detected in inner ear, olfactory bulbus and pineal gland. Furthermore it was shown that day/night differences exist in the rat pineal gland. These findings may lead to speculations as to whether all sensory receptors depend on vitamin A for perception process in the same way as the retina. Yet phenomenological results have to be confirmed by experiments which clearly demonstrate functional alterations of perceptive organs in relation to vitamin A metabolism.

We are able to lend support to Vinnikov's [1] hypothesis that some ciliated cells contain vitamin A but we are unable to conclude that it is essential to their function.

Acknowledgements: The author gratefully thanks Dr. H. Welker (melatonin determination) and Prof. Dr. L. Vollrath (Department of Anatomy, University of Mainz) for kind support and helpful discussions on pineal gland studies and Dres Weiser and Hanck (Hoffmann-La Roche, Basle) for their valuable support.

References

1 Vinnikov, J A: Principles of structural, chemical and functional organization of sensory receptors. Cold Spring Harbor Symp Quant Biol *30,* 243-299, 1965.
2 Wald, G: The molecular basis of visual excitation Nature *219,* 800-821, 1968.
3 Bernard, R A: The reversible effect of vitamin A on taste. Fed Proc *21,* 362, 1961.
4 Duncan, R B, Briggs, M: Treatment of uncomplicated anosmia by vitamin A. Arch Otolaryngol *75,* 116-124, 1962.
5 Escher, F, Rupp, F: Die Schutzfunktion des Vitamin A bei der Streptomycinintoxication. Acta Otol *43,* 311, 1953.
6 Rüedi, L: Wirkungen des Vitamin A im menschlichen und tierischen Gehörorgan. Schweiz Med Wschr *51,* 1411-14, 1954.
7 Tschirren, B: Die Schutzwirkung von Vitamin A bei der Streptomycin- und Neomycinvergiftung des Gehörorgans. Schweiz Med Wschr *51,* 1414-1415, 1954.
8 Videbech, H: Possibilities of treatment for deafness caused by streptomycin treatment with vitamin A. Ugeskr Laeg *120,* 708-709, 1958.
9 Willemse, C: Protection contre la surdité professionelle – rôle de la vitamine A. Acta med Belg *6,* 319, 1952.
10 Hume, E M, Krebs, H A: Vitamin A requirements of human adults. An experimental study of vitamin A deprivation in man. H M S O, p 124, London, 1949.

11 Sauberlich, H E, Hodges, R E: Vitamin A metabolism and requirements in the human studied with the use of labeled retinol. Vit Horm 32, 251–275, 1974.

12 Mellanby, E: The experimental production of deafness in young animals by diet. J Physiol 94, 380, 1938.

13 Loch, W E: Veränderungen der Labyrinthkapsel bei tierexperimentellen Avitaminosen. Mschr Ohrenhlkd 73, 542, 1939.

14 Chole, R A: Experimental studies on the role of vitamin A on the inner ear. Otol Head Neck Surg 86, 595–620, 1978.

15 Lawrence, M: Vitamin A deficiency and its relation to hearing. J Exp Psychol 29, 37–48, 1941.

16 Löhle, E: The influence of a chronic vitamin A deficiency on the acoustic sensory cells and the ganglion spirale cochleae of the rat. Arch Otorhinolaryngol 229, 45, 1980.

17 Covell, W P: Pathologic changes in peripheral auditory mechanism due to avitminosis. Laryngoscope 50, 632–647, 1940.

18 Lovino, M, Lecco, V: Avitaminosi 'A' experimentale ed orecchio. Arch Ital Otol 61, 177–188, 1950.

19 Ajodha, J M et al: Drug induced deafness and its treatment. Practitioner 216, 561–570, 1970.

20 Löhle, E: Unpublished data.

21 Bernard, R A et al: Effect of vitamin A deficiency on taste. Proc Soc Exptl Biol Med 108, 784–786, 1961.

22 Duncan, C J: The taste bud membrane and the role of vitamin A. Int J Vit Res 34, 410–414, 1964.

23 Vollrath, L: In: Oksche and Vollrath (eds) Handbuch der mikroskopischen Anatomie des Menschen, vol VI/7. Springer, Berlin 1981.

24 Vigh-Teichmann, I et al: Comparison of the pineal complex, retina and cerebrospinal fluid contacting neurons by immunocytochemical antirhodopsin. Z mikr anat Forsch 94, 623–640, 1980.

25 Vigh, B et al: Immunoreactive opsin in the pineal organ of reptiles and birds. Z mikr anat Forsch 96, 113–129, 1982.

26 Vigh, B, Vigh-Teichmann, I: Light and electronmicroscopic demonstration of immunoreactive opsin in the pinealocytes of various vertebrates. Cell Tissue Res 221, 451–463, 1981.

27 Hartwig, H G: Photolabile Substanzen im Pinealkomplex von Anuren. Verh Anat Ges 69, 439–441, 1975.

28 Hartwig, H G, Baumann, C: Evidence for photosensitive pigments in the pineal complex of the frog. Vision Res 14, 579–98, 1974.

29 Oksche, A, Hartwig, H G: Pineal sense organs – Components of photoneuroendocrine system. Progr Brain Res 52, 113–130, 1979.

30 Menaker, M, Oksche, A: The avian pineal organ. In: Farner and King (eds) Avian Biology, vol 4, pp 79–118. Academic Press, New York, 1974.

31 Collin, J P, Oksche, A: Structural and functional relationships in the nonmammalian pineal organ. In: Reiter (ed) The pineal gland, vol 1, pp 27–64. CRC Press, Boca Raton, 1981.

32 Rosner, J M et al: Direct effect of light on duck pineal explants. Life Sci 10, 1065–1069, 1971.

33 Rosner, J M et al: Direct action of light on serotonin metabolism and RNA biosynthesis in duck pineal explants. Life Sci 11, 829–836, 1972.

34 Deguchi, T: Circadian rhythm of serotonin N acetyltransferase-activity in organ culture of chicken pineal gland. Science 203, 1245–1247, 1979.

35 Wainwright, S D, Wainwright, L K: Chick pineal serotonin acetyltransferase: a diurnal cycle maintained in vitro and its regulation by light. Can J Biochem 57, 700–709, 1979.
36 Wainwright, S D, Wainwright, L K: The relationship between variations in levels of serotonin acetyltransferase activity and cGMP content in cultured chick pineal gland. Can J Biochem 59, 593–601, 1981.
37 Kasal, C A, Perez Polo, J R: In vitro evidence of photoreception in the chick pineal gland and its interaction with the circadian clock controlling N-acetyltransferase (NAT). J Neurosci Res 5, 579–585, 1980.
38 Deguchi, T: Rhodopsin like photosensitivity of isolated chicken pineal gland. Nature 290, 702–704, 1981.
39 Wurtman, R J et al: The pineal. Academic Press, New York, 1968.
40 Hubbard, R et al: Methodology of vitamin A and visual pigments. In: Mc Cormick and Wright (eds) Methods in enzymology, vol XVIII. Vitamins and coenzymes, part C. Academic Press, New York, 1971.
41 Krinski, N Y: The enzymatic esterification of vitamin A. J Biol Chem 232, 881–894, 1958.
42 Bridges, C D B: Storage, distribution and utilization of vitamin A in the eyes of adult amphibians and their tadpoles. Vision Res 15, 1311–1322, 1975.
43 Wald, G: The visual system and vitamin A of the sea lamprey. J Gen Physiol 25, 331–336, 1942.
44 Bridges, C D B et al: Vitamin A in human eyes: Amount, distribution and composition. Invest Ophthal 22, 706–714, 1982.
45 Futtermann, S, Andrews, J S: The fatty acid composition of human retinal vitamin A ester and the lipids of human retinal tissue. Invest Ophthal 3, 441, 1961.
46 Biesalski, H K, Welker, H: Distribution of melatonin and melatonin synthesis in the guinea pig inner ear. Acta Otolaryngol (in press).
47 Clabough, J W: Ultrastructural studies of pineal cytogenesis in fetal rats and hamsters. Anat Rec 166, 291, 1970.
48 Clabough, J W: Cytological aspects of pineal development in rats and hamsters. Am J Anat 137, 215–230, 1973.
49 Zimmermann, B L, Tso, M: Morphologic evidence of photoreceptor differentiation of pinealocytes in the neonatal rat. J Cell Biol 66, 60–75, 1975.
50 Pevet, P: The pineal gland of the mole (Talpa europaea L.) The fine structure of pinealocytes. Cell Tissue Res 153, 277–292, 1974.
51 Nadakavukaren, M J, Bucana, C D: Cone like structure in the pineal gland of the hamster. J Submicr Cytol 12, 691–693, 1980.
52 Wolfe, D E: The epiphyseal cell: an electronmicroscopic study of its intercellular relationship morphology in the pineal body of the albino rat. Progr Brain Res 10, 332–386, 1965.
53 Hakanson, D O, Bergstrom, W H: Phototherapy-induced hypocalcaemia in newborn rats: prevention by meltonin. Science 214, 807–809, 1981.
54 Zweig, M et al: Evidence for a non-retinal pathway of light to the pineal glands of newborn rats. Proc Natl Acad Sci USA 56, 515, 1966.
55 Bok, D: Autoradiographic studies on the incorporation of ^{3}H-11,12-retinol into rod photoreceptors of the frog. Assoc Res Vision Ophthal, No 5, p 32, Sarasota, 1982.
56 Bridges, C D B: Vitamin A and the role of pigment epithelium during bleaching and regeneration of rhodopsin in the frog eye. Exp Eye Res 22, 435–455, 1976.
57 Alvarez, R A: High pressure liquid chromatography of fatty acid esters of retinol isomers. Invest Ophthal 30, 304, 1981.
58 Dowling, J F: Chemistry of visual adaptation in the rat. Nature 188, 144, 1960.
59 Zimmermann, W F: The distribution and proportions of vitamin A compounds during the visual cycle in the rat. Vision Res 14, 795, 1974.

60 Daemen, F J M *et al:* On the rhodopsin cycle. Exp Eye Res *18,* 97–103, 1974.
61 Binkley, S *et al:* NAT responds to environmental lighting in the eye as well as in the pineal gland. Nature *281,* 479–481, 1979.
62 Binkley, S *et al:* N-acteyltransferase in the chick retina I. Circadian rhythms controlled by environmental lighting are similar to those in the pineal gland. J Comp Physiol (B) *139,* 103–108, 1980.

Dr. H.K. Biesalski, Physiologisch-chemisches Institut II, Universität Mainz, Saarstrasse 21, D-6500 Mainz, West Germany

Drug-Vitamin Interaction

T.K. Basu

Department of Foods and Nutrition, University of Alberta, Edmonton, Alberta, Canada

Key Words: Drugs · Ascorbate · Folacin · Vitamins · Risk groups · Aspirin · Anticonvulsants

Abstract: Most of the drugs in use today for the treatment of human diseases owe their activity to a selectively toxic effect on an infective or invasive agent, or to the selective inhibition of an enzyme system. It is increasingly being recognized that the vitamin status is one of the major factors capable of modifying the pharmacological effect of drugs. Conversely, the disease itself and drug treatment of a disease may impair the vitamin nutriture of a patient with consequent effects upon the body's response to drugs. This paper will be concerned with these aspects of drug-interaction with vitamins with particular references to ascorbic acid and folacin, the deficiencies of which are often encountered in risk groups, such as the elderly.

Introduction

During the last 50 years, medicine has experienced a profound transformation with the ability to cure most infectious diseases due to the discovery of the sulphonamides and antibiotics, the amelioration of mental disease by the use of phenothiazines, tricyclic drugs, barbiturates and benzodiazepines, the successful treatment of cardiovascular disease with diuretics and β-blockers, and of gastrointestinal disease with H_2-receptor antagonists and carbenoxolone, and the treatment of many more disease states by other new discoveries of the medicinal chemist. Together with the widespread use of drugs has come the gradual but increasing recognition of the significance of interactions between drugs [1]. One drug may interfere with the intestinal absorption or renal excretion of another drug, or block its binding to plasma proteins and tissue receptor sites, or one drug may accelerate or retard the metabolic transformations of another drug. Pharmacologists and clinicians have thus realized the importance of taking into account drug-drug interactions in order to obtain maximal therapeutic effectiveness as well as to minimize the incidence and severity of adverse reactions.

More recently, there has also been increasing recognition of the many physiological and pathological variables which influence the body's response to drugs [2]. Such factors as genetic, age, hormones, disease, heavy metals and nutrition, have profound effects upon the results of drug administration. As yet, however, relatively little consideration has been given to the effect of drugs upon nutrition or to that of nutritional alterations upon the pharmacological effect of drugs. Some drugs may affect the nutritional status [3] by decreasing appetite (e.g., amphetamines, mazindol and biguanides); some may increase appetite (e.g., insulin, steroids, sulphonylureas, psychotropic drugs and anti-histamines); some may impair the absorption of nutrients either by altering the morphology of the intestinal mucosa (e.g., neomycin, phenindione and p-aminosalicylic acid), by inhibiting the digestive enzymes (e.g., chlorotetracycline) or by causing nausea, vomiting and diarrhea (e.g., cytotoxic drugs); and some may affect electrolyte balance (e.g., diuretics, corticosteroids). Conversely, the nutritional status is one of the major factors capable of modifying the metabolism of drugs [4].

Drug and Vitamin Interactions

It may seem strange to suggest that drugs should enter into a consideration of the physiological requirements for vitamins. However, in adequate dietary vitamin intake is not the only way that deficiencies occur. A number of secondary mechanisms exist, not the least of which is drug-induced vitamin deficiency. Administration of drugs producing latent deficiencies in otherwise healthy populations may not be much of a problem, but administration of these drugs to patients with superimposed disease processes or to subjects with impaired nutritional status can result in hypovitaminosis with the respective symptoms. In view of the ready availability of drugs prescribed by the clinicians, combined with the ease with which many pharmaceutical preparations can be obtained over the counter without a prescription, drug-induced vitamin deficiencies deserve more attention than they have so far received.

The interaction between vitamins and drugs is influenced by the effects of drugs on the functions of vitamins and on the enzymes which they control. Drugs may also affect the bacterial synthesis in the gastrointestinal tract as well as the rates of absorption, utilization and elimination of vitamins [5]. A full discussion of all the vitamins that are affected by drug therapy would be too long for this presentation; only two vitamins, ascorbic acid and folic acid, will be discussed in some detail in relation to their interaction with drugs.

Ascorbic Acid

Several drugs listed in Table I have been reported to cause ascorbic acid deficiency by depleting tissue stores, as indicated by decreased leucocyte levels of the vitamin. Among these drugs, salicylate-containing agents such as aspirin are perhaps the most commonly and chronically used drugs, and hence impose a serious problem on our community at large. The interactions between aspirin and ascorbic acid have been the subject of many studies. Thus, administration of therapeutic doses of aspirin to healthy volunteers was found to decrease the metabolic availability of ascorbate [17]. Isolated reports indicate that rheumatoid arthritic patients who ingest high doses of aspirin have low plasma levels of ascorbic acid [18].

Tab. I: Drugs affecting ascorbate status

Drug	Possible mechanisms	References
Corticosteroids	increased oxidation	6
Calcitonin	increased utilization	7
Tetracycline	competitive blockage of intracellular metabolism interference with tubular reabsorption	8–10
Oral contraceptives	increased oxidation	11–13
Salicylates	decreased absorption	14–16

In order to highlight the possible mechanism for the ascorbate-aspirin interaction, the effect of soluble aspirin on the utilizable ascorbic acid in human subjects has been investigated [18]. In this study, the concentrations of ascorbate in plasma, leucocytes and urine were found to be markedly elevated at various intervals following administration of a single oral dose of 500 mg of the vitamin (Fig. 1). The ascorbate-associated increases appeared to be blocked, however, when vitamin C was given simultaneously with aspirin (900 mg).

The respiratory tract is the major route of elimination for ascorbic acid in guinea pigs. About 60–70% of a dose of vitamin C is metabolized to CO_2 and expired in the breath of these animals during the first 10 days following administration, half of which is eliminated during the first day. Exhalation of CO_2 provides, therefore, a good means by which the metabolism of ascorbate and its interactions with other agents may be studied. Using $(1-^{14}C)$ ascorbic acid, the rate of exhalation of CO_2 has been shown to be three times higher in

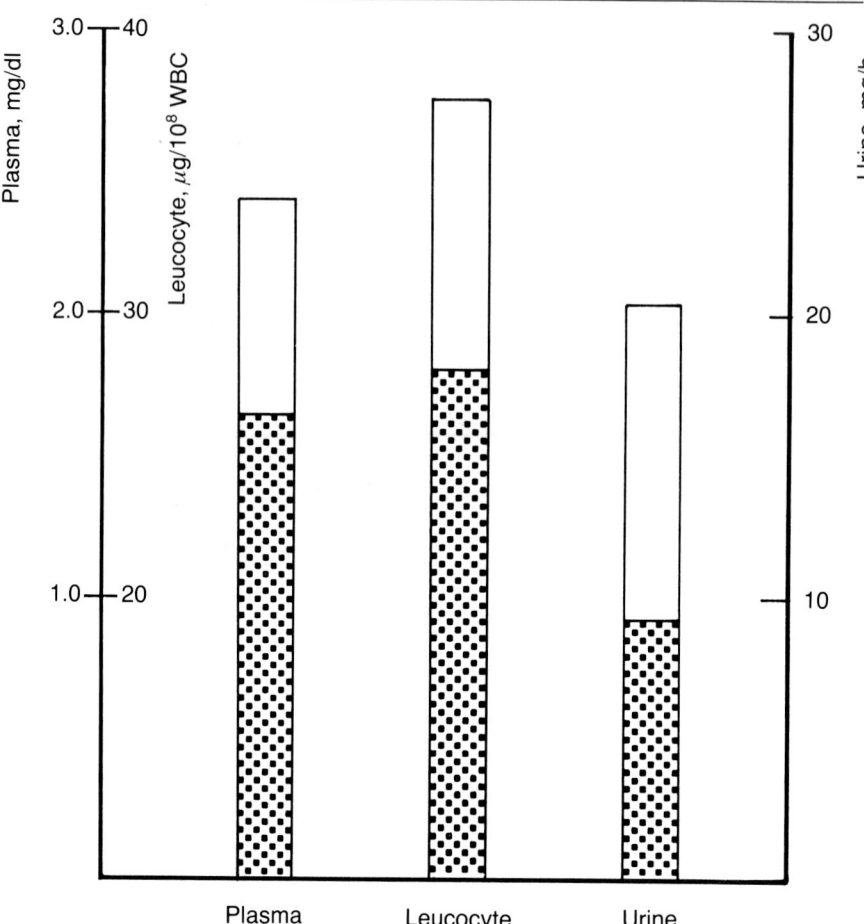

Fig. 1: Ascorbate levels in plasma, leucocytes and urine in female subjects 3 h following an oral dose of aspirin (900 mg) either alone (n = 7) or in combination (n = 7) with ascorbate (500 mg). Dotted columns = ascorbate + aspirin; open columns = ascorbate.

guinea pigs receiving ascorbic acid alone than in those given the vitamin simultaneously with sodium salicylate [16]. The rate of exhalation appeared to reach a peak at about 90 min in the animals given ascorbate alone, while in the presence of salicylate the peak exhalation time was approximately 160 min (Table II). The metabolic bioavailability of ascorbic acid during the first 400 min appeared to be reduced by half following simultaneous administration of salicylate. It is unlikely that aspirin interfered with the metabolism of ascorbic acid, since a decrease in the rate of CO_2 exhalation following aspirin administration was evident as early as 10 min after the administration of ascorbate when the rate of absorption was much higher than the rate of elimination. Furthermore, the rate of CO_2 exhalation, following the completion of absorption and the distribution phases, was the same in the animals taking ascorbate alone or ascorbate plus aspirin. These observations suggest that aspirin may impair the gastro-intestinal absorption of ascorbic acid.

Tab. II: Effect of Na-salicylate on the $^{14}CO_2$ exhalation following ingestion of L-(1-^{14}C)ascorbic acid in guinea pigs

Parameter	Ascorbic acid	Ascorbic acid + Na-salicylate
Initial rate of exhalation, dpm $\times$ 10^3/min	7.7	2.3
Peak exhalation rate, dpm $\times$ 10^3/min	9.1	3.0
Time taken to reach peak exhalation rate, min	87.5	157.0
Area under the curve (0–400 min), dpm/10^6	2.2	1.1

Folic acid

A volume of literature has accumulated in relation to the effects of a variety of drugs on folate metabolism (Table III). These studies range from case reports of megaloblastic anemia to studies of blood folacin levels. Of the drugs listed in Table III, barbiturates, phenytoin and primidone are the agents which are most chronically and extensively used to control seizures in epileptics, and barbiturates are taken as sleeping agents by all population groups. Although megaloblastic anemia in epileptics taking anticonvulsants is relatively rare, and occurs in less than 1 % [33], the incidence of low serum folate levels in this group was found in various studies to range from 27 to 91 % [34]. Lowered serum folate also appears to be significantly correlated with reduced red cell folate concentrations [35].

The mechanism by which the drugs induce folate deficiency is believed to be malabsorption of folic acid due to the inhibition of the intestinal conjugase enzyme, which promotes folate absorption by reducing dietary polyglutamate to the monoglutamate form [28]. Another theory holds that phenobarbital and phenytoin, both potent inducers of NADPH-dependent hepatic microsomal enzymes, compete for the folic acid coenzymes [36].

Correction of folate deficiency as a result of anticonvulsant therapy is an area of much debate. Folic acid supplementation was reported to provoke

Tab. III: Drugs affecting folacin status

Drug	Possible mechanism	References
Methotrexate Pyrimethamine Trimethoprim	inhibition of dihydro- folate reductase	19–22
Barbiturates Phenytoin Primidone	decreased absorption competitive inhibition of vitamin coenzymes enzyme induction	23–28
Sulfasalizine	decreased absorption	29
Oral contraceptives	increased synthesis of folate-binding macroglobulin	30–32

seizures in many case trial studies [37, 38]. The accelerated anticonvulsant metabolism resulting in lowered serum drug levels [39] and in an increased CSF folate level [40, 41] was implicated in such effects. However, numerous controlled studies revealed little or no effect on the seizure frequency of folate supplementation [42, 43].

The importance of folate especially in pregnancy is well established. It has been suggested that folate deficiencies in pregnant women may be related to premature babies, low birthweights, and complications during pregnancy [56]. Folate supplementation is believed to be a useful tool in the prevention of some cases of pre-term birth or of low birthweight. Much criticism, however, has been levelled against the indiscriminate use of folate therapy in pregnant epileptic women [44–46]. If teratogenesis of anticonvulsants is dose-dependent [47], the folate-associated lowering of serum anticonvulsant levels to concentrations still affording full protection against seizures could decrease the risk of congenital malformation. Insight into the mechanisms by which anticonvulsants exert their action on folate absorption and metabolism will hopefully lead to better prophylactic and therapeutic measures for epilepsy.

Risk Populations

Drug-mediated vitamin deficiency may be of clinical significance, especially in people with borderline intake and abnormal metabolism of vitamins, such as alcoholics, the ill and the aged. Indeed, a number of dietary surveys of people over 65 years of age have suggested that the intake of various nutrients with particular reference to vitamins is reduced with increasing age. The causes of malnutrition may be found in a variety of factors [66], including social isolation, physical disability, mental disturbances, impaired appetite, malabsorption, alcohol and drugs, increased requirement for certain vitamins. All these factors may not only affect the dietary intake but also the body-pool size of vitamins by altering their rates of absorption, utilization, catabolism and excretion.

Ascorbic acid is of concern for the elderly, since both plasma and tissue concentrations of this vitamin fall with increasing age [48]. There is substantial evidence based on studies carried out in the United Kingdom, suggesting that inadequate dietary intake may be the principal cause of the low ascorbic acid status in the elderly [49]. However, studies carried out in North America indicate that the elderly may have a higher requirement for ascorbic acid due to either impaired absorption or increased utilization [50]. In a recent study [51] involving 270 free-living, healthy elderly subjects (60 years of age and older), the average daily dietary intake of ascorbic acid was found to be 137 mg for women (n = 145) and 142 mg for men (n = 125). In addition, 156 of these subjects consumed more than 350 mg/day as ascorbic acid supplements. Despite the large daily intake, eleven subjects exhibited plasma levels below 0.4 mg/dl, representing a high risk group according to the criteria used in the Nutrition Canada Survey [52].

Folic acid deficiency is endemic in many parts of the world. It presents more acutely when an added folate stress is present. This occurs commonly in pregnancy, at times of rapid growth in early life, and in old age. In recent years, considerable attention has been paid to the folate status of the elderly. Dietary surveys in the United Kingdom revealed the existence of biochemical or clinical evidence of folate deficiency in 10–27% of an elderly population [53]. In developing countries the frequency of deficiency may exceed 90% in children and 50% in adults. A recent study carried out in the United States involving 270 free-living healthy men and women over 60 years of age showed that more than 37% of this group received dietary folic acid less than 50% of the recommended dietary allowance [54].

Drug Metabolism and Toxicity in Vitamin Deficiency

Vitamin malnutrition due to either shortage of food in the developing countries or wrong choice of food in the affluent communities, appears to be prevalent in a considerable segment of the world population, especially in the

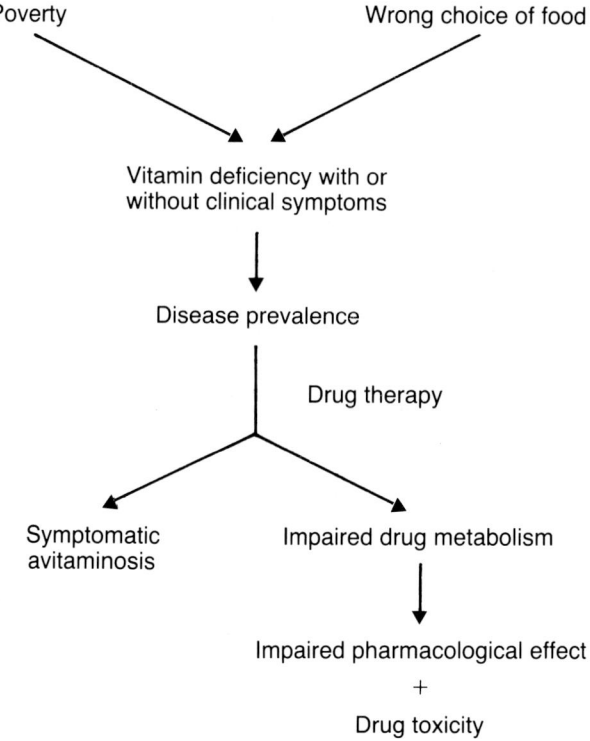

Fig. 2: Consequences of drug-induced vitamin deficiency.

elderly. The deficiency state is exacerbated when these subjects are treated with drugs, resulting in many cases in overt deficiency with clinical manifestations (Fig. 2). Such deficiencies may, in turn, result in drug toxicity by impairing the rates of drug metabolism.

The metabolism of drugs occurs in two phases, namely biotransformation (oxygenation, reduction and hydrolysis) or phase 1 metabolism, and conjugation (with glucuronic acid, glycine and sulphate) or phase 2 metabolism. Both phases of drug metabolism are brought about by a variety of enzymes, which are primarily located in the endoplasmic reticulum of the liver cells. The enzymes which catalyze the biotransformations are predominantly the microsomal mixed function oxidases (MFO), whereas those which catalyze the conjugations and the transferases are located in the endoplasmic reticulum or in the cytosol of the cell. The MFO system consists essentially of an electron transport chain extending from the reduced coenzyme (NADPH.H$^+$) through reductases to the terminal oxygen transferring enzyme, cytochrome

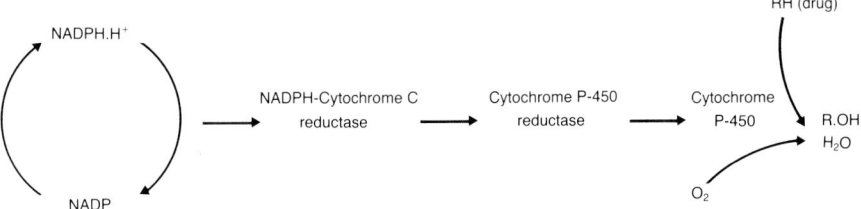

Fig. 3: The microsomal mixed-function oxidase system.

P–450 (Fig. 3). Molecular oxygen is required for the oxygenation, and one atom of the oxygen is inserted into the drug substrate; the other combines with two hydrogen atoms to form a molecule of water.

The activities of many of the enzymes involved in drug metabolism were shown to be dependent on the nutritional status including the vitamin status. Thus, there is increasing experimental evidence suggesting that the hepatic microsomal drug metabolizing enzyme system can be affected by the deficiency of various vitamins such as retinol [55], α-tocopherol [56], riboflavin [57], and ascorbate [58]. Among these vitamins, ascorbic acid has been most extensively studied in relation to drugs. In addition to the evidence linking changes in the activity of hepatic microsomal drug-metabolizing enzymes with changes in ascorbic acid status in guinea pigs [59], the excretion of ascorbic acid appeared to be markedly increased in rats receiving a variety of drugs [60]. The drug-induced ascorbic aciduria implies an induced biosynthesis of the vitamin, and this may be due to its increased requirement. It is, therefore, possible that in humans, who are unable to synthesize ascorbate when undergoing therapy with these drugs, ascorbic acid deficiency may be precipitated if the increased need is not met through either dietary intake or supplementation.

In man, 95 % of antipyrine is metabolized by the hepatic microsomal mixed function oxidase system. In a recent study in human volunteers given 500 mg of ascorbic acid daily for 12 months, the plasma half-life of antipyrine was shown to decrease, associated with an increased renal clearance [61]. These results indicate that ascorbate influences the ability to metabolize drugs not only in experimental animals, but also in humans.

Conclusions

The interrelationships between vitamins and the metabolism of drugs are important in view of the widespread occurrence of primary malnutrition in developing countries and of secondary malnutrition in certain disease states in more affluent countries. The study of this interrelationship may be viewed as an extension of the search for factors that modify drug action and dosage. A variety of drugs also appear to interfere with the availability and utilization of certain vitamins and may thus affect the vitamin nutriture of the patient. It may be necessary either to increase the intake of a vitamin or to decrease the dosage of a drug in order to counteract any detrimental effect of a drug upon vitamin status, and vice versa. Such considerations are of importance, especially in the risk groups, such as elderly, alcoholics, epileptics, arthritics, dieters and the children, where even the normal complex pharmacokinetics of drug metabolism may be further complicated by additional physiological factors. The ability to metabolize and dispose of active drugs in the elderly, for example, decreases progressively with age [62, 63], primarily due to impaired detoxication mechanisms, impaired kidney function, and primary or secondary deficiencies of vitamins. These factors may account for the known high incidence of adverse drug reactions in the elderly [64, 65].

References

1 IOANNIDES, C: Drug interactions. In: BASU (ed) Clinical implications of drug use p 31. CRC Press, Boca Raton, 1980.
2 BASU, T K: Principles of drug metabolism. In: BASU (ed) Clinical implications of drug use, p 1. CRC Press, Boca Raton, 1980.
3 BASU, T K: Interaction of drugs and nutrition. J Human Nutr 31, 449–458, 1977.
4 BASU, T K, DICKERSON, J W T: Interrelationship of nutrition and the metabolism of drugs. Chem Biol Interact 8, 193, 1974.
5 BASU, T K: Drug and vitamin interactions in adults. Int J Vit Nutr Res, suppl 26, pp 157–168, 1984.
6 BARTHOLOMEW, G: Rheumatoid arthritis and prednisone-treated scurvy. Postgrad Med J 48, 243, 1972.
7 BASU, T K: Ascorbic acid therapy for the relief of bone pain in Paget's disease. Acta Vitaminol Enzymol 32, 45–49, 1978.
8 SHAH, K V et al: Ascorbic acid levels in blood during tetracycline administration. J Ind Med Assoc 51, 127, 1968.
9 WINDSOR, A C M et al: Effects of tetracycline on leucocyte ascorbic acid levels. Br Med J 1, 214–215, 1972.
10 GOLDSMITH, G A: Current status of the clinical use of antibiotic-vitamin combinations. N Engl J Med 254, 165, 1956.
11 HARRIS, A B: Reduced ascorbic acid excretion and oral contraceptives. Lancet ii, 201, 1973.

12 RIVERS, J M, DEVINE, M M: Plasma ascorbic acid concentrations and oral contraceptives. Am J Clin Nutr 25, 684, 1972.

13 CARRUTHERS, M E et al: Raised serum copper and ceruloplasmin levels in subjects taking oral contraceptives. J Clin Pathol 19, 498, 1966.

14 LOH, H S, WILSON, C W M: The interactions of aspirin and ascorbic acid in normal men. J Clin Pharmacol 15, 36, 1975.

15 SAHUD, M A, COHEN, R J: Effect of aspirin ingestion on ascorbic acid levels in rheumatoid arthritis. Lancet i, 937, 1971.

16 IOANNIDES, C et al: Impairment of absorption of ascorbic acid following ingestion of aspirin in guinea pigs. Biochem Pharmacol 31, 4035–4038, 1982.

17 LOH, H S et al: The effects of aspirin on the metabolic availability of ascorbic acid in human beings. J Clin Pharmacol 13, 480, 1973.

18 BASU, T K: The influence of drugs with particular reference to aspirin on the bioavailability of vitamin C. In: COUNSELL and HORNIG (eds). Vitamin C (ascorbic acid), pp 273–289. Applied Science, London, 1981.

19 BORRIE, P, CLARK, P A: Megaloblastic anaemia during methotrexate treatment of psoriasis. Br Med J 1, 1339, 1966.

20 WAXMAN, S et al: Drugs, toxins, and dietary amino acids affecting vitamin B_{12} or folic acid absorption or utilization. Am J Med 48, 599, 1970.

21 JEWKES, R F et al: Hematological changes in a patient on long-term treatment with a trimethoprim-sulphonamide combination. Postgrad Med J 46, 723, 1970.

22 TENPAS, A, ABRAHAM, J P: Hematological side effects of pyrimethamine in the treatment of ocular toxoplasmosis. Am J Med Sci 249, 448, 1965.

23 BERNSTEIN, L H: The absorption and malabsorption of folic acid and its polyglutamates. Am J Med 48, 570, 1971.

24 FEHLING, C et al: The effect of anticonvulsant therapy upon the absorption of folates. Clin Sci 44, 595, 1973.

25 HAGHSHENASS, M, RAO, D B: Serum folate levels during anticonvulsant therapy with diphenylhydantoin. J Am Geriat Soc 21, 275, 1973.

26 JENSEN, O N, OLESEN, O V: Subnormal serum folate due to anti-convulsive therapy. Arch Neurol 22, 181, 1970.

27 REYNOLDS, E H: Iatrogenic nutritional effects of anticonvulsants. Proc Nutr Soc 33, 225, 1974.

28 STRAUM, W et al: Intestinal folate absorption. N^5-methyltetrahydrofolic acid. J Clin Invest 50, 1910, 1971.

29 FRANKLIN, J L, ROSENBERG, I H: Impaired folic acid absorption in inflammatory bowel disease: effects of salicylazosulfapyridine. Gastroenterology 64, 517, 1973.

30 SHOJANIA, A M, HORNADY, G J: Oral contraceptives and folate absorption. J Lab Clin Med 82, 869, 1973.

31 LINDENBAUM, J et al: Oral contraceptive hormones, folate metabolism and cervical epithelium. Am J Clin Nutr 28, 346, 1975.

32 DACOSTA, M, ROTHENBERG, S P: Appearance of folate binder in leucocytes and serum of women who are pregnant or taking oral contraceptives. J Lab Clin Med 83, 207, 1974.

33 REYNOLDS, E H: Anticonvulsants, folic acid and epilepsy. Lancet i, 1376, 1973.

34 REYNOLDS, E H: Neurological aspects of folate and vitamin B_{12} metabolism. Clinics Hematol 5, 661, 1976.

35 PREECE, J et al: Relation of serum to red cell folate concentrations in drug-treated epileptic patients. Epilepsia 12, 335, 1971.

36 MAXWELL, J D et al: Folate deficiency after anticonvulsant drugs: an effect of hepatic enzyme induction. Br Med J 1, 297, 1972.

37 CHAMARIN, I et al: Megaloblastic anemia due to phenobarbitone. Br Med J 1, 1099, 1960.

38 WELLS, D G: Folic acid and neuropathy in epilepsy. Lancet i, 146, 1968.

39 BAYLISS, E M et al: Influence of folic acid on blood-phenytoin levels. Lancet i, 62, 1971.
40 SPECTOR, R G: Influence of folic acid on excitable tissues. Nature 240, 247, 1972.
41 BAXTER, M G et al: Some studies on the convulsant action of folic acid. Br J Pharmacol 48, 350P, 1973.
42 NORRIS, J W, PRATT, R F: A controlled study of folic acid in epilepsy. Neurology 21, 659, 1971.
43 GIBBERD, F B et al: The influence of folic acid on the frequency of epileptic attacks. Eur J Clin Pharmacol 19, 57, 1981.
44 WAZIRI, J et al: Teratogenic effect of anticonvulsant drugs. Am J Dis Child 130, 1022, 1976.
45 DEVORE, G R, WOODBURY, D M: Phenytoin: an evaluation of several potential teratogenic mechanisms. Epilepsia 18, 387, 1977.
46 STUMPF, D A, FROST, M: Seizures, anticonvulsants, and pregnancy. Am J Dis Child 132, 746, 1978.
47 HARBISON, R D, BECKER, B A: Diphenylhydantoin teratogenicity in rats. Toxicol Appl Pharmacol 22, 193, 1972.
48 BROOK, M, GRIMSHAW, J J: Vitamin C concentrations of plasma and leucocytes as related to smoking habit, age and sex of humans. Am J Clin Nutr 21, 1254, 1968.
49 BASU, T K, SCHORAH, C J: In: Vitamin C in health and disease. Croom Helm, London, 1982.
50 IRWIN, M I, HUTCHINS, B K: A conspectus of research on vitamin C requirements of man. J Nutr 106, 821–879, 1976.
51 GARRY, P J et al: Nutritional status in a healthy elderly population: vitamin C. Am J Clin Nutr 36, 332–339, 1981.
52 Nutrition Canada Interpretive Standards, National Survey, p 46. Information Canada, Ottawa, 1973.
53 CHANARIN, I: The folate. In: BARKER and BENDER (eds). Vitamins in medicine, vol 1. Heinemann, London, 1980.
54 GARRY, P J et al: Nutritional status in a healthy elderly population: dietary and supplemental intakes. Am J Clin Nutr 36, 319, 1983.
55 BECKING, G C: Vitamin A status and hepatic drug metabolism in the rat. Can J Physiol Pharmacol 51, 6, 1973.
56 HORN, L R et al: Drug metabolism and hepatic heme proteins in the vitamin E-deficient rat. Arch Biochem Biophys 172, 270, 1976.
57 CATZ, C S et al: Effects of iron, riboflavin and iodide deficiencies on hepatic drug-metabolizing enzyme system. J Pharmacol Exp Ther 174, 197, 1970.
58 ZANNONI, V G, LYNCH, M M: The role of ascorbic acid in drug metabolism. Drug Metabol Rev 2, 57–69, 1973.
59 BASU, T K: Effects of protein malnutrition and ascorbic acid levels on drug metabolism. Can J Physiol Pharmacol 61, 295–301, 1983.
60 WILSON, C W M: Vitamins and drug metabolism with particular reference to vitamin C. Proc Nutr Soc 33, 231–238, 1974.
61 GINTER, E, VEJMOLOVA, J: Vitamin C status and pharmacokinetic profile of antipyrine in man. Br J Clin Pharmacol 12, 256–258, 1981.
62 O'MALLEY, K et al: Effect of age and sex on human drug metabolism. Br Med J 3, 607, 1971.
63 BASU, T K: Pharmacological response as a function of age. In: BASU (ed). Clinical implications of drug use, pp 98. CRC Press, Boca Raton, 1980.
64 HURWITZ, N: Admissions to hospitals due to drugs. Br Med J 1, 549, 1969.
65 GREENBLATT, D J et al: Toxicity of high dose flurazepam in the elderly. Clin Pharmacol Ther 21, 355, 1977.
66 EXTON-SMITH, A N: Nutritional deficiency in modern society. In: HOWARD and McLEAN (eds) Nutritional deficiencies in modern society. Newman, London, 1973.

Dr. T.K. Basu, Professor, Department of Foods and Nutrition, Faculty of Home Economics, The University of Alberta, Edmonton, Canada, T6G-2M8

Oxidation, Monosubstitution and Industrial Synthesis of Ascorbic Acid

A Review[1]

P.A. SEIB

Department of Grain Science and Industry, Kansas State University, Manhattan, Kansas, USA

Key Words: L-Ascorbic acid · Synthesis · Oxidation · Monoesters · Monoethers · Derivatives

Abstract: Established and proposed methods to synthesize L-ascorbic acid on a commercial scale are presented. The preparation and properties of L-ascorbate free radical and dehydroascorbic acid are reviewed. Conditions needed to selectively monoesterify and monoetherify L-ascorbic acid are illustrated, along with the significance of its C-2 and C-4 carbanions.

Introduction

L-ascorbic acid is a fine chemical used in pharmaceuticals, food, feed, and a variety of minor products [1]. In 1972 the production of L-ascorbic acid in the United States was estimated to be 16×10^6 kg/y [2]. An estimate of present world production might be 35×10^6 kg/y. Because of its vitamin C potency, strong reducing power, low toxicity, and other useful properties, L-ascorbic production will continue to grow in the future. Derivates of L-ascorbic acid also will be used in increasing quantities.

The chemistry of L-ascorbic acid has challenged and fascinated chemists for over 50 years. In this paper current methods of commercial synthesis of L-ascorbic acid and speculation on possible enzymic methods of preparation are reviewed. The oxidation of L-ascorbic acid, and methods to selectively monoetherify and monoesterify (organic and inorganic) the molecule at its 0-1, 0-2, 0-3, 0-5, and 0-6 positions are presented. The significance of carbanions at C-2 and C-4 is illustrated.

---

[1] Contribution No. 84-378A, Department of Grain Science and Industry, Kansas State Agricultural Experiment Station, Manhattan, KS 66506, USA.

Structure

L-ascorbic acid (1) is the trivial name for L-*threo*-2-hexenono-1,4-lactone; it is one of four diastereomeric, 6-carbon ascorbic acids. The enantiomer of L-ascorbic acid (1) is D-ascorbic acid (2). The other two stereoisomers, D-and L-*erythro*-2-hexenono-1,4-lactones (3 and 4), are designated with one of three trivial names, D- and L-araboascorbic, isoascorbic, and erythorbic acid. The *erythro* and *threo* configurations can be interconverted [3] through racemization at C-4 in hot methanolic alkali.

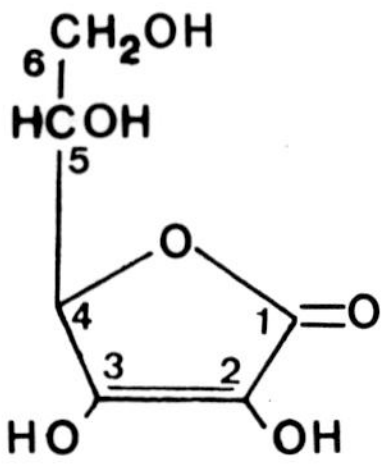

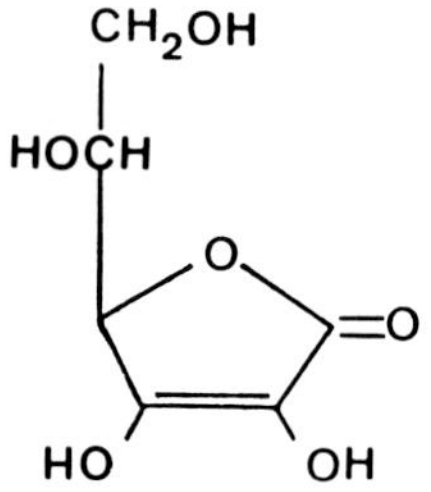

L-Ascorbic acid may exist in at least five tautomeric forms [4, 5], three of which (1, 5 and 6) are shown here. Crystalline L-ascorbic acid [m.p. 192°, $[\alpha]_D^{18} + 22°$ (c1.0, water)] has been shown to be tautomer (1) by x-ray crystallography [6]; tautomer (1) also predominates in aqueous solution at pH 2 as shown by ^{1}H- and ^{13}C-nuclear magnetic resonance (nmr) spectroscopy [7]. Tautomer (5) has been isolated in derivative form either as 2-*C*-benzyl-L-*xylo*-3-hexulosonic acid lactone (7) [8] or as ascorbigen (8) [9]. Tautomer (6) is found [10, 11] in 1-*0*-methyl-L-ascorbic acid (9).

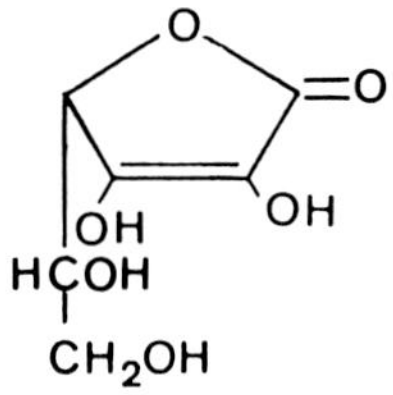

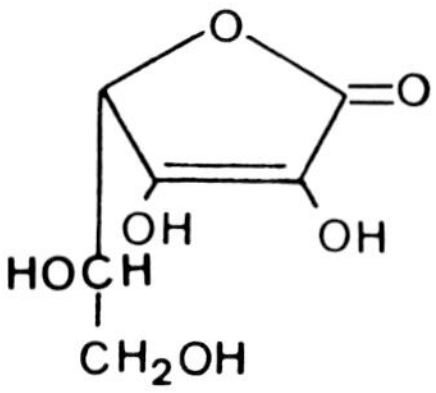

L-ascorbic acid is soluble in water (33 % at 25°) but only slightly soluble in ethanol (2 %), acetonitrile (0.05 %), and acetic acid (0.2 %). In aqueous solu-

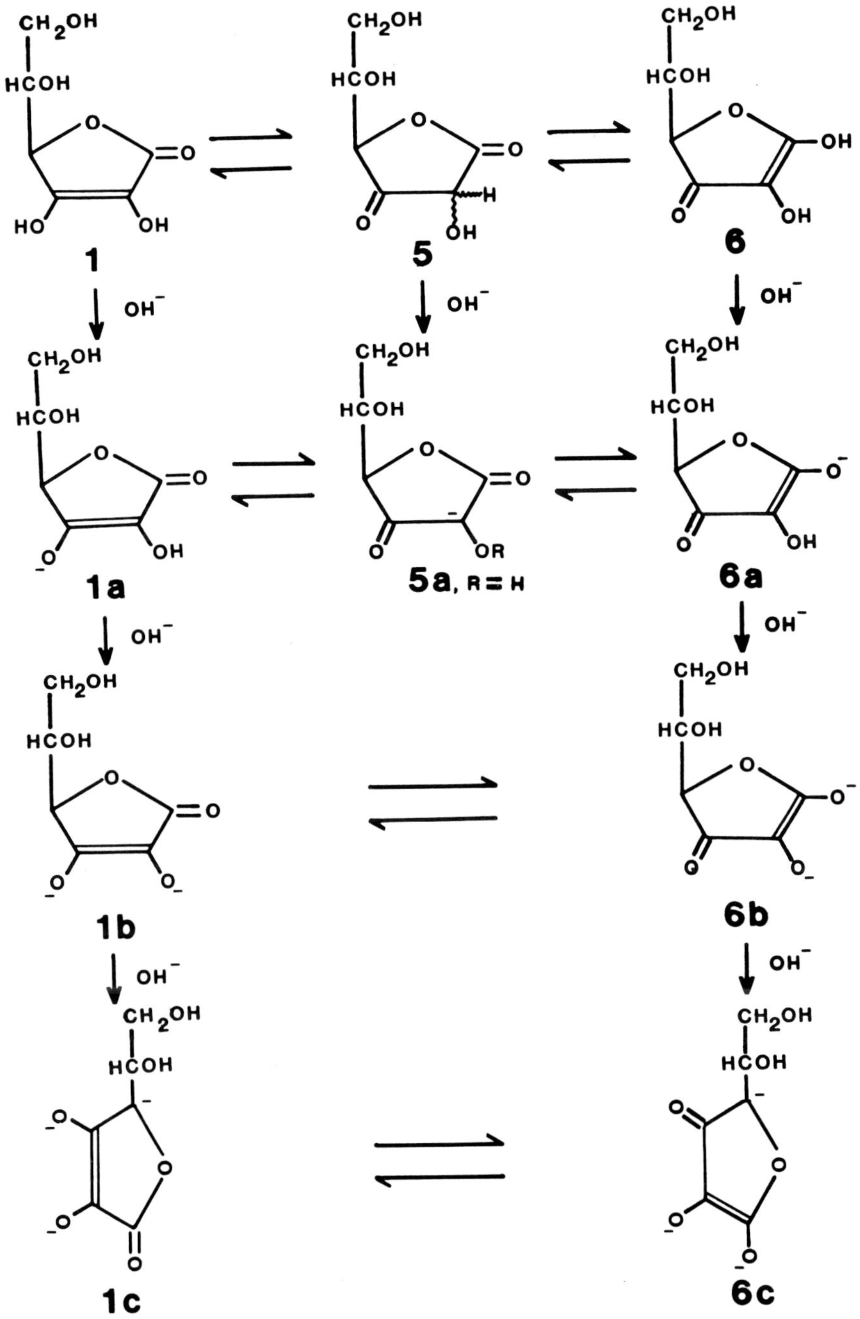

CH₂OH
HCOH
=O
HO OH
1

CH₂OH
HCOH
=O
O H OH
5

CH₂OH
HCOH
OH
O OH
6

OH⁻

OH⁻

OH⁻

CH₂OH
HCOH
=O
⁻O OH
1a

CH₂OH
HCOH
=O
O OR
5a, R = H

CH₂OH
HCOH
O⁻
O OH
6a

OH⁻

OH⁻

CH₂OH
HCOH
=O
⁻O O⁻
1b

CH₂OH
HCOH
O⁻
O O⁻
6b

OH⁻

OH⁻

CH₂OH
HCOH
⁻O
O⁻
O
1c

CH₂OH
HCOH
O
O⁻
O⁻
6c

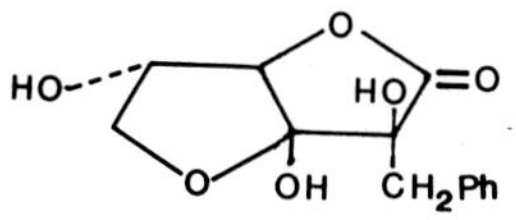

7 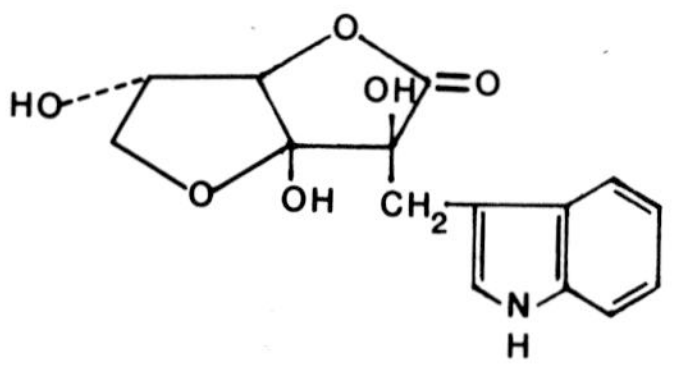   **8** 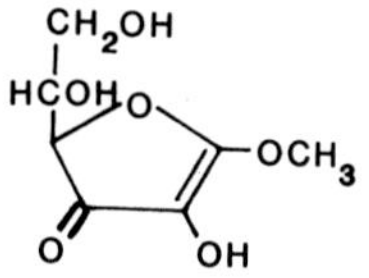   **9**

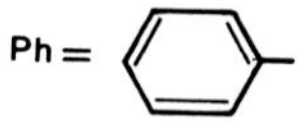

Ph = (benzene ring)

tion, the 3-OH and 2-OH have ionization constants of pK_1 4.17 and pK_2 11.79, respectively [5]. The monobasic salts of L-ascorbate are readily isolated, but the dibasic salts are unstable. The crystal structures of sodium and calcium L-ascorbate show [6] the metal is associated with 0–3. The optical absorbance spectrum as other physical properties of **1**, is pH-dependent [12]. Under carefully controlled conditions the undissociated acid at pH 1.5 gave λ_{max} 224 nm with ε 10 500 M^{-1} cm^{-1}, while the ascorbate ion at pH 7.4 gave λ_{max} 265 nm with ε 20 400 M^{-1} cm^{-1}.

Proton coupling constants obtained from the ^{1}H-nmr spectrum of L-ascorbic acid at 600.2 MHz indicate [7] the conformation of **1** is the same in aqueous solution as it is in the crystalline solid. The 5-OH is positioned above the top of the practically flat, lactone ring, and 0–5 is in a *gauche* conformation with 0–4. Furthermore, rotation around the C-5:C-6 bond is restricted, and 0–5 is *anti* to 0–6. In solid sodium ascorbate, 0–6 changes to a *gauche* orientation with respect to 0–5 as determined by x-ray analysis. However, in aqueous solution 0–5 of sodium L-ascorbate remains *anti* to 0–6 since the vicinal coupling constants between H-5 and H-6, H-6' do not change [7] when a solution of **1** is neutralized with sodium hydroxide. No intramolecular hydrogen bonds are observed in crystalline **1** or its salts [6].

Synthesis

At least twenty schemes have been devised to synthesize L-ascorbic acid [5, 13]. All the methods are useful in labeling **1** with isotopes [5], but only the Reichstein-Grüssner synthesis [14] is used industrially to produce L-ascorbic acid. In the Reichstein-Grüssner synthesis, the 6-carbon chain of D-glucose, the starting material, is inverted so that C-6 of D-glucose becomes C-1 of

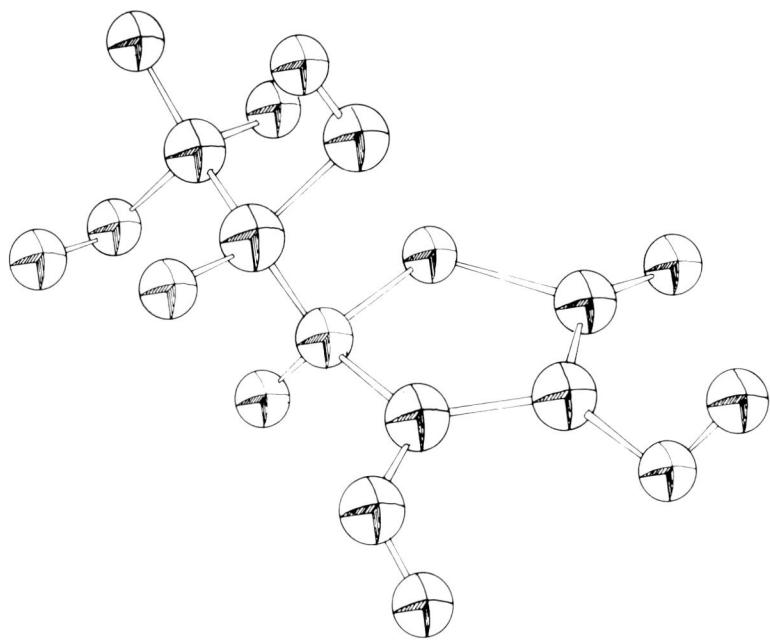

L-ascorbic acid. The essence of the synthesis is to reduce C-1 of D-glucose, ox-
idize C-5 and C-6, and preserve the chirality at C-2 and C-3 to give the L-*threo*
configuration at C-4 and C-5 of L-ascorbic acid. In the five-step synthesis,
D-glucose (**10**) is reduced to sorbitol (**11**) and the alditol (**11**) is then oxidized
to L-sorbose (**12**) by aerobic fermentation. Reaction of L-sorbose with
acetone and acid gives 2,3;4,6-di-*0*-isopropylidene-L-*xylo*-2-hexulofuranose
(**13**). The free primary alcohol group of the diacetone derivative (**13**) is oxidized to 2,3:4,6-di-*0*-isopropylidene-L-*xylo*-2-hexulosonic acid (**14**), which is
then heated with an acid in a non-aqueous medium. Heating **14** one hour at
110° C in a mixture of toluene with catalytic amounts of concentrated
hydrochloric acid results in crystallization of 90–95 % L-ascorbic acid as a
separate phase [5]. The over-all yield of **1** from **10** is ~ 50 %.

Currently, a second industrial method of producing L-ascorbic acid is being
developed [15], which entails two fermentation steps. The method begins with
D-glucose (**10**) and the carbon chain of **10** is converted to **1** without inversion.
The chirality of C-4 in D-glucose is preserved, C-1, C-2 and C-5 are oxidized,
and C-5 is then reduced selectively and stereospecifically to give the desired
L-*threo* configuration at C-4 and C-5 of **1**.

The two-stage fermentative process begins with a mutant strain of *Erwinia*
sp. that converts D-glucose (**10**) in 94 % yield to calcium D-*threo*-2,5-hexodiu-

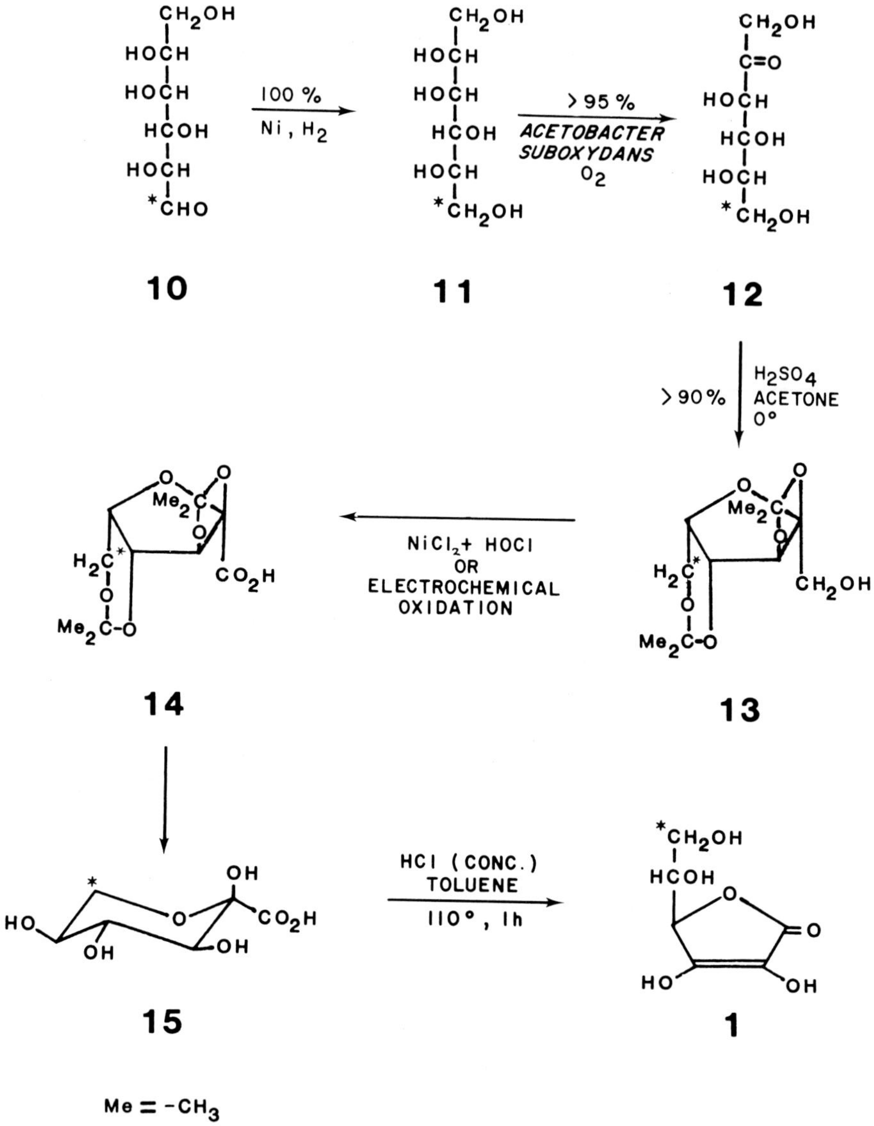

$$
\begin{array}{ccc}
\text{CH}_2\text{OH} & \text{CH}_2\text{OH} & \text{CH}_2\text{OH} \\
\text{HOCH} & \text{HOCH} & \text{C=O} \\
\text{HOCH} & \text{HOCH} & \text{HOCH} \\
\text{HCOH} & \text{HCOH} & \text{HCOH} \\
\text{HOCH} & \text{HOCH} & \text{HOCH} \\
{}^{*}\text{CHO} & {}^{*}\text{CH}_2\text{OH} & {}^{*}\text{CH}_2\text{OH}
\end{array}
$$

10    $\xrightarrow[\text{Ni, H}_2]{100\%}$ 11 $\xrightarrow[\substack{\text{ACETOBACTER}\\ \text{SUBOXYDANS} \\ O_2}]{>95\%}$ 12

$\xrightarrow[\substack{\text{H}_2\text{SO}_4 \\ \text{ACETONE} \\ 0^\circ}]{>90\%}$

14   $\xleftarrow[\substack{\text{OR} \\ \text{ELECTROCHEMICAL} \\ \text{OXIDATION}}]{\text{NiCl}_2 + \text{HOCl}}$ 13

14 → 15

15   $\xrightarrow[110^\circ,\ 1h]{\substack{\text{HCl (CONC.)} \\ \text{TOLUENE}}}$ 1

Me = -CH₃

losonate (16) (calcium 2,5-diketo-D-gluconate). The diketo intermediate (16) is unstable and is not isolated. Instead, the cells in the first broth are inactivated by adding sodium dodecyl sulfate, and without removal of the cells, the broth is then treated with a mutant strain of *Corynebacterium* sp. In the second fermentation step D-glucose is fed to the bacterium as a source of electrons to reduce 16 stereospecifically to L-*xylo*-2-hexulosonic acid (2-keto-L-gulonic acid) (15) in 92 % yield. The overall conversion of D-glucose (10) is 73 %, which is approximately the same as achieved in the Reichstein-Grüssner synthesis. Compound 15 is converted to 1 as described previously.

10   **16**   **15**

A 1981 patent [16] describes the direct O_2-oxidation of L-sorbose (12) to 2-keto-L-gulonic acid (15) in 87 % yield using a catalyst comprised of a mixture of platinum (or palladium) and lead (or bismuth). This route to 15 is attractive because of the high yield (~ 83 %) of 15 directly from 10 without the isolation of intermediate compounds.

Synthesis of L-Ascorbic Acid Using Enzymes or Direct Fermentation

Most eukaryotic organisms contain enzymes that synthesize L-ascorbic acid from D-glucose [17, 18]. In the future, it is probable that L-ascorbic acid will be manufactured using enzymes produced by way of recombinant DNA. Enzymatic synthesis of 1 offers advantages over current microbiological-chemical methods. Enzyme reactions are specific; few by-products would be present and isolation and purification of 1 would be facilitated, provided the substrates are stable in a reaction medium and the enzymic reactions proceed to completion.

Two enzymic routes to 1 appear feasible; both routes require one or two enzymes. The starting material for the first route is pectic acid (17) which can be hydrolyzed enzymically [19, 20] with polygalacturonases [E.C.3.2.1.15 and 3.2.1.67] to give 86 % D-galacturonic acid (18). Chemical reduction [21] of D-galacturonic acid followed by lactonization gives L-galactono-1,4-lactone (19). The lactone (19) can be converted to L-ascorbic acid using L-galactonolactone oxidase (E.C.1.3.2.3) [22, 23].

In the other enzymic route to **1** the key intermediate is D-glucuronic acid
(**21**). The acid (**21**) is chemically reduced [24] to L-gulono-1,4-lactone (**22**),
and **22** is oxidized to **1** in the presence of L-gulono-lactone oxidase
(E.C.1.1.3.8.) [25–27]. In 1957 ISHERWOOD and MAPSON [28] first reported the
use of L-gulono-lactone oxidase to prepare **1** from **22** in up to 60–70 % yield [26].

D-Glucuronic acid can be prepared by one of several methods. *Myo*-inositol
(**20**) is oxidized to **21** in the presence of *myo*-inositol oxidase (E.C.1.13.99.1)
[29, 30]. An exocellular microbial polysaccharide can be hydrolyzed [31] to
give 27% of **21** in its lactone form. MEHLTRETTER [32] used a platinum
catalyst to prepare the lactone of **21** in 38 % yield from D-Glucose. HEYNS and
GRAEFE [33] oxidized starch with a mixture of nitric acid and nitrogen tetrox-
ide to obtain 26% of **21** after acid-hydrolysis. Another chemical route [34]
yields 20–40% of **21** by successive oxidation of methyl α-D-glucopyranoside
with NO_2 followed by acid hydrolysis.

Since yeasts [5, 22], fungi [5] and algae [35, 36] contain L-ascorbic acid (**1**),
it is theoretically possible to produce **1** directly by fermentation. However, the

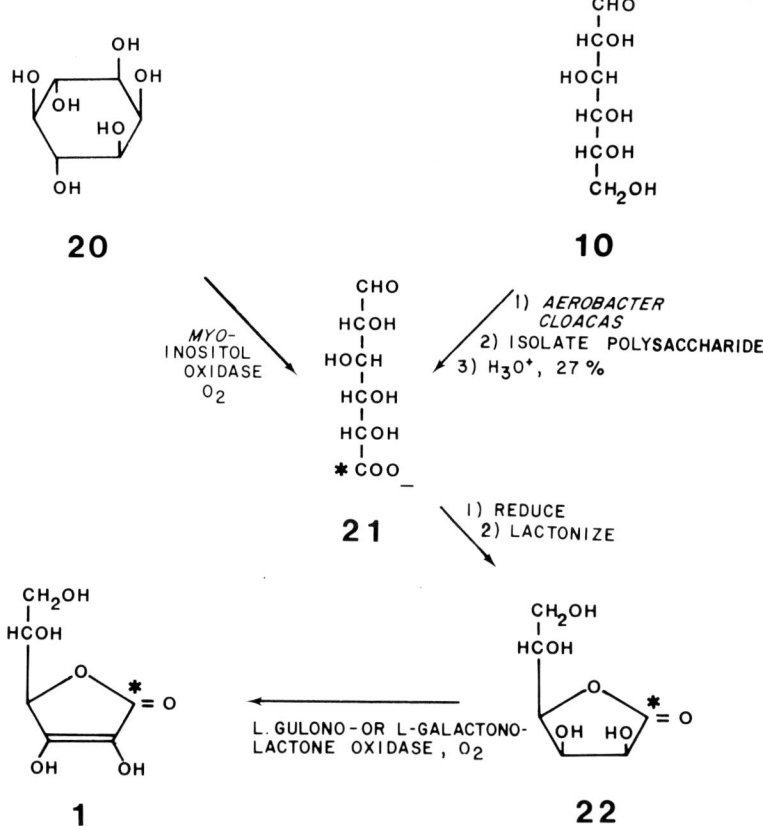

yield and concentration of **1** are low in fermentations reported to date. For example [35], the algae *Ochromonas danica* converts a 1% solution of D-glucose to **1**, and secretes the vitamin into the medium, in which **1** is stable. The conversion of D-glucose to **1** was ~ 1%, which fixes the concentration of **1** in the broth at ~ 0.001%.

Oxidation of L-Ascorbic Acid

Perhaps the most important property of L-ascorbic acid (**1**) is that it can undergo a two-step oxidation to give dehydroascorbic acid (**25**) by way of the intermediate ascorbate free radical (**23**), which is also called monodehydro-ascorbic acid or semidehydroascorbic acid [37, 38]. In nature the combination of reduced L-ascorbic acid, monodehydroascorbic acid, and dehydroascorbic acid constitutes a redox buffer system. The vitamin C redox system contains

CH$_2$OH

HCOH

1a

23

mostly **1** and **25**. Monodehydroascorbic acid concentration is very low because it is both a potent oxidizing and a potent reducing agent; thus **23** decomposes to give **1** and **25** [39].

In aerobic organisms L-ascorbic acid (**1**) protects biological tissue against activated species of oxygen ($HO_2\cdot$, O_2^{-}, and $HO\cdot$) and other radicals; **1** readily reduces these radicals to give the ascorbate radical (**23**). Furthermore, **1** quenches singlet oxygen [39a]. The ascorbate radical also reduces free radicals to give dehydroascorbic acid. In living cells the vitamin C redox cycle is complete when dehydroascorbic acid is reduced back to **1** by enzymes such as glutathione reductase [39].

The ascorbate free radical appears to exist [38] in the bicyclic form (**23**). It is a strong acid (pK = 0.45) that absorbs in the ultraviolet with λ_{max} 380 nm and $\varepsilon = 3\,300\ M^{-1}\ cm^{-1}$ at pH 8. Electron spin resonance showed [38] a 1 M aqueous solution of sodium L-ascorbate was $\sim 0.7 \times 10^{-6}$ M in **23** when the solution was saturated with O_2.

Monodehydroascorbic acid (**23**) is a relatively unreactive radical that is generally regarded as innocuous [37]. When **23** does react, it prefers to react with itself or other free radicals thereby terminating radical reactions and preventing damage to sensitive components of tissue or food flavour [40, 41]. The dismutation of **23** is a rapid second-order disproportionation [42] that results in a 1:1 mixture of dehydroascorbic acid (**25**) and L-ascorbate (**1**). The dimeric peroxide (**24**) may explain the second order dependence of **23** on the rate of dismutation.

The reaction of L-ascorbate with molecular oxygen in the presence of transition metal ions is important in aerobic systems found in tissue, pharmaceuticals, and foods. The instability of L-ascorbic acid in aqueous solution is widely recognized; an illustration [43] of the oxidative loss of **1** can be seen in Figure 1. In the absence of catalysts, however, L-ascorbic acid reacts slowly with dioxygen at pH 4–10 [44, 45].

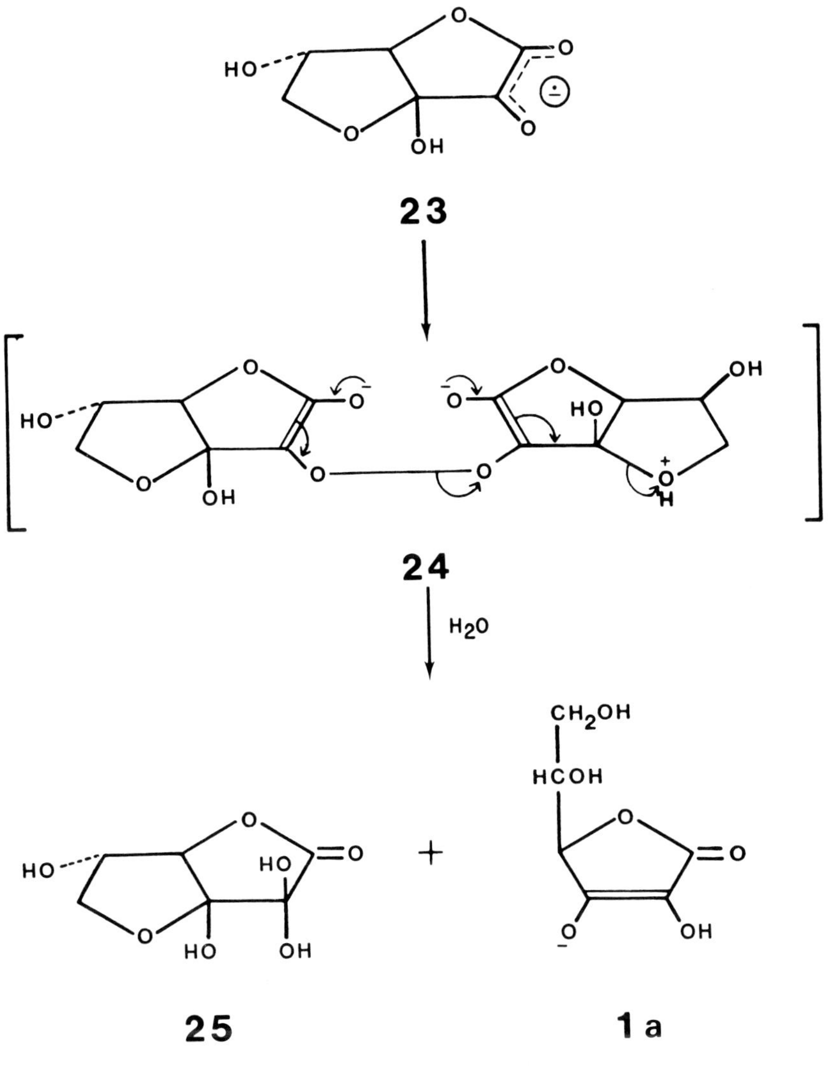

23

24

H_2O

25   **1 a**

Transition metals catalyze the autoxidation of L-ascorbate by forming an intermediate ternary complex between metal, ascorbate and dioxygen. The ternary complex is proposed to account for the much more rapid oxidation of 1 in the presence of oxygen and metal ion as opposed to its oxidation by stoichiometric quantities of the metal ion alone [46]. The ternary complex, which is illustrated with ferric ion in **26** is thought to undergo a single two-electron transfer to yield dehydroascorbic acid (**25**) and H_2O_2 [46, 47]. However, one cannot rule out a two-step oxidation with an initial, slow, one-

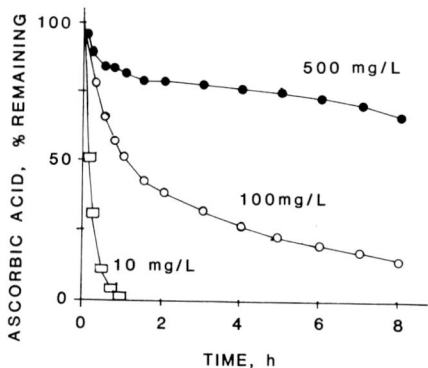

Fig. 1: Loss of L-ascorbic acid at various concentrations in tap water [43].

electron transfer to give the intermediate ascorbate free radical (23) and the hydroperoxyl radical (HO$_2$·), which then react together [48] very rapidly (k $\cong$ 5 × 10^{9}M^{-1}s^{-1}) to give 25 and H$_2$O$_2$. Reaction of L-ascorbic acid (1) with the HO$_2$· formed in the rate-controlling step is two orders of magnitude slower than the reaction between HO$_2$· and the ascorbate free radical [48].

The rate of autoxidation of 1 accelerates as acidity is decreased from pH 1.5 to 3.5 in the presence of Cu(II) or Fe(III) [46, 49]. Apparently below pH 7, the mono-anion of L-ascorbate is the form of 1 that is chelated in the intermediate ternary complex. Furthermore, as the pH moves from the acid towards neutral pH, superoxide ion (O$_2^-$) is the initial reduction product of dioxygen because the perhydroxyl radical (HO$_2$·) has pK 4.7 [49]. CABELLI and BIELSKI [48] showed that O$_2^-$ reacts with the ascorbate radical (23) with a rate constant of 2.6 × 10^8 M^{-1} s^{-1}, but O$_2^-$ reacts 10^4 times slower with L-ascorbate (k = 5 × 10^{4}M^{-1}s^{-1}). Thus, the two-step mechanism for autoxidation of L-ascorbate may still occur at pH 4–7. In agreement with results on polyunsaturated fatty acids [50], the perhydroxyl radical (HO$_2$·) reacted faster with L-ascorbate than did the superoxide radical (0$_2^-$), i.e. k = 5 × 10^{9}M^{-1}s^{-1} *vs* 0.26 × 10^{9}M^{-1}s^{-1} [48].

PUGET and MICHAELSON [51] reported that superoxide dismutase (SOD) inhibited autoxidation of L-ascorbate at pH 7.8. The enzyme SOD catalyzes the reaction 2O$_2^-$ + 2H$_3$O$^+$ → H$_2$O$_2$ + O$_2$ + 2H$_2$O. Inhibition of autoxidation of 1 by SOD may be due to competition between the enzyme and ascorbyl radical (23) for O$_2^-$, or SOD may specifically or nonspecifically chelate the metal ions. Autoxidation of 1 is much slower in the presence of chelated Fe(III) or Cu(II) than when the metal ion is free [46, 49, 52–54]. A variety of chelating agents inhibit autoxidation of 1, including ethylenediaminetetraacetate, nitrilotriacetate, hydroxyethyliminodiacetate, oxalate, acidic polysaccharides, flavonoids, proteins, and some amino acids, to name but a few. Figure 2 shows that albumin and catalase inhibited autoxidation of 1 in tap water, but that lysozyme had no effect [55]. Borenstein [56] showed that myoglobin greatly stabilized a 1 mM solution of 1 at pH 6.8. Lysozyme may be too small a protein to complex non-specifically with the metal ions.

Taqui-Khan and Martell [57] reported that hydrogen peroxide disappears rapidly during autoxidation of 1. It is possible that H_2O_2 is destroyed by the combined reactions given in Figure 3 [58]. Ferric ion is first reduced by 1 to ferrous ion plus ascorbate radical (23) [46], and the ferrous ion then undergoes the Fenton reaction with H_2O_2 [59]. The hydroxyl radical (HO·) released by the net reaction can then react with L-ascorbate radical or excess

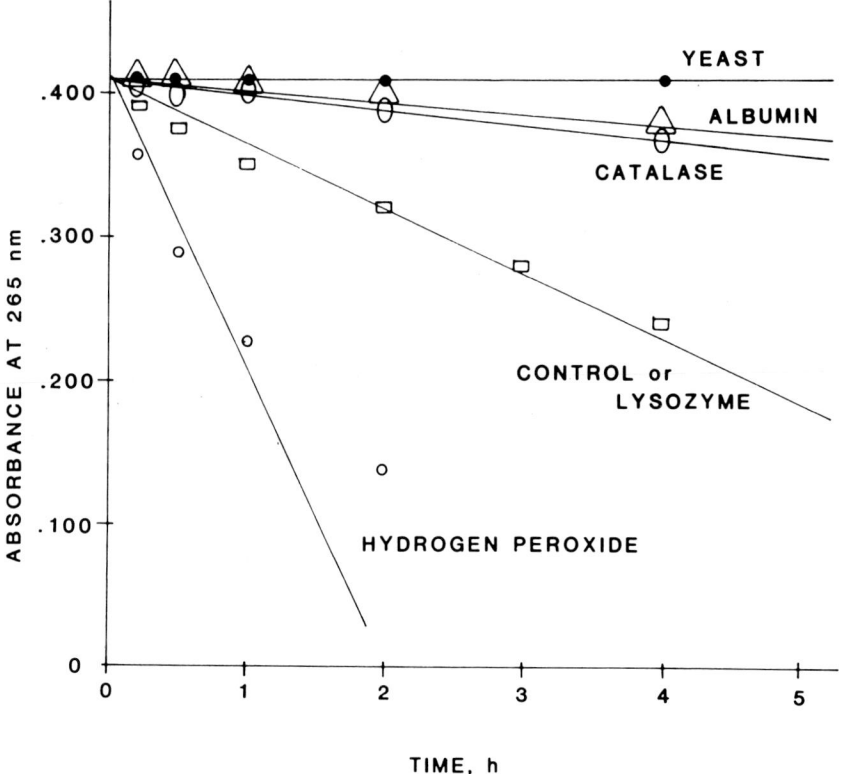

TIME, h

Fig. 2: Loss of L-ascorbic acid (initially 1.42 mM) in the presence of bakers' compressed yeast (50 g/l), various proteins (0.25 g/l), and hydrogen peroxide (1.42 mM) [55].

L-ascorbate to generate dehydroascorbic acid (**25**) or ascorbate radical (**23**). The generation of OH· by the reactions shown in Figure 3 explains the seemingly contradictory nature of L-ascorbate; that is, **1** is an antioxidant that accelerates the bleaching of pigments [60] and the oxidative depolymerization of polysaccharides [61] and proteins [62].

Methods used to prevent autoxidation of **1** depend on inhibiting formation of the ternary complex (**26**). Addition of chelating agents such as metaphosphoric acid [63], inhibit autoxidation by competing for metal ions. High hydrogen ion concentration (~ pH 1) suppresses ionization of **1**, and the fully protonated molecule (**1**) is slowly attacked by oxygen [44]. However, cold acid should be used to avoid dehydration of L-ascorbic acid. Oxygen may be excluded from the ternary complex by boiling, purging with nitrogen, and evacuating the medium, or by addition of sodium hydrosulfite, dithiothreitol,

$$Fe^{+3} + AH^- \longrightarrow Fe^{+2} + A^{\overline{\cdot}} + H^+$$

$$Fe^{+2} + H_2O_2 \longrightarrow Fe^{+3} + HO^- + HO^{\cdot}$$

Net: $AH^- + H_2O_2 \longrightarrow A^{\overline{\cdot}} + HO^{\cdot} + H_2O$

$AH^- = L-ascorbate$ **(1a)**

$A^{\overline{\cdot}} = L-ascorbate\ free\ radical$ **(23)**

Fig. 3: Mechanism postulated to explain the destruction of hydrogen peroxide during O_2-oxidation of L-ascorbic acid in the presence of ferric/ferrous ions [58].

glucose oxidase, and yeast (Fig. 2). Foods and biological preparations may contain enzymes that accelerate the destruction of ascorbic acid, in particular ascorbic acid oxidase [64] and ascorbate-specific peroxidase [65–67]. These enzymes should be inactivated to prevent oxidative loss of **1**.

L-Ascorbate may be protected from oxidation by coating its crystals with a thin film of fat or polymer that slowly dissolves. Such coated forms of **1** are available commercially. Chemical substitution on the ene-diol hydroxyls stabilizes the molecule against oxygen. L-ascorbate 2-sulfate [68], 2-phosphate [69], and the 2-methyl and 3-methyl ethers [11] react with oxygen at 1/10th – 1/20th the rate of **1**. Even 1-0-methyl-L-ascorbic acid is ten times more stable to oxygen at 25° and pH 7–10 than is L-ascorbate [11].

Dehydroascorbic acid (25)

The purity of dehydroascorbic acid prepared by oxidation of L-ascorbic acid depends on the choice of oxidant, solvent, and reaction time. Halogens, quinones, iodate, and oxygen have been used in water, alcohols and dipolar aprotic solvents [6, 70, 71].

Ohmori *et al* [72] developed a facile preparation of highly pure dehydroascorbic acid by O_2-oxidation of **1** in methanol containing activated charcoal. After oxidation, removal of the charcoal and solvent gave syrupy dehydroascorbic acid as a methanol adduct. Tolbert and Ward [70], on the other hand, found that 95 % ethanol as reaction medium did not lead to an alcohol adduct; they obtained pure syrupy **25** after evaporating ethanol from the reaction mixture. Refluxing syrupy **25** in methyl ethyl ketone gave a colorless, crystalline dimer (**27**) in 64 % yield [72]. The dimer was prepared in one step by oxidization of **1** in dimethylformamide or dimethylsulfoxide [71]. X-ray crystallography showed the dimer is a symmetrical molecule having a system of five-fused rings [6]. A dissymmetric dimer of **25** also has been isolated [71]. When dimer **27** is dissolved in water the dioxane ring of **27** is split, and two molecules of monomeric dehydroascorbic acid (**25**) are released.

In aqueous solution dehydroascrobic acid exists in the bicylic structure (**25**) having a 6,3-furanose ring, a 1,4-lactone ring, and a C-2 *gem*-diol [38, 70, 77]. The bicyclic ring can be capped by methylation of **25** with diazomethane in methanol [73] to give 20% of methyl 2,2-di-*O*-methyl-β-L-*threo*-3-hexulosidono-1,4-lactone (**28**). The 3,5-*bis*-*O*-(trimethylsilyl) dervative of **25** has also been prepared [74]. When 0–6 derivatives of **1** are oxidized with oxygen over charcoal, they form dehydro derivatives having a 2,3-dihydrated-γ-lactone ring and an open side-chain [38, 70].

Dehydroascorbic acid is stable for several days at 4°C in aqueous solution at pH 2.5–5.5. However, in buffered solution at neutral or alkaline pH, both rings of **25** open rapidly to give L-*threo*-2,3-hexodiulosonic acid (2,3-diketogulonic acid) (**29**) in a straight-chain structure [70, 75]. Upon standing 14 hours in water at pH 7 and 27° compound (**29**) decarboxylates to give L-*threo*-2-pentulose (**30**). L-ascorbic acid (**1**) and L-*glycero*-2-pentenono-1,4-lactone (**32**) then form due to oxidation of **30** by **29**. Compound (**30**) is an α-

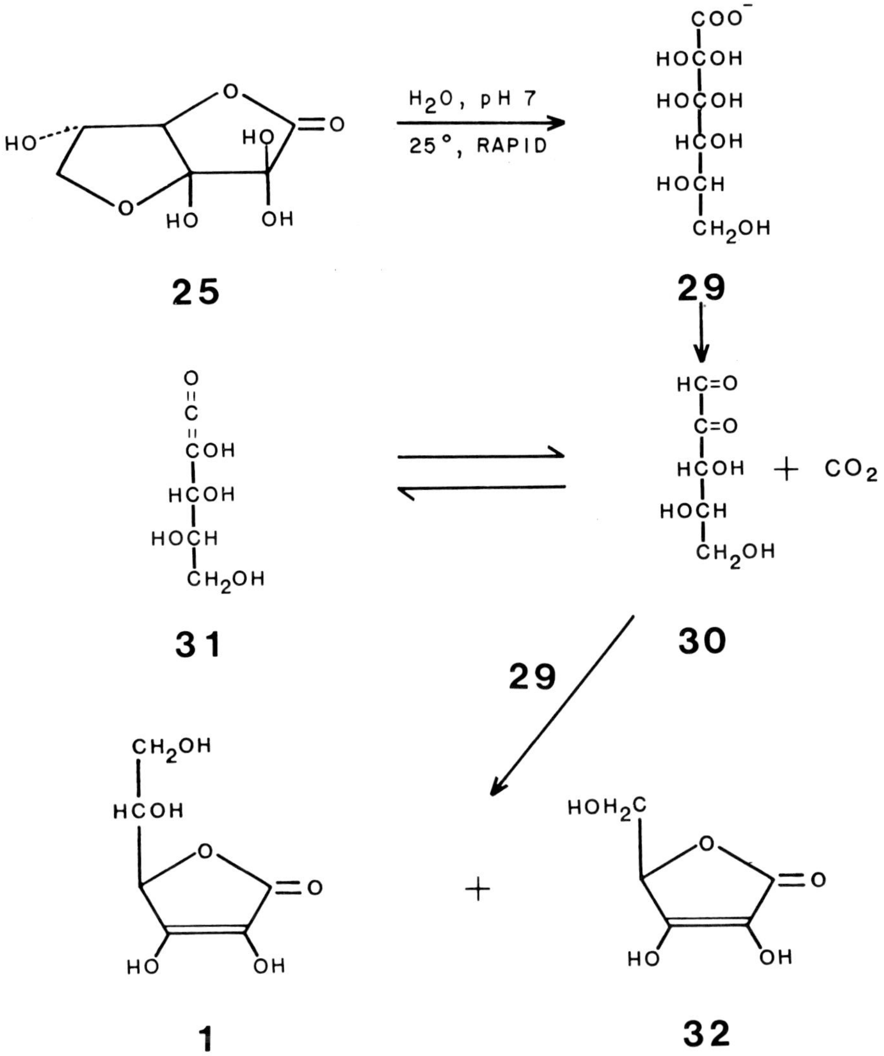

25 → (H$_2$O, pH 7, 25°, RAPID) → **29**

$$
\begin{array}{l}
COO^- \\
HOCOH \\
HOCOH \\
HCOH \\
HOCH \\
CH_2OH
\end{array}
\quad \mathbf{29}
$$

29 →
$$
\begin{array}{l}
HC=O \\
C=O \\
HCOH \\
HOCH \\
CH_2OH
\end{array}
+ CO_2 \quad \mathbf{30}
$$

31
$$
\begin{array}{l}
O \\
\parallel \\
C \\
\parallel \\
O \\
COH \\
HCOH \\
HOCH \\
CH_2OH
\end{array}
$$

29 → **1** + **32**

ketoaldehyde with the tautomeric structure (**31**). The facile formation of **30–31** from diketogulonic acid and dehydroascorbic acid possibly explains their inhibitory effect on cell growth [75].

Dehydroisoascorbic acid, freshly prepared by oxidation of **3** in water, assumes the bicyclic structure with a furanose and lactone ring [70, 76]. When placed in water at 28°, dehydroisoascorbic acid hydrolyzes rapidly at its lactone ring as evidenced by the decline in pH. The products after hydrolysis are a mixture of α- and β-pyranoses. Under similar conditions, **25** shows no hydrolysis of its lactone ring [76]. Hvoslef and Pedersen [76] suggest that the non-bonded interaction between oxygen atoms 0–4 and 0–5, which are in a *gauche* conformation in dehydroisoascorbic acid, introduces strain in the lactone ring. The strain is absent in **25** where 0–4 and 0–5 are disposed *anti* to each other. Consequently, the lactone ring of **25** is relatively stable in water, which facilitates the redox system involving L-ascorbic acid, monodehydroascorbic acid and dehydroascorbic acid. Dehydroascorbic acid, as previously mentioned, is relatively stable in water between pH 2.4–5.5; the hydrolytic effect of the hydroxyl ion on the lactone ring of **25** is 10 times stronger than the effect of the hydronium ion [77].

Dehydroascorbic acid is thought to be an intermediate in the facile preparation of L-threonic acid (94% yield of lithium salt) by treatment of **1** with alkaline hydrogen peroxide [61] or hypoiodite [78]. The other product of the oxidation is oxalic acid. Extensive decomposition of **25** in water gives a complex mixture of products [79].

Dehydroascorbic acid (**25**) can be reduced to L-ascorbic acid by hydrogen sulfide, reduced nicotinamide adenine dinucleotide, reduced glutathione, and reduced dithiothreitol. Compound (**25**) has been reacted with a number of amines to produce a variety of nitrogen derivatives [80]. These include mono-

33   **34**   **35**

36   **37**   **38**

and bis-hydrazones (33 and 34), the monoamino (35) [64] and diamino (36) analogs of 1, and the triazole (37) and imidazoline (38) derivatives of dehydroascorbic acid.

It has long been known that 25 deaminates amino acids to give ammonia, carbon dioxide and an aldehyde [80]. In the early stages of the reaction pink, yellow, red, blue, and brown chromophores can be separated by thinlayer chromatography [81–83]. When dehydroascorbic acid (25) is reacted with L-phenylalanine in hot 95 % ethanol containing L-ascorbic acid (1), 6 % of tris(2-deoxy-2-L-ascorbyl)-amine (39) is isolated as a yellow powder after

purification on Sephadex LH-20 and paper chromatograms [84, 85]. The amine is oxidized reversibly by two one-electron steps. The first product (40) is a blue-colored anion radical that is unusually stable in water. Oxidation of 40 in the second step gives an unstable intermediate that slowly loses an ascorbyl residue to yield the oxidized form of bis(2-deoxy-2-L-ascorbyl)-amine (41). The oxidized amine (41) is red (λ_{max} 515 nm), which is the characteristic color of the early reaction between 25 and amino acids.

Determining Positions of Esterification or Etherification on L-Ascorbic Acid

Beginning with the earliest work on the chemistry of vitamin C (**1**), ester and ether derivatives of L-ascorbic acid (**1**) have been important to determine structure and biological role, and to modify solubility and stability [52, 86, 87]. But the structures of some derivatives, particularly those with a 2- or 3-O-substituent, were often uncertain due to their instability and conditions of synthesis. Now, nuclear magnetic resonance (nmr) spectroscopy, ultraviolet (uv) spectroscopy, and x-ray crystallography permit rapid structural determination of L-ascorbate derivatives [6, 7, 88, 89].

The ^{13}C-nmr method is based on changes in chemical shifts induced by ionization of the 3-OH while maintaining the 2-OH in unionized form. The 3-OH in a 2-O-derivative of **1** generally has pK 2–3, whereas the 2-OH in a 3-O-derivative has pKa 6–8 [11, 89–92]. To illustrate, the 2-methyl ether of **1** with pK 3.2 shows a + 16 ppm and a – 3.2 ppm change in the chemical shifts of C-3 and C-2, respectively, on going from pH 2 to 7. On the other hand, the 3-methyl ether with pK 7.9, when subjected to the same pH change, shows a –0.9 ppm and a + 0.8 ppm for its C-3 and C-2 resonances, respectively. Ionization of the 3-methyl ether at pH 9.3 causes C-2 to shift + 9.9 ppm and C-3 to shift –7.3 ppm from their values at pH 7 [11, 88]. In the ^{1}H-nmr spectra of **1** or its derivatives, the signal of H-4 shifts upfield ∼0.5 ppm when the 3-OH ionizes [7].

Uv spectroscopy can be used to verify structural assignments based on nmr. Substitution at either O-2 or O-3 shifts the uv absorption maximum ∼10 nm toward shorter wavelength (hypsochromic shift) compared to the λ_{max} of the unsubstituted chromophore at the same pH. Upon ionization at either the 2-OH or 3-OH, the λ_{max} of either derivative shifts to longer wavelength (a bathochromic shift) by 20–30 nm [7, 91]. However, the anion of a 3-O derivative of **1** bears a cross-conjugated chromophore, while the anion of a 2-O-derivative carries a linear conjugated chromophore. Consequently, the absorption intensity (ε) of a 3-O-derivative decreases upon ionization, whereas the intensity of a 2-0-derivative increases [89].

Esterification or etherification at O-5 or O-6 of **1** is readily determined by nmr using well known changes [93–95] in the chemical shifts of H-5, H-6, C-5 and C-6 with reference to the unsubstituted molecule. Acylation of an OH group deshields the α-carbon (∼2 ppm) and its α-hydrogens (∼0.5 ppm), while etherification deshields the α-carbon (∼10 ppm) but shields the α-hydrogen (∼0.3 ppm). Changes at the β-atoms are lower in magnitude than those at the α-atoms. The uv properties of a 5- or 6-O-derivative are the same as those of **1**.

Selective Esterification and Etherification at O-3 and O-1 of L-Ascorbic Acid

Several conditions appear important to selectively esterify or etherify O-3 of **1**. First, oxygen must be excluded from the reaction for obvious reasons. Second, O-3 should be ionized but not O-2, and the electron density on O-3 should be maximal. This is accomplished using a reaction medium of moderate to low dielectric, such as a ketone, ether, alcohol or a dipolar aprotic solvent with or without addition of a base. Sometimes, instead of starting with the free acid (**1**), the mono-anion form (**1a**) is the starting material. The ascorbate nucleophile (**1a**) is known [96] to react 40–300 times faster than predicted from its pKa. Third, the temperature during reaction and isolation of product is kept low to prevent loss or migration of a 3-O substitutent. Fourth, reactive electrophiles are used because of low reaction temperatures and delocalization of the charge on O-3. Fifth, the starting material in some reactions is blocked at O-6 to enhance selectivity and to prevent O-6 from forming a hemiacetal ring at C-3. Removal of the 6-blocking groups is not always possible without loss of the 3-O-substituent. Examples of 6-blocked derivatives include 5,6-*O*-isopropylidene-L-ascorbic acid (**42**) and 2,6-*O*-bis[(*t*-butyldimethyl)-silyl]-L-ascorbic acid (**43**).

42   **43**

The classical studies on the chemistry of vitamin C in the laboratories of Haworth [97] and Reichstein [98] first demonstrated selective substitution at 0–3 and 0–1 of **1**. Methylation of **1** with diazomethane in methanol at 0° gave 50% of the 3-methyl ether (**44**) and 8% of the 1-methyl ether (**9**) by reaction of tautomers (**1a**) and (**6a**), respectively. 1-*O*-Methyl-L-ascorbic acid is easily separated from **44** by fractional crystallization.

Compound (**9**) is unique in that it is the only known O-1 derivative of **1**. Compound (**9**) has high vitamin C activity probably because of its ease of hydrolysis in acid and alkali. The 3-methyl ether (**44**), on the other hand, gives

5–10% vitamin C, and is stable for hours at pH 1.6 and 25° [99] and for days at pH 10 [11]. The 3-methyl ether (44) has also been prepared in low yield by methylation of the sodium salt of 42 with methyl iodide in methyl sulfoxide followed by removal of the 5,6-acetal [100]. The 3-butyl ether (40% yield) was synthesized in the same way starting from 1 [101].

The 1-methyl ether (9) possesses an unusually acidic methine proton at C-4. Apparently, the 3-keto group adjacent to H-4 in 9 increases the acidity of H-4 to the same degree as does the 5-keto group in 5-keto ascorbic acid (45) [87]. The H-4 in 9 ionizes with pKa 9.1 to give the conjugated di-ene (9aa).

3-O-Benzoyl-5,6-O-isopropylidene-L-ascorbic acid (46) can be prepared [102, 103] in 71% yield by reaction of the acetonide (42) with benzoyl chloride at −78° C in a mixture of acetone and pyridine. Adding the benzoyl chloride at −20° and allowing the mixture to stand overnight at 25° gave mainly the 2-benzoate (48) and only 14% of the 3-benzoate (46). Stirring 46 overnight with a strongly acidic cation-exchange resin [H⁺] in methanol/water removed the 5,6-acetal and catalyzed acyl migration from O-3 to give 6-O-benzoyl-L-ascorbic acid (47). The same migration occurred during hydrolysis of 3-O-benzoyl-5,6-O-isopropylidine-2-O-methyl-L-ascorbic acid to give 6-O-benzoyl-2-O-methyl-L-ascorbic acid (49) as the sole product in 90% yield. De-benzoylation of 49 yielded 2-O-methyl-L-ascorbic acid (50).

3-O-Palmitoyl-L-ascorbic acid (52) was obtained in 20% yield by reaction of N-palmitoylimidazole (51) with 1 in N,N-dimethylformamide (DMF) at room temperature [104]. No base is present to start the reaction, but imidazole is released as the reaction proceeds. Such conditions favor 2- or

3-esterification. The 3-palmitate ester was not characterized, but its melting point was lower than that reported for the isomeric 2-palmitate [104].

PAULSSEN et al [90] examined the reaction of L-ascorbic acid with acetic anhydride in water at 25° and pH 4–7. Addition of the anhydride immediately changed the optical rotation at 350 nm which was interpreted as formation of the kinetic product 3-O-acetyl-L-ascorbic acid (53). The 3-acetate (53) was not stable and in a matter of minutes rearranged at pH 4–7 to the 2-acetate (54).

Neither the 2 or 3-acetate (53 or 54) was isolated, but the 2-acetate was indicated by the following observations; the reaction product did not react with 2,6-dichlorophenol-indophenol, its λ_{max} at 254 nm was hypso-chromically shifted 9 nm from that of 1 at pH 4.7, and the uv properties of the reaction products did not change when 42 was acetylated in place of 1. The half-life of the 2-acetate at pH 4.5 and 25° C was estimated to be ~24 h [90].

Migration of the 3-acetate to O-2 was accelerated as the pH of the acetyla-tion reaction was increased from 4 to 7 [90]. In acidic solution, the 3-acetate would be expected to migrate to O-6 [102]. Thus, the formation of 2,6-diesters of 1 using two equivalents of acylating agent in the presence of pyridine [105] indicates esterification at O-3 and O-6 followed by migration of an acyl group from O-3 to O-2.

In 1944 synthesis of 3-O-acetyl-5,6-O-isopropylidene-L-ascorbic acid (m.p. 115–116° C, yield 56%) was reported [106] by reaction of **42** with ketene at 25° in acetone. Paulssen and coworkers [90] repeated the synthesis; however, they found the product with m.p. 113–115° is the 2,3-diacetate (**55**). Perhaps selective 3-acetylation could be achieved using ketene at a lower temperature than 25° C.

3-O-Phospho-derivatives of **1** and **42** have been prepared. In DMF the thallium salt of (**42a**) reacted with bis-morpholinophosphinyl chloride (**56**) to give 63% of 3-O-[bis-(morpholino)-phosphinate]-5,6-O-isopropylidene-L-ascorbic acid (57) [89]. In acetone, the pyridinium salt of 42a reacted slowly with 56, but gave a high yield (95%) of 57.

The structure of 57 was determined by x-ray crystallography [6]. Removal of the morpholino blocking groups from 57 by acid-catalyzed hydrolysis gave 25% of L-ascorbate 2-phosphate (58) as its crystalline tricyclohexyl-ammonium salt. It seems during the hydrolysis reaction a cyclic 2,3-O-(morpholinophosphonyl) ester may form, which undergoes further hydrolysis to give the acid-stable 2-phosphate (58) rather than the labile 3-phosphate ester of L-ascorbic acid [92, 107]. It is not clear why in acid a 3-O-phospho group migrates to O-2 while under the same condition a 3-O-acyl group migrates to O-6.

Treatment of 42 in pyridine with monophenylphosphoric acid and dicyclohexylcarbodiimide (DCC) gave 25% and 50% of the 3- and 2-phenylphosphoryl esters (59 and 60), respectively [108]. The esters (59 and 60) were isolated in pure form by column chromatography on diethylamino-ethylcellulose.

Monosodium L-ascorbate (1a) reacted at 25° with 2,3,4,6-tetra-O-acetyl-α-D-glucopyranosyl bromide (61) in DMF to give 22% of the 3-O-β-acetogluco-sylated conjugate (62). No 2-O-conjugate of 1 was isolated from the reaction mixture. The syrupy conjugate (62) was unstable, but methylation of its ascor-byl residue's 2-OH followed by acetylation of the 5-OH and 6-OH gave a stable molecule (63). The hypsochromic shift in the λ_{max} of 63 from 243 nm (unsubstituted chromophore) to 229 nm was consistent with 2- or 3-O-substi-

$$Ac = -\overset{\overset{\textstyle O}{\|}}{C}CH_3$$

tution. Glucosidation was assigned to the 3-O position of L-ascorbic acid because of the dissimilarity of 63 compared with 5,6-di-O-acetyl-3-O-methyl-2-O-(2,3,4,6-tetra-O-acetyl-β-D-glucopyranosyl)-L-ascorbic acid (64), prepared in three steps from the known [11, 97] 3-O-methyl-L-ascorbic acid (44).

The monosodium salt of L-ascorbate (1a) reacted with benzyl chloride in dimethylsulfoxide (DMSO) to produce a 3:1 mixture of 3-O-benzyl-L-ascorbic acid (65) and 2-C-benzyl-L-xylo-3-hexulosonic acid lactone (7) [8]. The reaction mixture was treated with ammonia, and the 3-benzyl ether (65) purified as a syrup in 50% yield from the amide of (7) using cellulose column chromatography. The structure of the 3-benzyl ether (65) was deduced by its conversion in two steps to crystalline 3-O-benzyl-5,6-O-isopropylidene-2-O-methyl-L-ascorbic-acid (66), which was different from crystalline 2-O-benzyl-

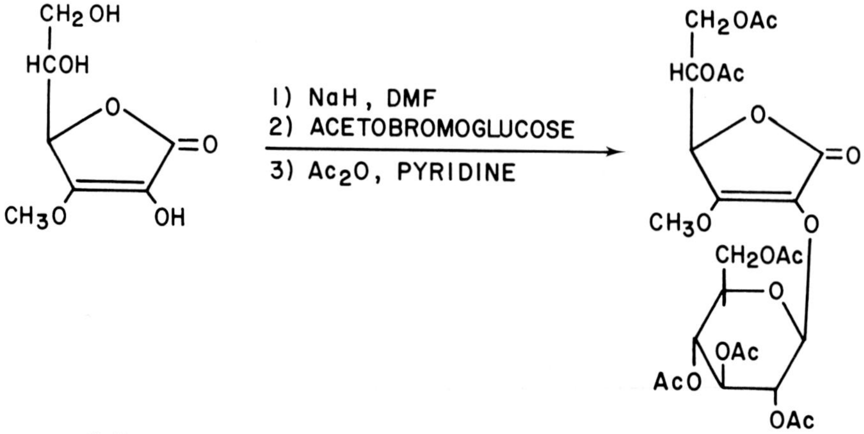

CH2OH
|
HCOH

(structure **44**)

CH3O   OH

44

1) NaH, DMF
2) ACETOBROMOGLUCOSE
———————————————→
3) Ac2O, PYRIDINE

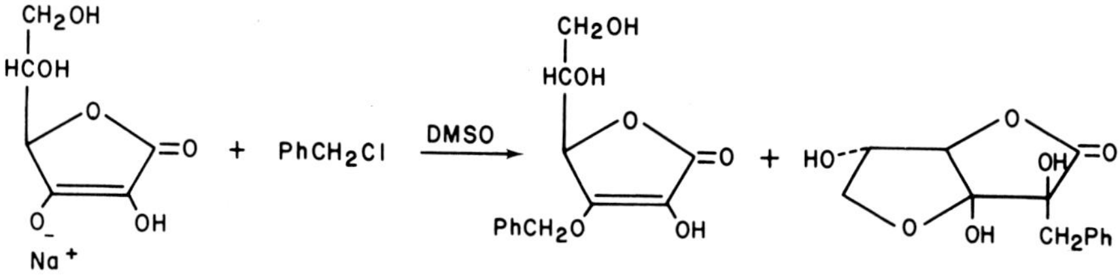

CH2OAc
|
HCOAc

(structure **64**)

CH3O

CH2OAc

AcO   OAc

OAc

64

CH2OH
|
HCOH

(structure **1a**)

O⁻
|
Na⁺   OH

1a

+ PhCH2Cl

DMSO
————→

CH2OH
|
HCOH

(structure **65**)

PhCH2O   OH

65

+ HO

(structure **7**)

OH   OH   CH2Ph

7

Ph = ⟨benzene ring⟩

H2C-O   CH3
| ╳
HC-O   CH3

(structure)

R1O   OR2

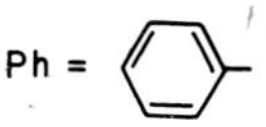

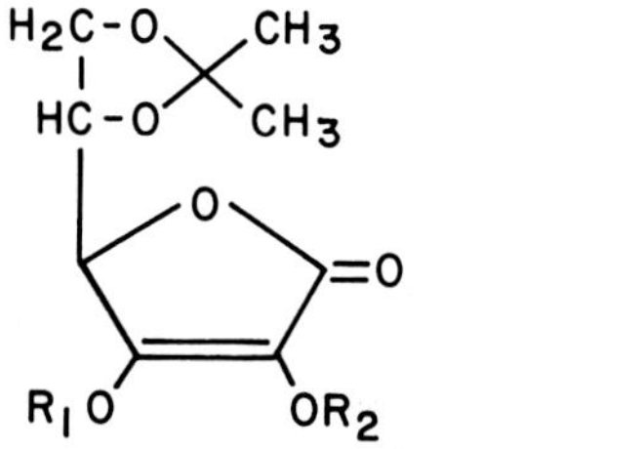

66 R1 = −CH2Ph, R2 = −CH3
67 R1 = −CH3 , R2 = −CH2Ph

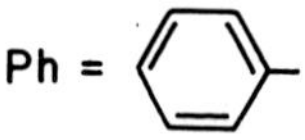

Ph = ⟨benzene ring⟩

5,6-*O*-isopropylidene-3-*O*-methyl-L-ascorbic acid (**67**) prepared from 3-*O*-methyl-L-ascorbic acid (**44**).

The structure of the *C*-benzyl ether (**7**) was determined by x-ray crystallography of its methyl glycoside [6]. It is not known whether the 3-keto-group in **7** forms a 6,3-furanose ring or remains free. The configuration originally assigned to **7** appears to be in error; the configuration is L-*xylo* instead of L-*lyxo*. It seems likely that compound (**7**) forms directly by reaction of the 2-carbanion (**5a**) with benzyl chloride. Other reactions of the 2-carbanion (**5a**) are discussed under the next subtitle.

Selective Esterification and Etherification at O-2

To prepare 2-monoesters or 2-monoethers of L-ascorbic acid, the acid (**1**) should be reacted in its dianion (**1b**) form, and the derivative must be stable in the reaction medium. Moreover, in etherifications, O-6 should be blocked to prevent MICHAEL addition of O-6 to the etherified 2,3-enediol.

L-Ascorbate 2-sulfate (**69**) has been synthesized in practically quantitive yield by reaction of **1b** with trimethylamine-sulfur trioxide (**68**) in alkali (pH 9.5–10.5) at 70° [68]. It is assumed that sulfation occurs at the 2-oxyanion of **1b** due to its high nucleophilicity compared to that of the 3-oxyanion whose charge is dispersed. The 2-sulfate ester (**69**) was also obtained in 75 % yield by sulfation of 5,6-*O*-isopropylidene-L-ascorbic acid (**42**) with pyridine-sulfur trioxide (**70**) in DMF/pyridine followed by hydrolytic removal of the 5,6-blocking group [68]. Other workers have prepared the 2-sulfate ester by similar schemes [87, 109].

L-Ascorbate 2-sulfate occurs in animals, but its vitamin C potency is species-dependent; it is active in finfish [110, 111] but not in insects [112] or mammals [113]. Ascorbate 2-sulfate (**69**) is poorly absorbed and rapidly eliminated except in fish. Fish appear to use **69** as a storage form of vitamin C [114]. L-Ascorbate 2-sulfate is approximately 20X more stable than L-ascorbate towards oxygen in boiling water. Formulated feeds for growing trout, salmon and catfish require 50–100 mg of L-ascorbate per kilogram of feed. Processing and storage of feed invariably exposes the vitamin to oxygen, which requires an excess of **1** in feed. L-Ascorbate 2-sulfate (**69**), which is equivalent to **1** in vitamin C potency in finfish, can be added in lower amounts to fish diets than **1**.

5,6-*O*-Isopropylidene-L-ascorbate 2-phosphate (**71**) was prepared in almost quantitative yield when phosphoryl chloride reacted with **42b** at 0–5° in alkali (pH 12–13) containing a high concentration of pyridine [116, 117]. After

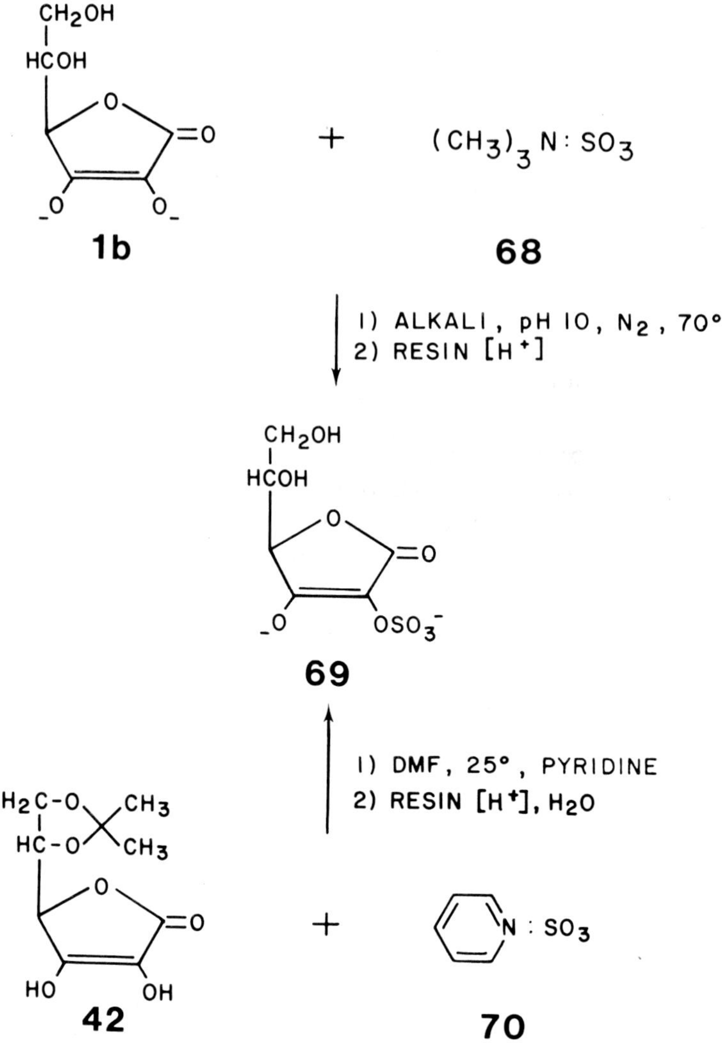

CH$_2$OH
|
HCOH

(structure 1b) + (CH$_3$)$_3$N : SO$_3$

1b   **68**

1) ALKALI, pH 10, N$_2$, 70°
2) RESIN [H$^+$]

CH$_2$OH
|
HCOH

(structure 69 with OSO$_3^-$)

69

1) DMF, 25°, PYRIDINE
2) RESIN [H$^+$], H$_2$O

H$_2$C–O   CH$_3$
| X
HC–O   CH$_3$

(structure 42 with HO, OH) + (pyridine) N : SO$_3$

42   **70**

hydrolytic removal of the 5,6-acetal group, L-ascorbate 2-phosphate (**58**) was isolated in 70% yield as a crystalline amine salt. When no pyridine was present in the reaction mixture, **42b** was converted to a mixture of (**71**) and bis-(5,6-O-isopropylidene-L-ascorbate) 2,2'-phosphate, which after removal of the 5,6 protecting group, gave the phosphoric diester (**72**). The diester was obtained free of (**58**) in 32% yield by fractional crystallization of its barium salt.

Recently, L-ascorbate 2-phosphate (**58**) was prepared in four steps (53% yield) starting from fully trimethylsilylated L-ascorbic acid [74]. The

2-phosphate ester (58) also was synthesized, as discussed above, by acid treatment of 3-O-[(bis-morpholino)-phosphinate]-5,6-O-isopropylidene-L-ascorbate (57) [89]. The 2-diphenyl-phosphinyl ester (73) was reported in 1984 [96].

The role of pyridine in the reaction between **42b** and phosphoryl chloride has not been investigated. It appears that **42b** reacts rapidly with $POCl_3$ to give the intermediate 5,6-O-isopropylidene-2-O-(dichlorophospho)-L-ascorbate, and pyridine then displaces the chloride from that intermediate. Without pyridine, the 2-O-(dichlorophospho)-ester reacts with the 2-oxyanion of a second molecule of **42b** to give the phosphodiester **(72)**.

L-Ascorbate 2-phosphate **(58)** has been shown to be an active source of vitamin C in the rhesus monkey and guinea pig [118]. The 2-phosphate ester, like the 2-sulfate ester **(69)**, is much more stable to air than L-ascorbic acid [119]. In foods and feeds the 2-phosphate **(58)** might be used as a stable source of vitamin C, provided the ingredients are free of phosphatase activity. In the field of medicine, the 2-phosphate **(58)** improves the performance of stored red blood cells from humans by enhancing their ability to release oxygen [120].

5,6-O-isopropylidene-L-ascorbic acid **(42b)** was 2-methylated by dimethyl sulfate **(74)** at pH 10.5 and 60° C. Removal of the 5,6-blocking group gave 85% 2-O-methyl-L-ascorbic acid **(50)** [11]. Methylation of L-ascorbate **(1b)** with **74** (1.6 eq) at pH 10–11 gave predominantly **50** (70% yield), but the reaction was complicated by a side-reaction that produced the methyl β-furanoside **(75)** of 2-O-methyl-L-*xylo*-3-hexulosonic acid in ~15% yield. Compound **75** is identical to "isodimethylascorbic acid" which is produced when 2,3-di-O-methyl-L-ascorbic acid **(76)** is treated with aqueous barium hydroxide [11], first described by HAWORTH and coworkers in 1937 [10].

The methyl β-L-furanoside **(75)** is probably formed by an intramolecular Michael addition of the 6-oxyanion at C-3 when both the 2-OH and 3-OH are methylated. After formation of the furanoside ring, the lactone ring saponifies, but it reforms during isolation of **75**. In support of that mechanism, the yield of **75** from **1** increased as more sulfating agent **(74)** was used [11]. Furthermore, 2-O-methyl-L-ascorbic acid **(50)**, which is the first product in the methylation of **1** with **74** in alkali, does not undergo the

Michael addition reaction when placed in alkali. Neither does the 1- or 3-monoethyl ether (9 or 44). In alkali all the monomethyl ethers have ionized enolic hydroxyls, and some of the negative charge is dispersed to C-3 which appears to repulse the 6-oxyanion.

In spite of formation of two new asymmetric centers when the 2,3-dimethylether (76) undergoes the intramolecular addition reaction, only one isomer (75) was detected by ^{13}C-nmr [11]. Jones [121] showed that 75 has the L-xylo configuration. Apparently, the L-xylo isomer (75) is the kinetic product, since the thermodynamic product would be expected to have the L-lyxo-configuration wherein the 2-OCH$_3$ is disposed exo to the bicyclic ring system. In the mechanism proposed here for the formation of 75 from 50, the solvent molecule approaches the C-2 carbanion (77) exo to the bicyclic ring system, forming the L-xylo configuration.

It is interesting to note that 2-O-methyl-L-ascorbic acid (50) can be prepared quantitatively from the methyl furanoside (75) by methanolic hydrogen chloride [10, 11]. Since glycosides normally form in hot methanolic hydrogen chloride, the bicyclic furanoside-lactone (75) is less stable than the isomeric monocyclic structure (50) with an ionizable 2,3-ene-lactone.

However, the formation of **75** from **76** is favored due to saponification of the lactone ring to give the carboxylate anion (**77a**).

2-O-Methyl-L-ascorbic acid has been found in urine from the rat, guinea pig and humans, but it has little antiscorbutic activity in the guinea pig or insects [11]. It may be a by-product of catechol-O-methyltransferase [122].

The ambident nature of the L-ascorbate anion (**1a**, **5a** and **6a**) is now well recognized. Reactions are known in which the C-2 carbanion (**5a**) reacts with electrophiles to produce C-alkalylated derivatives of L-ascorbate [8, 9, 123]. JACKSON and JONES [8] were the first to demonstrate C-2 alkylation of **1** when they reacted potassium L-ascorbate in water with benzyl chloride in acetone. Approximately equal quantities of 3-O-benzyl-L-ascorbic acid (**65**) and 2-C-

Ph = (phenyl ring structure)

benzyl-L-*xylo*-3-hexulosonic acid lactone (7) were isolated [8]. The L-*xylo*-configuration in 7 is consistent with benzyl chloride approaching the C-2 carbanion (5a) from the side opposite to the C-5, C-6 side-chain.

Ascorbigen, which is a C-2 bound form of L-ascorbic acid found in ground cabbage, has been synthesized chemically by reaction of 3-hydroxymethyl-indole (78) with L-ascorbic acid in water at pH 4 [9]. In the mechanism proposed for synthesis of ascorbigen, the protonated form of 78 loses a molecule of water to form a carbonium-immonium ion (79) that combines with the 2-carbanion (5a) to give ascorbigen (8) in 50–60% yield. The structure of 8 was deduced from its ir and ^{1}H-nmr spectra, and from the ease of its conversion to a methyl furanoside (80) and an amide (81). The configuration of 8 was assumed to be L-*xylo*. A small amount (2%) of the L-*lyxo* isomer of 8 was purified from the reaction mixture, but no O-skatyl derivatives of

L-ascorbate were detected. L-ascorbic acid was slowly released [9] by hydrolysis of ascorbigen at pH 2 and 37° C.

L-Ascorbyl 2-palmitate (**83**) can be prepared in 38 % yield by reaction of a pyridine-acetone solution of 5,6-*O*-isopropylidene-L-ascorbic acid (**42**) with palmitoyl chloride followed by deacetonation of **82** in methanolic hydrogen chloride [124].

R = $C_{15}H_{31}-$

Selective Esterification and Etherification at O-6

Selective esterification of O-6 on L-ascorbic acid occurs readily in strong acid [86, 87]. A high yield (85%) of 6-O-palmitoyl-L-ascorbic acid (88) is realized when 1 is dissolved in concentrated sulfuric acid (98–99%) containing 30% excess palmitic acid [124]. The 6-ester (88) is the thermodynamic product when equilibrium is reached in the strongly acidic medium. Other 6-fatty acid esters of 1 are prepared in the same manner.

At first, esterification of 1 in concentrated sulfuric acid appears to be inconsistent with the decomposition of low-molecular weight carbohydrates in strong acid. Indeed, in hot acid L-ascorbic acid decarboxylates and dehydrates to give almost quantitative yields of furfural and carbon dioxide [125, 126]. But in 95–98% sulfuric acid at 25° the skeletal structure of 1 remains intact after 46 days as shown by uv and optical rotation [124]. Apparently, L-ascorbic acid is protonated in concentrated sulfuric acid to a stable hydroxyallyl cation (84); the cation (84) gives λ_{max} 265 nm, and ^{13}C-nmr shows that all carbons of 84 are deshielded by 3–16 ppm with reference to the signals of 1 in water at pH 2.

When L-ascorbic acid (1) dissolves in concentrated H_2SO_4, its 6-OH is sulfated immediately to give intermediate (84). Then, the fatty acid in the reaction mixture displaces the weakly nucleophilic sulfate ion to form intermediate (87), which is converted to 88 as the reaction mixture is added to a large excess of ice-water. The 6-sulfate ester (85, 85% yield) and the 5-sulfate ester (86, 4% yield) were isolated after 1 was dissolved in concentrated sulfuric acid. No 2-sulfate (69) was detected [127].

The non-oxidation degradation of L-ascorbic acid in acid is the second most important reaction responsible for loss of vitamin C in foods, feeds and phar-

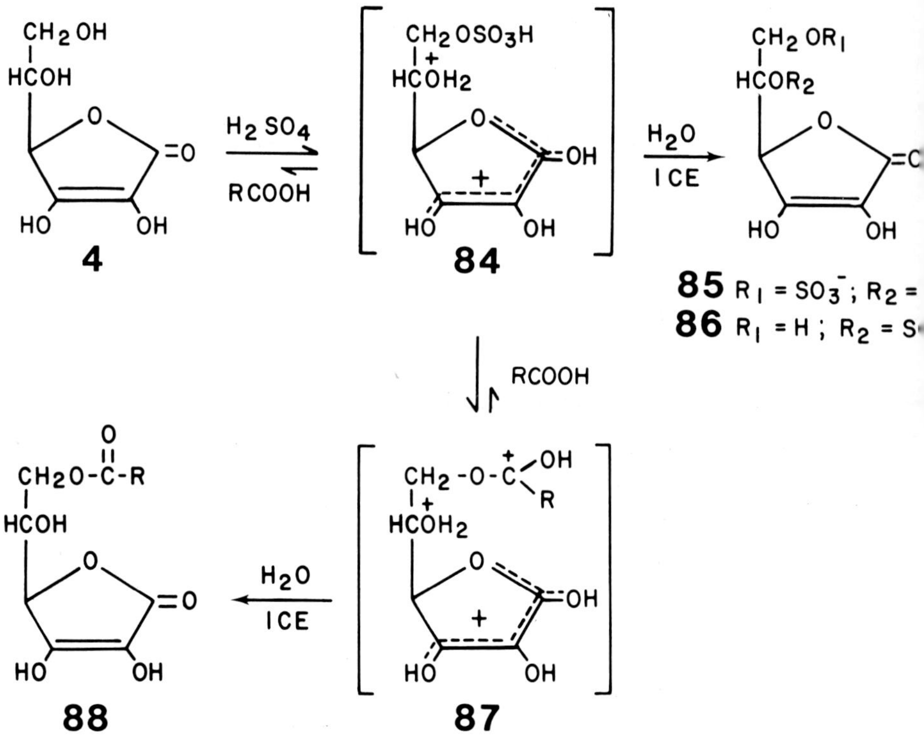

$$\begin{array}{c} CH_2OH \\ | \\ HCOH \end{array} \quad \xrightarrow[RCOOH]{H_2SO_4} \quad \begin{array}{c} CH_2OSO_3H \\ |+ \\ HCOH_2 \end{array} \quad \xrightarrow[ICE]{H_2O} \quad \begin{array}{c} CH_2OR_1 \\ | \\ HCOR_2 \end{array}$$

4

84

85 $R_1 = SO_3^-$; $R_2 =$

86 $R_1 = H$; $R_2 = S$

↓ RCOOH

$$\begin{array}{c} O \\ || \\ CH_2O-C-R \\ | \\ HCOH \end{array} \quad \xleftarrow[ICE]{H_2O} \quad \begin{array}{c} +\;OH \\ CH_2-O-C \\ |+ \quad\quad R \\ HCOH_2 \end{array}$$

88   **87**

$R = CH_3(CH_2)_{14}-$

maceuticals. It is important to digress here briefly to examine this reaction. Furfural (90), 3-deoxy-L-2-pentosulose (91) and 2-oxalylfuran (89) have been identified in reaction mixtures of 1 in acid. Goshima and coworkers [126] have explained the occurrence of 89 and 91 as by-products of the intermediates involved in the main pathway of 1 to 90 in hot acid. The intermediates shown in the mechanism herein are slightly modified from those given by Goshima et al [126].

6-Acyl esters of L-ascorbic acid can also be prepared by esterification initially at O-3 on 5,6-O-isopropylidene-L-ascorbic acid (42) followed by removal of the 5,6-blocking group in aqueous acid with simultaneous migration of the 3-O-acyl group to O-6 [102]. This method was discussed previously under the subtitle dealing with 3-O substitution.

6-Tosylation of 2-O-palmitoyl-L-ascorbic acid (83) was not successful when 83 was reacted with p-tolylsulfonyl chloride in pyridine [128]. However, 6-O-p-tolylsulfonyl-2-O-palmitoyl-L-ascorbic acid [m.p. 72–74°] (92) was formed smoothly if the reaction was done in ethyl ether with only small amounts of pyridine. This approach might be useful in synthesizing 6-O trityl and 6-O-(t-butyldimethylsilyl) ethers in O-2 blocked derivatives of **1**.

6-Phenoxy and 6-thiophenoxy ethers of L-ascorbic acid have been prepared by nucleophilic attack at the epoxide ring of 5,6-anhydro-L-ascorbic acid **(95)** [129]. The epoxide derivative **(95)** was generated as a reactive intermediate from 6-bromo-6-deoxy-L-ascorbic acid **(94)**, which was prepared in two steps by treatment of **1** with hydrogen bromide in acetic or formic acid followed by hydrolytic removal of the 5-acyl group from **93**. The reaction of halogen acids

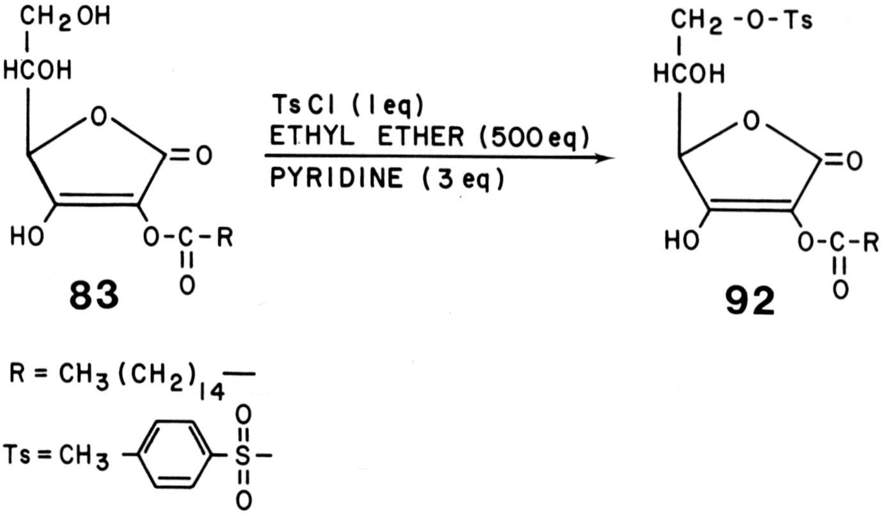

CH$_2$OH
|
HCOH

83

TsCl (I eq)
ETHYL ETHER (500 eq)
PYRIDINE (3 eq)
⟶

CH$_2$-O-Ts
|
HCOH

92

R = CH$_3$(CH$_2$)$_{14}$—

Ts = CH$_3$—⟨ ⟩—S—

in acetic or formic acid is a general method of producing 6-deoxy-6-halo derivatives of **1** and **3** [87, 130]. The epoxide intermediate (**95**) was too labile to isolate, but it could be generated in aqueous solution and then reacted with moderately basic nucleophiles, such as phenoxide, thiophenoxide, and azide ion. Attempts to add more basic nucleophiles to **95**, such as sodium methoxide/methanol, were not successful [128]. The 6-azido-6-deoxy derivative was reduced to give 6-amino-6-deoxy-L-ascorbic acid (**97**).

Selective Sulfation at O-5

L-Ascorbate 5-sulfate (**86**) is the only known O-5 monosubstituted derivative of **1**. Reaction of **1** with two equivalents of *t*-butyldimethylsilyl chloride in pyridine followed by sulfation with pyridine-sulfur trioxide gave 2,6-bis-*O*-(*t*-butyldimethylsilyl)-L-ascorbate 5-sulfate (**98**). Hydrolytic removal of the silyl blocking groups with 80% acetic acid followed by purification on diethylaminoethylcellulose gave 60% of **86** as its barium salt [127].

The strong electronegativity of the 5-sulfate ester facilitates formation of the C-4 carbanion in **86**. When an aqueous solution of the barium salt of **86**

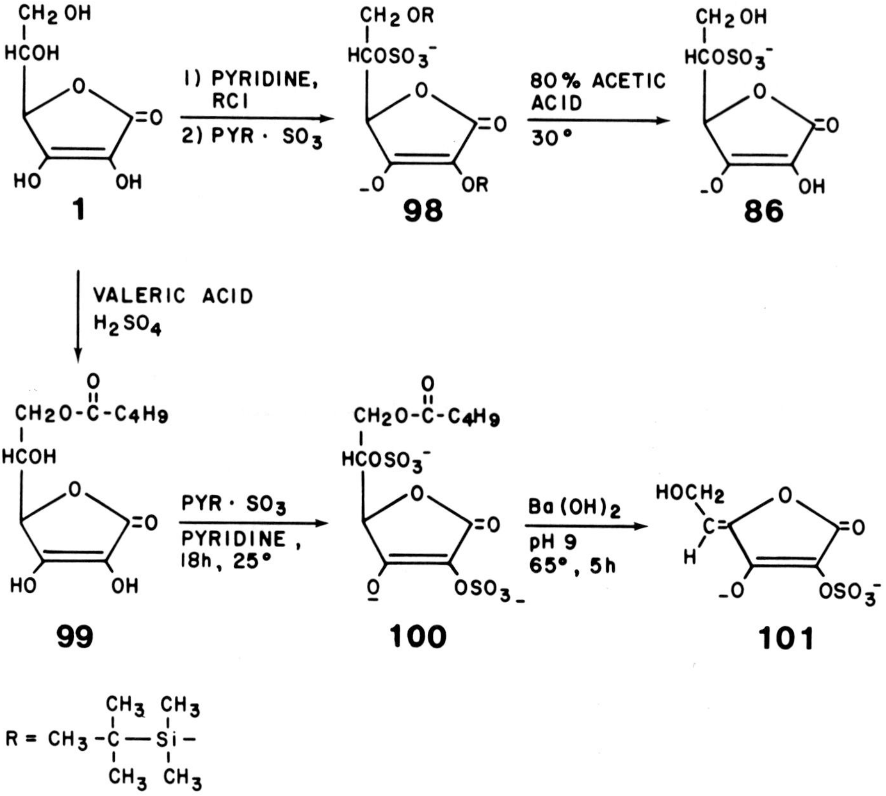

CH2 OH
|
HCOH
      1) PYRIDINE,
        RCl
      2) PYR · SO3
              =0
HO   OH
1

CH2 OR
|
HCOSO3⁻
      80% ACETIC
      ACID
      30°
              =0
₋0   OR
98

CH2 OH
|
HCOSO3⁻
              =0
₋0   OH
86

VALERIC ACID
H2SO4

       O
       ‖
CH2O-C-C4H9
|
HCOH
      PYR · SO3
      PYRIDINE,
      18h, 25°
              =0
HO   OH
99

       O
       ‖
CH2O-C-C4H9
|
HCOSO3⁻
      Ba(OH)2
      pH 9
      65°, 5h
              =0
₋O   OSO3₋
100

HOCH2
    C=
H
              =0
₋0   OSO3⁻
101

        CH3 CH3
         | |
R = CH3-C—Si-
         | |
        CH3 CH3

was allowed to stand at room temperature, barium sulfate precipitated due to elimination of sulfuric acid between C-4 and C-5. Facile elimination of sulfuric acid at C-4 and C-5 also occurred when 6-O-valeroyl-L-ascorbate 2,5-disulfate (**100**) was treated with barium hydroxide. The 4,5-ene product (**101**) is optically inactive and is thought to have the Z-configuration [7].

Other derivatives with an acidic H-4 include 1-O-methyl-L-ascorbic acid (**9**), 5-keto-L-ascorbic acid (**45**), and L-*threo*-2,3-hexodiulosono-1,4-lactone 2-(phenylhydrazone); cf. (**33**, R = phenyl).

Note added in proofs. G. M. Jaffe reported [131] U.S. production of

L-ascorbic acid is 11×10^6 kg/year, and world production 30×10^6 kg/year. Stable transition-metal complexes of (**1**) have been prepared [132], and X-ray crystallography showed the C-2 of tautomer (**5a**) formed a metal-carbon bond in the complex.

Acknowledgments: The author thanks Drs G.C. Andrews and G.A. Iacobucci for preprints, and Mr Ming-Long Liao for searching the recent literature.

References

1 BAUERNFEIND, J: Ascorbic acid technology in agricultural, pharmaceutical, food and industrial applications. In: SEIB and TOLBERT (eds). Ascorbic acid: chemistry, metabolism, and uses. Adv Chem Ser No 200, pp 395–497. American Chemical Society, Washington, 1982.

2 Anonymous: Vitamin C expansion may pose problem. Chem Eng News 50(49), 4, Dec. 4, 1972.

3 BRENNER G S et al: Isomerization of the ascorbic acids. J Org Chem 29, 2389–2392, 1964.

4 HIRST, E L et al: The structure of ascorbic acid. Chem Ind. (London) 11, 221–222, 1933.

5 CRAWFORD, T C, CRAWFORD, S A: Synthesis of L-ascorbic acid. Adv Carb Chem 37, 79–155, 1980.

6 HVOSLEF, J: Crystallography of the ascorbates. In: SEIB and TOLBERT (eds): Ascorbic acid: chemistry, metabolism, and uses. Adv Chem Ser No 200, pp 37–57. American Chemical Society, Washington, 1982.

7 PAUKSTELIS, J V et al: Nmr spectroscopy of ascorbic acid and its derivatives. In: SEIB and TOLBERT (eds). Ascorbic acid: chemistry, metabolism, and uses. Adv Chem Ser No 200, pp 125–151. American Chemical Society, Washington, 1982.

8 JACKSON, K G A, JONES, J K N: The O- and C-benzylation of L-ascorbic acid. Canad J Chem 43, 450–457, 1965.

9 KISS, G, NEUKOM, H: Concerning the structure of ascorbigen. Helv Chim Acta 49, 989–992, 1966.

10 HAWORTH, W N et al: Isomerization of 2,3-dimethyl ascorbic acid. J Chem Soc 829–834, 1937.

11 LU, P W et al: Synthesis of the 2-methyl ether of L-ascorbic acid: Stability, vitamin activity, and carbon-13 nuclear magnetic resonance spectrum compared to those of the 1- and 3-methyl ethers. J Agric Food Chem 32, 21–28, 1984.

12 LEWIN, S: Vitamin C: Its molecular biology and medical potential, pp 6–9. Academic Press, New York, 1976.

13 CRAWFORD, T C: Synthesis of L-ascorbic acid. In: SEIB and TOLBERT (eds). Ascorbic acid: chemistry, metabolism, and uses. Adv Chem Ser No 200, pp 1–36. American Chemical Society, Washington, 1982.

14 REICHSTEIN, T, GRÜSSNER, A: A good synthesis of L-ascorbic acid (vitamin C). Helv Chim Acta 17, 311–328, 1934.

15 SONOYAMA, T et al: Production of 2-keto-L-gulonic acid from D-glucose by two-stage fermentation. Appl Environ Microbiol 43, 1064–1069, 1982.

16 Mitsui Toatsu Chemicals. 2-Keto-L-gulonic acid. Jap Kokai Tokkyo Koho JP 57, 163, 340 [82, 163, 340] 1982. Chem Abst 98, 107688f, 1983.

17 LOEWUS, F A: L-Ascorbic acid: metabolism, biosynthesis, function. In: PREIS (ed). The biochemistry of plants, vol 3, Carbohydrates: structure and function, pp 77–99. Academic Press, New York, 1980.

18 CHATTERJEE, I B et al: Synthesis and some major functions of vitamin C in animals. Ann NY Acad Sci 258, 24–47, 1975.

19 STRAND, L L et al: Characterization of two endopolygalacturonase isozymes produced by Fusarium Oxysporum f. sp. Lycopersici. Biochim Biophys Acta 429, 870–883, 1976.

20 PILNIK, W, ROMBOUTS, F M: Pectic enzymes. In: BLANSHARD and MITCHELL (eds). Polysaccharides in food, pp 109–126. Butterworths, Boston, 1979.

21 ISBELL, H S: Interpretation of some reactions in the carbohydrate field in terms of consecutive electron displacement. J Res Nat Bureau Stand 33, 45–59, 1944.

22 NISHIKIMI, M et al: Occurrence in yeast of L-galactonolactone oxidase which is similar to key enzyme for ascorbic acid biosynthesis in animals, L-gulonolactone oxidase. Arch Biochem Biophys 191, 479–486, 1978.

23 Nishikimi, M et al: Redox properties of L-galactono-lactone oxidase purified from bakers' yeast. Biochem Int 1, 155–161, 1980.

24 Crawford, T C, Breitenback, R: New syntheses of L-ascorbic acid (vitamin C). J Chem Soc (D) 388–389, 1979.

25 Nishikimi, M et al: Purification and characterization of L-gulonolactone oxidase from rat and goat liver. Arch Biochem Biophys 175, 427–435, 1976.

26 Isherwood, F A et al: Synthesis of L-ascorbic acid in rat-liver homogenates. Conversion of L-gulono- and L-galactono-γ-lactone and the respective acids into L-ascorbic acid. Biochem J 76, 157–171, 1960.

27 Sato, P H, Grahn, I V: Administration of isolated chicken L-gulonolactone oxidase to guinea pigs evokes ascorbic acid synthetic capacity. Arch Biochem Biophys 210, 609–616, 1981.

28 Isherwood, F A, Mapson, L W: Biosynthesis of ascorbic acid from γ-lactones. British Pat 763,055, 1956. Chem Abstr 51, 8387b, 1957.

29 Loewus, F A, Loewus, M W: Myo-Inositol: its biosynthesis and metabolism. Ann Rev Plant Physiol 34, 137–161, 1983.

30 Hanninen, O et al: Biosynthesis of L-ascorbic acid from myo-inositol. Carb Res 16, 343–351, 1971.

31 Teramoto, S, Mizaki, A: Glucuronic acid. Japan Pat 15,119, 1962. Chem Abst 59, 2136b, 1964.

32 Mehltretter, C L: D-Glucuronic acid: α-D-glucofuranurono-6,3-lactone by catalytic air oxidation of 1,2-O-isopropylidene-α-D-glucofuranose. Methods Carb Chem 2, 29–31, 1963.

33 Heyns, K, Graefe, G: Oxidative conversion of carbohydrates. Part VII. Synthesis of D-glucuronic acid by way of carboxyl-starch. Chem Ber 86, 646–650, 1953.

34 Corn Products Refining Co. Glucuronic acid. British Patent 676, 567, July 30, 1952. Chem Abst 47, 935li, 1953.

35 Helsper, J P et al: L-ascorbic acid biosynthesis in Ochromonas danica. Plant Physiol 69, 465–468, 1982.

36 Shigeoka, S et al: The biosynthetic pathway of L-ascorbic acid in Euglena gracilis Z. J Nutr Soc Vitaminol 25, 299–307, 1979.

37 Bielski, B H J: Chemistry of ascorbic acid radicals. In: Seib and Tolbert (eds). Ascorbic acid: chemistry, metabolism, and uses. Adv Chem Ser No 200, p 81–100. American Chemical Society, Washington, 1982.

38 Sapper, H et al: ^{1}H-NMR and ESR investigations on the structures of dehydroascorbic acid and the semidehydroascorbate radical. Z Naturforsch 37C, 129–131, 1982.

39 Sapper, H et al: The reversibility of the vitamin C redox system: Electrochemical reasons and biological aspects. Z Naturforsch 37C, 942–946, 1982.

39a Chou, P T, Khan, A U: L-Ascorbic acid quenching of singlet delta molecular oxygen in aqueous media: generalized antioxidant property of vitamin C. Biochem Biophys Res Commun 115, 932–937, 1983.

40 Bielski, B H J et al: Some properties of the ascorbate free radical. Ann NY Acad Sci 258, 231–237, 1975.

41 Packer, J E et al: Direct observation of a free radical interaction between vitamin E and vitamin C. Nature 278, 737–738, 1979.

42 Bielski, B H J et al: Mechanism of disproportionation of ascorbate radicals. J Am Chem Soc 103, 3516–3518, 1981.

43 Hornig, D H, Moser, U: The safety of high vitamin C intakes in man. In: Counsell and Hornig (eds). Vitamin C; ascorbic acid, p 226. Applied Science Publishers, London, 1981.

44 Weissberger, A et al: Oxidation processes. XVI. The autoxidation of ascorbic acid. J Am Chem Soc 65, 1934–1939, 1943.

45 Blaug, S M, Hajratwala, B: Kinetics of aerobic oxidation of ascorbic acid. J Pharm Sci 61, 556–562, 1972.

46 MARTELL, A E: Chelates of ascorbic acid; formation and catalytic properties. In: SEIB and TOLBERT (eds). Ascorbic acid: chemistry, metabolism, and uses. Adv Chem Ser No 200, pp 153–178, American Chemical Society, Washington, 1982.

47 YAMAZAKI, I, PIETTE, L H: Mechanism of free radical formation and disappearance during the ascorbic acid oxidase and peroxidase reactions. Biochim Biophys Acta 50, 62–69, 1961.

48 CABELLI, D E, BIELSKI, B H J: Kinetics and mechanism for the oxidation of ascorbic acid/ascorbate by HO_2/O_2^- radicals. A pulse radiolysis and stopped-flow photolysis study. J Phys Chem 87, 1809–1812, 1983.

49 GEBICKI, J, BIELSKI, B H J: Comparison of the capacities of the perhydroxyl and superoxide radicals to initiate chain oxidation of linoleic acid. J Am Chem Soc 103, 7020–7021, 1981.

50 BIELSKI, B H et al: A study of the reactivity of HO_2/O_2^- with unsaturated fatty acids. J Biol Chem 258, 4759–4761, 1983.

51 PUGET, K, MICHELSON, A M: Iron curtaining superoxide dismutase from luminous bacteria. Biochimie 56, 1255–1267, 1974.

52 HAY, G W et al: In: SEBRELL and HARRIS (eds). The vitamins, 2nd Ed, vol 1, pp 307–336. Academic Press, New York, 1967.

53 SCAIFE J F: The catalysis of ascorbic acid oxidation by copper and its complexes with amino acids, peptides and proteins. Canad J Biochem Physiol 37, 1049–1067, 1959.

54 FLEMING, J E, BENSCH, K G: Effects of amino acids, peptides and related compounds on the autoxidation of ascorbic acid. Int J Pept Protein Res 22, 355–351, 1983.

55 LIANG, Y T, SEIB, P A: Unpublished results.

56 BORENSTEIN, B: Potentiation of the ascorbate effect in cured meat pigment development. J Food Sci 41, 1054–1055, 1976.

57 TAQUI KHAN, M M, MARTELL, A E: Metal ion and metal chelate catalyzed oxidation of ascorbic acid by molecular oxygen. II. Cupric and ferric chelate catalyzed oxidation. J Am Chem Soc 89, 7104–7111, 1967.

58 ROWLEY, D A, HALLIWELL, B: Superoxide-dependent and ascorbate-dependent formation of hydroxyl radicals in the presence of copper salts: a physiologically significant reaction? Arch Biochem Biophys 225, 279–284, 1983.

59 WALLING, C: Fenton's reagent revisited. Accounts Chem Res 8, 125–131, 1975.

60 IACOBUCCI, G A, SWEENY, J G: The chemistry of anthocyanins, anthocyanidins, and related flavylium salts. Tetrahedron 39, 3005–3038, 1983.

61 ISBELL, H S, FRUSH, H L: Oxidation of L-ascorbic acid: preparation of L-threonic acid. Carb Res 72, 301–304, 1979.

62 ROBINSON, A B, REICHHEIMER, S L: Instability and functions: Ascorbic acid and glutaminyl and asparaginyl residues. Ann NY Acad Sci 258, 314–316, 1975.

63 MORSE, R E: Ascorbic acid and sequestered copper. Food Res 18, 48–56, 1953.

64 KRONECK, P M H et al: Ascorbate oxidase: molecular properties and catalytic activities. In: SEIB and TOLBERT (eds). Ascorbic acid: chemistry, metabolism, and uses. Adv Chem Ser No 200, pp 223–248. American Chemical Society, Washington, 1982.

65 HALLIWELL, B: Ascorbic acid and the illuminated chloroplast. In: SEIB and TOLBERT (eds). Ascorbic acid: chemistry, metabolism, and uses. Adv Chem Ser No 200, pp 263–274. American Chemical Society, Washington, 1982.

66 NAKANO, Y, ASADA, K: Hydrogen peroxide is scavenged by ascorbate-specific peroxidase in spinach chloroplasts. Plant Cell Physiol 22, 867–880, 1981.

67 GRODEN, D, BECK, E: H_2O_2 destruction by ascorbate-dependent systems from chloroplasts. Biochim Biophys Acta 546, 426–435, 1979.

68 SEIB, P A et al: Synthesis and stability of L-ascorbate 2-sulfate. J Chem Soc 1220–1224, 1974.

69 LEE, C H et al: Chemical synthesis of several phosphate esters of L-ascorbic acid. Carbohydr Res 67, 127–138, 1978.

70 Tolbert, B M, Ward, J B: Dehydroascorbic acid. In: Seib and Tolbert (eds). Ascorbic acid: chemistry, metabolism, and uses. Adv Chem Ser No 200, pp 101–123. American Chemical Society, Washington, 1982.

71 Hvoslef, J, Pedersen, B: The structure of dehydroascorbic acid in solution. Acta Chem Scand Ser B 33, 503–511, 1979.

72 Ohmori, M et al: Pure dehydro-L-ascorbic acid prepared by O_2-oxidation of L-ascorbic acid with active charcoal as catalyst. Agric Biol Chem 47, 607–608, 1983.

73 Egge, H: Bicyclic derivative of dehydroascorbic acid. Tetrahedron Letters 801–803, 1969.

74 Sekine, M et al: Silyl phosphites, 21. A new method for synthesis of L-ascorbic acid 2-O-phosphate by utilizing phosphoryl rearrangement. J. Org Chem 47, 3453–3456, 1982.

75 Kang, S O et al: The oxidative degradation of L-ascorbic acid via an α-ketoaldehyde. Z Naturforsch 37C, 1064–1069, 1982.

76 Hvoslef, J, Pedersen, B: Structure of dehydroisoascorbic acid isomers in solution. Carb Res 92, 9–20, 1981.

77 Velisek, J et al: On the behaviour of L-dehydroascorbic acid in aqueous solutions. Coll Czech Chem Comm 37, 1465–1470, 1971.

78 Herbert, R W et al: The constitution of ascorbic acid. J Chem Soc 1270–1290, 1933.

79 Velisek, J et al: Volatile degradation products of L-dehydroascorbic acid. Z Lebensm Unters Forsch 162, 285–290, 1976.

80 El Ashry, E S H: Nitrogen derivatives of L-ascorbic acid. In: Seib and Tolbert (eds). Ascorbic acid: chemistry, metabolism, and uses. Adv Chem Ser No 200, pp 179–197. American Chemical Society, Washington, 1982.

81 Kurata, T et al: Red pigment produced by the oxidation of L-scorbamic acid. J Agric Food Chem 21, 676–680, 1973.

82 Kurata, T, Fujimaki, M: Monodehydro-2,2'-iminodi-2(2')-deoxy-L-ascorbic acid, a radical product from the reaction of dehydro-L-ascorbic acid with an α-amino acid. Agric Biol Chem 38, 1981–1988, 1974.

83 Yano, M et al: Formation of free radical products by the reaction of dehydroascorbic acid with amino acids. Agric Food Chem 24, 815–819, 1976.

84 Hagashi, T, Namiki, M: Tri(2-deoxy-2-L-ascorbyl)amine: a novel compound related to a fairly stable free radical. Tetrahedron Letters 46, 4467–4470, 1979.

85 Tsuji, K et al: Redox reaction of tri(2-deoxy-2-L-ascorbyl)amine. Formation of a persisting radical species in water. Electrochim Acta 25, 605–611, 1980.

86 Tolbert, B M et al: Chemistry and metabolism of ascorbic acid and ascorbate sulfate. Ann N Y Acad Sci 258, 48–69, 1975.

87 Andrews, G C, Crawford, T: Recent advances in the derivatization of L-ascorbic acid. In: Seib and Tolbert (eds). Ascorbic acid: chemistry, metabolism, and uses. Adv Chem Ser No 200, pp 395–497. American Chemical Society, Washington, 1982.

88 Radford, T et al: Ascorbic acid derivatives. Structure determination by carbon-13 nuclear magnetic resonance. J Org Chem 44, 658–659, 1979.

89 Jernow, J et al: Structural determination of ascorbic acid 2-O-phosphate formed via acid hydrolysis of an ascorbic acid 3-O-phosphinate. Tetrahedron 35, 1483–1486, 1979.

90 Paulssen, R B et al: Acylation of ascorbic acid in water. J Pharm Sci 64, 1300–1305, 1975.

91 Bond, A D et al: Ascorbic acid 2-sulfate of the brine shrimp Artemia salina. Arch Biochem Biophys 153, 207–214, 1972.

92 Lee, C H et al: Chemical synthesis of several phosphoric esters of L-ascorbic acid. Carbohydr Res 67, 127–138, 1978.

93 Kotowycz, G, Lemieux, R U: Nuclear magnetic resonance in carbohydrate chemistry. Chem Rev 73, 669–698, 1973.

94 Pople, J A et al: High resolution nuclear magnetic resonance, pp 271–280. McGraw-Hill, New York, 1959.

95 Bock, K, Pedersen, C: Carbon-13 nuclear magnetic resonance spectroscopy of monosaccharides. Adv Carb Chem *41*, 27–66, 1983.

96 Shaskus, J, Haake, P: Ascorbic acid. 2. Nucleophilic reactivity of ascorbate anion toward acyl carbon and phosphorus. J Org Chem *49*, 197–199, 1984.

97 Haworth, W N *et al:* Methyl ethers of ascorbic acid. J Chem Soc 1556–1560, 1934.

98 Reichstein, T *et al:* Synthesis of ascorbic acid and related compounds by the ozone-hydrogen cyanide method. Helv Chim Acta *17*, 510–520, 1934.

99 Vestling, C S, Rebstock, M C: The antiscorbutic properties of 3-methyl ascorbic acid. J Biol Chem *164*, 631–637, 1946.

100 Sato, T: L-Ascorbic acid derivatives. Japan Kokai Tokkyo Koho JP *58*, 57, 373 [83, 57, 373]. Chem Abstr *99*, 38782p, 1983.

101 Eli Lilly, & Co: Ascorbic acid ethers. Jpn Kokai Tokkyo Koho JP *58*, 131, 978 [83, 131, 978]. Chem Abstr *100*, 34783f, 1984.

102 King, G A *et al:* The acylation of 5,6-isopropylidene ascorbic acid. Synthesis of 2-0-acyl and 2-0-methyl ascorbic acid. Abstr Pap 181st Nat Meet Am Chem Soc, Div Org Chem, March 29 – April 3, 1981. Abstr 230.

103 Iacobucci, G A: Private communication, 1984.

104 Staab, H A, Mannschreck, A: Synthesis of carboxylate esters using the imidazole method. Chem Ber *95*, 1284–1297, 1962.

105 Tanaka, H, Yamamoto, R: Pharmaceutical studies on ascorbic acid derivatives. I. Syntheses of esters of ascorbic acid and their physicochemical properties. Yakugaku Zasshi *86*, 376–83, 1966. Chem Abstr *65*, 5515a, 1966.

106 Vestling, C S, Rebstock, M C.: 3-Acetyl-5,6-isopropylidene ascorbic acid. J Biol. Chem *152*, 585–591, 1944.

107 MacDonald, D L: Phosphates and other inorganic esters. In: Pigman and Horton (eds). The carbohydrates, vol 1A, pp 256–257. Academic Press, New York, 1972.

108 Clark, V M *et al:* The oxidative dephosphorylation of phosphoryl esters derived from L-ascorbic acid. Experientia *22*, 425, 1966.

109 Kumiai Chemical Industry Co., Ltd. L-Ascorbic 2-sulfate ester salts. Jap Tokkyo Koho JP *57*, 52,346 [82, 52,346]. Chem Abstr *99*, 22303X, 1983.

110 Benitez, L V, Halver, J E: Ascorbic acid sulfate sulfohydrolase (C2-sulfatase): the modulator of cellular levels of L-ascorbic acid in rainbow trout. Proc Nat Acad Sci USA *79*, 5445–5449, 1982.

111 Murai, T *et al:* Use of L-ascorbic acid, ethocel coated ascorbic acid and ascorbate 2-sulfate in diets for channel catfish, *Ictalurus punctatus*. J Nutr *108*, 1761–1766, 1978.

112 Kramer, K J, Seib, P A: Ascorbic acid and the growth and development of insects. In: Seib and Tolbert (eds). Ascorbic acid: chemistry, metabolism, and uses. Adv Chem Ser No 200, pp 275–292. American Chemical Society, Washington, 1982.

113 Machlin, L J *et al:* Lack of antiscorbutic activity of ascorbate 2-sulfate in rhesus monkey. Am J Clin Nutr *29*, 825–831, 1976.

114 Tucker, B: Studies on vitamin C metabolism in rainbow trout; doct diss. University of Washington, Seattle, 1983.

115 Sato, M *et al:* Nonessentiality of ascorbic acid in the diet of carp. Bull Soc Sci Fish *44(10)*, 1151–1156, 1969.

116 Nomura, H *et al:* Studies on L-ascorbic acid derivatives. II. L-Ascorbic acid 3-phosphate and 3-pyrophosphate. Chem Pharm Bull *17*, 381–386, 1969.

117 Lee, C H *et al:* Chemical synthesis of several phosphoric esters of L-ascorbic acid. Carbohydr Res *67*, 127–138, 1978.

118 Machlin, L J *et al:* Antiscorbutic activity of ascorbic acid phosphate in the rhesus monkey and the guinea pig. Am J Clin Nutr *32*, 325–331, 1979.

119 Lee, C H: Synthesis and characterization of L-ascorbate phosphates and their stabilities in model systems; doct diss Kansas State University, Manhattan, 1976.

120 Moore, G L et al: Improved red blood cell storage using optional additive systems (OAS) containing adenine, glucose and ascorbate 2-phosphate. Transfusion 21, 723–731, 1981.

121 Jones, J K N: The synthesis of 3-hexuloses. Part 1. 2-O-Methyl-L-xylo-3-hexulose. J Am Chem Soc 78, 2855–2857, 1956.

122 Bowers-Komro D M et al: Confirmation of 2-O-methyl ascorbic acid as the product from the enzymatic methylation of L-ascorbic acid by catechol-O-methyltransferase. Int J Vit Nutr Res 52, 186–193, 1982.

123 Brimacombe, J S et al: An investigation of the use of L-ascorbic acid and its derivatives in the synthesis of spirolactones. Carbohydr Res 45, 45–53, 1975.

124 Cousins, R C et al: Synthesis of 6-fatty acid esters of L-ascorbic acid. J Am Oil Chem Soc 54, 308–312, 1977.

125 Feather, M S, Harris, J F: Dehydration reactions of carbohydrates. Adv Carb Chem 28, 161–224, 1973.

126 Goshima, K et al: A novel degradation pathway of L-ascorbic acid under non-oxidative conditions. Bull Chem Soc Japan 46, 902–904, 1973.

127 Lillard, D W, Seib, P A: Monosulfate esters of L-ascorbic acid. In: Sweiger (ed). Carbohydrate sulfates. ACS Symp Ser No 77, pp 1–18. American Chemical Society, Washington, 1978.

128 Lu, P W, Seib, P A: Unpublished results, 1982.

129 Andrews, G: 5,6-Anhydro-L-ascorbic acid. A reactive intermediate for the formation of 6-deoxy-6-substituted derivatives of L-ascorbic acid. Carbohydr Res (submitted).

130 El Ashry, E S, El Kilang, Y: Bromodeoxy-isoascorbic acid and derivatives thereof. Carb Res 80, C25–27, 1980.

131 Jaffe, G M. Ascorbic acid. In: Encyclopedia of chemical technology; 3rd ed. Vol 24, pp 8–40. Wiley, New York, 1984.

132 Anonymus. Platinum complexes of vitamin C show anticancer potential. Chem Eng News 62 (38), 29–30, Sept 17, 1984.

P.A. Seib, Department of Grain Science and Industry, Kansas State University, Manhattan, Kansas 66506, USA

Antioxidant Function of L-Ascorbic Acid in Food Technology

J. C. BAUERNFEIND

Gainesville, Florida, USA

Key Words: L-Ascorbic acid · Ascorbyl palmitate · Sodium ascorbate · Tocopherol · Oxygen scavenger · Antioxidant · Synergist · Fats · Oils · Heat processed foods · Frozen foods · Cured foods · Fermented or cultured foods · Carbonated foods

Abstract: L-Ascorbic acid, its sodium salt and palmitoyl ester are indeed unique and versatile chemical compounds. Ascorbic acid, a naturally occurring compound, is vitamin C. All three compounds are biologically active and hence can serve as vitamin C dietary sources. Due to the molecular structure, particularly at the 2- and 3-carbon atoms sites, the compounds possess the faculty of acting as oxygen scavengers, antioxidants and synergists. Thus when added to fat-base or water-base foods they serve a technological role by themselves. In the presence of the tocopherols, another class of natural commmpounds, in fatty type foods they inhibit or retard deteriorative changes and extend palatability and appearance of the food supply.

Introduction

Nearly a half century has passed since the synthesis and commercial production of L-ascorbic acid. Over this period of time L-ascorbic acid, its salts and esters, in addition to being sources of dietary vitamin C in pharmaceutical dosage forms and in processed foods [1], have found antioxidant application as additives [1–3, 112, 113] in a variety of circumstances because of their special chemical properties.

L-ascorbic acid, a six-carbon, water-soluble, white, crystalline compound is vitamin C (the antiscorbutic vitamin). Ascorbic acid ($C_6H_8O_6$) resembles the sugars in structure (Fig. 1). Some of the unusual properties of the molecule (mol. wt. 176.13) are due to the enediol grouping. It is a moderately strong reducing agent and is sufficiently acidic to form neutral salts with bases such as with sodium hydroxide. Description, identification, specifications and tests of L-ascorbic acid and sodium L-ascorbate (Fig. 1) are given in the US Pharmacopoeia and the Food Chemicals Codex. Similar information on ascorbyl palmitate (Fig. 1) is contained in the Codex and the National Formulary.

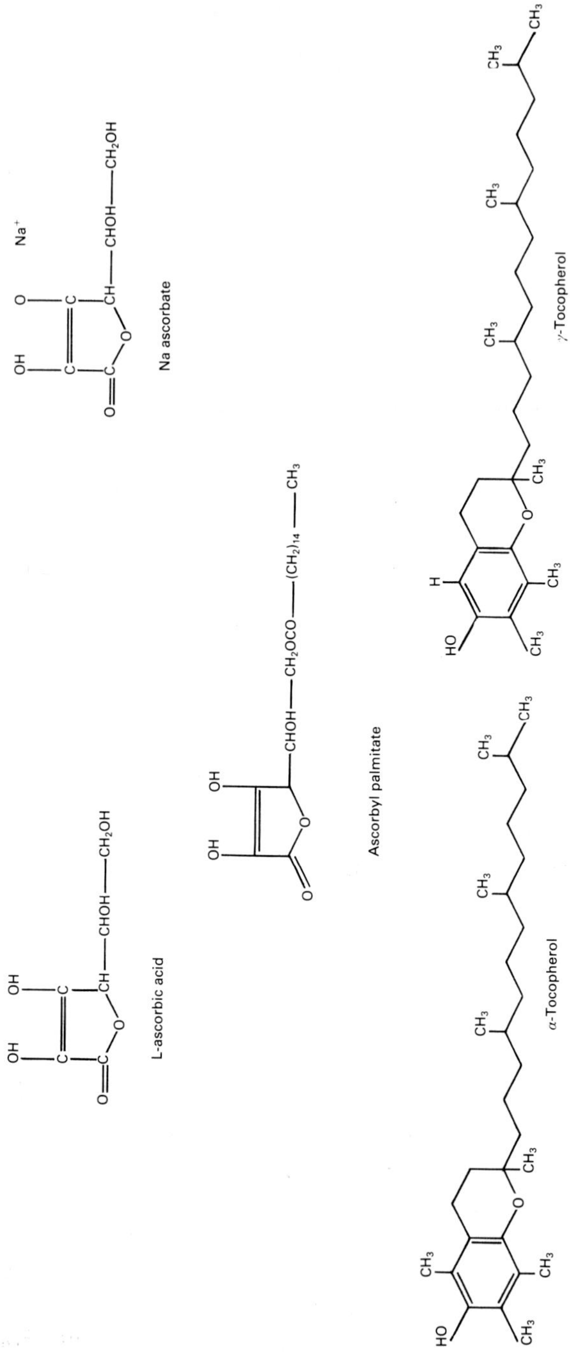

Fig. 1: Structural formulae of five chemical compounds.

Sodium ascorbate is more soluble in water (89 g in 100 ml) than is ascorbic acid (33 g in 100 ml). Ascorbyl palmitate is soluble in ethanol (25°C) at 12.5 %, in hot (80°C) glycerine or propylene glycol to 10 %, in vegetable oils (25°C) at 0.01–0.1 %, and in water (70°C) at 0.2 %. Sodium ascorbate and ascorbyl palmitate have 100 % of the biological activity of pure ascorbic acid on a molecular basis.

Not only does L-ascorbic acid have quite unusual chemical characteristics, it also has unique biological properties in that it is an essential nutrient for humans and must be present in the diet in adequate amounts [4]. L-ascorbic acid is a natural compound, widely distributed in the plant kingdom comprising many fruits and vegetables. Another compound, α-tocopherol (Fig. 1), although fat soluble, also possesses antioxidant properties [5], is well distributed in nature and is an essential nutrient (vitamin E). The antioxidant role of these two compounds [6,7] extend beyond their food preserving role as when consumed and absorbed within the body they continue to function in stress situations of life and maintenance of health [4].

Oxygen Scavenger

The scavenging effect of oxygen by ascorbic acid in solution under controlled conditions has been observed by BAYES [8]. Aqueous standardized solutions containing ascorbic acid (100 mg) were prepared with varied but known dissolved and headspace oxygen contents and stored (6 weeks, 35°C). Theoretically, 1 cm^3 of oxygen reacts with 15.7 mg ascorbic acid (one mole of ascorbic acid combining with one atom of oxygen). This would be equivalent to a reaction of approximately 3.3 mg with 1 cm^3 air. Data secured in this storage trial (Table I) show the experimental and theoretical values to agree fairly well, indicating that, under the conditions employed, the destruction of ascorbic acid is directly proportional to the amount of available oxygen in the containers.

Tab. I: Oxygen scavenging by ascorbic acid in sealed aqueous solutions; according to BAYES [8]

Test No.	Available oxygen			Final ascorbic acid content, mg/pt	Ascorbic acid loss	
	solution ml/100 ml	headspace	total, ml		experimental, mg	theoretical, mg
1	0.53	Air	6.6	0	100	103.6
2	0.53	Nitrogen	2.4	58	42	37.7
3	0.01	Air	4.2	38	62	65.9
4	0.01	Nitrogen	0.0	97	3	0

* Conditions of trial: initial ascorbic acid, 100 mg/pt; storage period 6 weeks at 35°C.

More recently CORT [9] conducted experiments in all glass bottles to observe the ability of added L-ascorbic acid in solution to scavenge oxygen from headspace air. From the data (Table II) collected, 3.4–3.6 mg ascorbic acid was required per cubic centimeter of headspace, close to the theoretical value. In a subsequent trial metal caps were inserted inside the glass equipment which caused faster oxygen removal but more ascorbic acid per cubic centimeter to be utilized. This oxygen scavenging ability is responsible for better flavor and color retention in sealed containers of oxygen sensitive foods treated with added ascorbic acid prior to sealing and heat processing. Ascorbic acid has been declared to have the property to scavenge superoxide and hydroxyl radicals as well as singlet oxygen [10].

Tab. II: Oxygen scavenging by ascorbic acid with reduced metal contamination in sealed containers; according to CORT [9]

Ascorbic acid, mg	Oxygen, ppm	Residual ascorbic acid, mg	Ascorbic acid consumed mg
0	8.0	0.0	0.0
3	0.4	1.3	1.7
6	0.0	4.2	1.8
9	0.0	7.2	1.8

Note: 0.5 cm^3 headspace, glass flasks and stopper; shaken 24 h at room temperature.

Oxidative Deterioration

The gathering or growing of food and the preservation of it for times of scarcity has occupied humans for millennia. It was and is highly desirable to have stored foods which have acceptable appearances, aromas, flavors and nutritive values. Oxidative deterioration results from the action of atmospheric oxygen upon the unsaturated, double bond linkages of fat, oil, sterol, phospholipid, color, flavor or fragrance component of the food bringing about chemical changes, thus unfavorably influencing palatability and nutritive value [11,12]. The oxidative mechanism may be stimulated by enzymes, light, heat and trace minerals such as cobalt, copper, iron, manganese, etc. As the oxidative mechanism proceeds there is formation of free radicals, of increased peroxides, of altered oxygen states leading to chain reactions whose duration is determined by the supply of energy available. Eventually degradation products, volatile carbonyl compounds such as short chain aldehydes, ketones, fatty acids appear and their presence is responsible for the offensive odors and flavors. Only a small quantity need to be produced for initial perception [13] of oxidation.

Protective measures [14] from oxidation include (a) use of high-quality ingredients and good manufacturing practices, (b) avoiding introduction or contact with pro-oxidant trace metals, (c) inactivation of oxidative enzymes, (d) elimination or reduction of dissolved and/or headspace oxygen, (e) protection from undue exposure to light, (f) employing low temperatures where practical, (g) adding chelating agents to remove trace minerals, if pertinent, and (h) adding antioxidants and synergists. For a fatty type food product to be successfully stabilized the antioxidant (and synergist and/or chelating agent) should be added before the initiation of oxidative deterioration.

Antioxidants and Synergists

Most primary antioxidants are aromatic compounds with one or more hydroxyl groups such as the tocopherols. Antioxidants act by furnishing hydrogen atoms or by reacting with free radicals to break chain reactions and by decomposing peroxides. Synergists are frequently used with antioxidants, markedly enhancing antioxidant action by supplying hydrogen atoms regenerating the phenolic state of the antioxidant and/or deactivating trace minerals. Synergists are usually polyhydroxy-acidic aliphatic structures. Chelating agents or sequestrants deactivate trace minerals such as iron and copper and hence remove their prooxidative influence in the oxidative phenomenon. L-ascorbic acid, sodium ascorbate and ascorbyl palmitate can be considered multi-functional types as they have some chelating action and some characteristics of synergists and primary antioxidants [15–17]. Contrary to the phenolic aromatic fat soluble primary antioxidants, the ascorbates have oxygen scavenging action, either for dissolved or headspace oxygen. In addition to producing off-flavor foods, oxidizing lipids are capable of reacting with amino acids, colors, enzymes, proteins and vitamins [16].

When incorporating antioxidants into water-base or fat-base food products the solubilities of antioxidants and synergists within the product must be considered for maximum effectiveness. L-ascorbic acid is readily water soluble. Ascorbyl palmitate is poorly soluble in oils or fats. α- or γ-tocooherols (Fig. 1) are readily soluble in oils and fats. In water-base foods tocopherols can be incorporated in water-dispersible emulsions. Ascorbyl plamitate should be first dissolved in hot oil [18]. In preparing a hot oil premix ascorbyl palmitate (20–50 g) is dissolved in heated (100° C) oil or fat (5 kg) and the premix immediately added to the remaining melted fat or oil (95 kg) to be treated.

Ascorbyl palmitate can be dissolved in hot glycerides or in a phospholipid-tocopherol premix formulation. One such formulation offered commercially (Roche, Basle) is Ronoxan A.

Fats and Oils

Ascorbyl palmitate, a biological form of vitamin C [19, 20], is an effective antioxidant for vegetable oils [21] as is evidenced by laboratory trials (Table III). The effectiveness of ascorbyl palmitate in vegetable oils is attributed to its strong synergistic action to the natural tocopherols present. In the case of lard, relatively devoid of natural tocopherols, high levels of ascorbyl palmitate are required, but better control is obtained in lard, butterfat, chicken fat, pork fat and beef fat with an ascorbyl palmitate-tocopherol combination (Tables IV and V) [18, 22].

To illustrate further the synergistical action of ascorbate and tocopherol, liquid lard (120° C) with additives was aerated in an automatically registering apparatus (Racimat, Metrohm) wherein the volatile breakdown products are collected, and their electrical conductivity measured and recorded. The interaction [21] of lecithin, ascorbyl palmitate and tocopherol is observed and as Ronoxan A (Table VI). Ronoxan A has been studied by Battna et al [23] for the stabilization of fats in a Czechoslovak infant formula and found to have significant retardation on autoxidation. The quality of lecithin is an important factor for increasing the potency of ascorbic acid esters [18, 21]. An antioxidant formulation of ascorbyl palmitate, α-tocopherol and phospholipids (200:100:700 ppm) was found to be quite effective by BOURGEOIS and CZORNOMAZ [24].

Tab. III: Antioxidative effect of increasing amounts of ascorbyl palmitate in various oils at 80°C; according to KLÄUI and PONGRACZ [21]

Ascorbyl palmitate, mg/kg oil	Peroxide values after x days				
	sunflower oil 1 day	peanut oil 2 days	soya-bean oil 2 days	palm oil 3 days	lard 5 days
0 (control)	46.2	17.2	100.0	29.5	> 400
100	12.7	7.6	43.2	23.6	> 400
200	15.4	6.5	12.5	14.2	> 400
300	10.0	4.9	3.2	13.3	> 400
400	13.7	4.3	2.5	13.0	186
500	14.2	3.7	2.0	9.9	1.2

Tab. IV: Antioxidant effect in various animal fats at 80°C;
according to PONGRACZ [18]

Antioxidants, mg/kg fat	Peroxide values	
	butterfat 3 days	lard 7 days
0 (control)	265	> 400
500 ascorbyl palmitate (AP)	74	> 400
200 α-tocopherol (TL)	9.9	28.5
500 AP + 100 α-TL	2.8	4.3
500 AP + 200 γ-TL	1.8	2.4

Tab. V: Comparative antioxidant activity, Schaal oven, thin layer, 45° C, according to CORT [22]

Antioxidant, 0,02% each	Days to reach 20 meq PV/kg fat		
	chicken fat	pork fat	beef fat
None (Control)	8	3	10
dl-α-Tocopherol	13	15	24
dl-γ-Tocopherol	29	37	40
Butylated hydroxyanisole (BHA)	20	28	36
Butylated hydroxytoluene (BHT)	15	18	24
dl-α-Tocopherol + ascorbyl palmitate	28	28	38
dl-γ-Tocopherol + ascorbyl palmitate	53	67	70
Ascorbyl palmitate	10	9	12

PV = peroxide value

Tab. VI: Antioxidant effect in lard at 120° C; according to KLÄUI and PONGRACZ [21]

Antioxidant, mg/kg fat	Induction time, h	Protection factor (PF value)
0 (control)	0.5	—
1400 lecithin (L)	0.8	1.5
100 α-tocopherol (TL)	2.7	5.3
500 ascorbyl palmitate (AP)	2.0	4.0
100 TL + 1400 L	4.4	8.8
500 AP + 1400 L	2.9	5.7
100 TL + 500 AP	7.1	14.2
100 TL + 500 AP + 1400 L (2000 Ronoxan A)	10.7	21.3

Both ascorbic acid and ascorbyl palmitate have antioxidant properties and synergistic activity to the tocopherols. CORT [9] in studying the effect of altering the ascorbate molecule found that substitutions in the 2- or 3-position make it no longer active as an antioxidant. Substitutions in the 6- or

5,6-positions have no influence and such compounds are active antioxidants. Ascorbyl palmitate addition (levels of 0.01–0.05 %) provides a useful increase in the shelf life of vegetable oils. Alone it is better than butylated hydroxyanisole (BHA) and butylated hydroxytoluene (BHT). In combination with the known antioxidants, shelf life of vegetable and animal fats is improved. MATTIL et al [25], in 1944, were earlier investigators of ascorbyl palmitate.

Ascorbyl palmitate (or in some cases ascorbic acid) has been added to a variety of fatty type foods. Using various evaluative criteria such as taste, odor, peroxide number, acid, color, viscosity and specific gravity observations, an improvement in oxidative retardation was noted. These food products include: oils, namely almond [26], corn [27], olive [26, 28, 29], peanut [29, 30], and sunflower [31]; butter [29, 32–35, 36]; cocoa butter [37]; shortening [38] and salad dressings, mayonnaise, cheese spreads and margarine [36].

PRIVETT and QUACKENBUSH [17] reported that 0.025 % ascorbic acids substantially delayed the rate of peroxide accumulation during the induction period of lard which contained low levels of α-tocopherol. These observations were substantiated by PYSZNIAK [39] who found that the addition of vitamins C and E to lard (0.01 to 0.05 %) in combination were effective antioxidants for lard stored at room temperature for long periods. BROWN et al [40] studied the catalytic effect of the hematins in fish flesh on the oxidation of oil by determining the oxygen uptake. From various combinations of antioxidants, they found a mixture of tocopherol, ascorbic acid and citric acid to be about 80 times as effective as ascorbic acid used alone in retarding the oxidation. Similar type studies and findings were observed, namely synergism by tocopherol and ascorbic acid, by TAPPEL et al [41]. Investigators continue currently to demonstrate efficacy of the tocopherol-ascorbate combinations in retarding oxidation of unsaturated lipid structures [42, 43]. KLÄUI [44] has reviewed the use of vitamins C and E as practical antioxidants in food processing applications.

The addition of ascorbic acid to animal fat low in tocopherols may even accelerate oxidation. Raising the concentration of tocopherol, or other phenolic antioxidants in the presence of ascorbic acid retards this action. The idea has been advanced that a copper-ascorbic acid complex may be the agent responsible for the pro-oxidant effect of ascorbic acid in aqueous fat systems. WATTS and coworkers [45, 46] found that this pro-oxidant effect could be eliminated when chelating or sequestering agents such as ethylenediamine tetraacetic acid or polyphosphates are added together with the ascorbic acid.

Heat-Processed Foods

Some fruits, such as peaches, apples, plums and pears, in their normal fresh condition possess a relatively low natural ascorbic acid content. When these fruits are home canned in either glass jars or tin cans, the canned product undergoes color and flavor changes which alter the appearance and taste characteristics during storage. These changes are brought about by the action of the oxygen in the air trapped in the headspace of the container.

Over 70 years ago oxygen was recognized as the causative agent in flavor alterations. In canning, while it is recognized that the headspace should remain small in an effort to reduce trapped air, it cannot be eliminated entirely as some headspace is necessary to permit expansion of the food and for good sealing operation. Since the enzymes are already destroyed by the heat treatment, the type of oxidation encountered in home canned fruit can be regarded as non-enzymatic or autocatalytic.

From theoretical aspects and experience in laboratory tests and early production trials, if added ascorbic acid is to function in a protective manner to an oxidizable processed food in hermetically sealed containers during storage, a sufficient amount of ascorbic acid must be initially present to (a) overcome any heat processing loss, (b) scavenge dissolved and headspace oxygen with time and (c) protect flavor and appearance with storage.

Sliced apples, applesauce, sliced peaches, halved pears and halved plums were canned by accepted canning methods. Headspace areas were found to vary from 45 to approximately 80 cubic centimeters per container. Crystalline ascorbic acid may be added by various procedures (Table VII) in the canning

Tab. VII: Adding ascorbic acid to canned fruit; according to Bauernfeind et al [47]

Method of ascorbic acid addition[1]	Product packed	Added ascorbic acid per jar, mg	Appearance of fruit after 5 months storage
Ascorbic acid mixed with one teaspoon of sugar and sprinkled over the top surface of the sauce	applesauce hot-packed in Ball pint jars	150	normal color (like freshly canned)
Ascorbic acid in one teaspoon of sugar blended throughout the sauce	ideal pint jars, $^{11}/_{16}$ in headspace	150	normal color
Ascorbic acid in water solution poured over top surface of the sauce	15 minutes processing	150	normal color
Ascorbic acid in water solution mixed with the upper half of jar contents	(water bath)	150	normal color

[1]Addition made just before jar was closed prior to processing.

Tab. VIII: Color and flavor of canned fruit; according to Bauernfeind et al [47]

Trial	Added ascorbic acid per jar, mg	Color after 5–6 months' storage	Flavor after 5–6 months' storage
		Canned sliced apples	
1	0	dark throughout	—
	67	slightly dark throughout	—
	135	normal (like freshly canned)	—
	200	normal	—
2	0	darkened top layer	poor flavor, oxidized
	100	darkened surface	preferred
	125	normal	preferred
	150	very slightly darkened top	preferred
		Applesauce	
1	0	dark	—
	67	slightly dark on top	—
	135	very slight darkening on top	—
	200	very slight darkening on top	—
2	0	darkened surface	oxidized
	100	normal	fair, slight off-flavor
	125	normal	fair, slight oxidized flavor
	150	normal	preferred
	200	normal	preferred
		Peaches	
1	0	darkened throughout	—
	67	dark on top	—
	135	slightly dark on top	—
	200	slightly dark on top	—
		Pears	
	0	dark on top	—
	67	slightly dark on top	—
	135	normal	—
	200	normal	—
2	0	darkened surface	poor pear flavor, oxidized
	100	normal	slight oxidized flavor
	125	normal	good
	150	normal	fair
		Plums, Italian	
1	0	darkened surface	—
	67	darkened surface	—
	135	lighter surface	—
	200	lighter surface	—
2	0	slight color	slight oxidized flavor
	100	differences	fair
	150	between jars	preferred

operation. Flavor and color comparisons and vitamin C analyses were made during the study (Table VIII).

Color and flavor improvement resulted from ascorbic acid addition [47] where 200 mg L-ascorbic acid was added initially, about 100 mg was still present per pint (473 ml) at the end of the six-month storage period. Thus by this operation a dual advantage was secured: improved quality of the product and an improved vitamin C content.

U.S. agricultural college extension departments have long recommended L-ascorbic acid addition to small-scale processed foods [48]. For example the Cornell bulletin on canning of fruits and vegetables states «the addition of 150 mg ascorbic acid (vitamin C) to a pint (473 ml) of applesauce, pears, peaches, plums or sweet corn and 250 mg of ascorbic acid for mushrooms tend to prevent surface darkening and off-flavors in the top layers of the canned food. The ascorbic acid itself is not detectable by flavor, odor or appearance and is not a preservative.»

Canned cherry pie filling [49] when treated with ascorbic acid (75-150 mg/lb sugared cherries) before the commercial canning operation maintained better color during storage than the control product. Ciupercescu and Marinescu [50] also reported a favorable effect of ascorbic acid (350 mg/kg) on color and taste of apricots and cherries packed in sugar syrup.

On a larger scale applicable to commercial processing, three varieties of apples [51] were peeled, cored, halved, packed in tin cans (20 oz or 600 ml), covered with sugar syrup (25% at 93°C), sealed, processed (10 min, 100°C) and cooled. Apples contain intracellular oxygen and unless it is removed by vacuum or otherwise before sealing, it reacts with the interior of the can during storage causing corrosion and leakage. To some cans, ascorbic acid (300 mg/454 g fruit) was added, before sealing and compared to control (no addition). Ascorbic acid treatment (Table IX) lowered oxygen content. Color and flavor were improved over the controls after processing and storage. Furthermore, there was no detectable corrosion of the containers with the treatment. A significant level of vitamin C was present following storage.

Tab. IX: Headspace oxygen and ascorbic acid values of canned apples; according to Hope [51]

Antioxidant	Cortland[1]		McIntosh[1]		Delicious[1]	
	headspace oxygen, volume %	ascorbic acid, mg/100 g	headspace oxygen, volume %	ascorbic acid, mg/100 g	headspace oxygen, volume %	ascorbic acid, mg/100 g
None	12.1	1.8	10.8	0.8	11.3	2.8
L-Ascorbic acid (300 mg/lb fruit)	0.3	23.5	0.4	18.8	0.6	24.6

[1] Name of apple variety.

In apple juice production, added ascorbic acid can function two ways [52] depending upon the type of juice desired. Enzymatic browning of the peeled fruit can be delayed by spraying with ascorbic acid solution during the pulping operation. The pulp quickly pressed, pasteurized, filled hot into cans or bottles and cooled yields light colored opalescent juice with fragrance and flavor of fresh fruit. If the pulp is not pressed but finely comminuted, one obtains an opaque light colored suspension with fresh fruit characteristics. In the cider or clarified cider type juice the browning of the juice has already occurred and only partial color reversal will take place if ascorbic acid is added before the canning operation. Added ascorbic acid, however, would still serve the function of reacting with dissolved and headspace oxygen for product quality protection during storage and confer a nutritional advantage to the product.

Color deterioration of pear juice and concentrate during processing, storage and marketing is a major industrial problem. The initial color deterioration during processing is caused by oxidation of endogenous pear phenolics by polyphenol oxidase. MONTGOMERY and PETROPAKIS [53] succeeded in preparing a light colored pear juice by applying ascorbic acid (300 ppm) to the fruit during grinding and quickly heating pulp and juice (to 90°C) during the continued processing operations.

ESSELEN et al [54] processed apple juice by flash heating, cooling, filtering, hot filling (88°C) into bottles, sealed with Vapor-Vacuum caps and water cooled. Ascorbic acid was added (50 mg/100 g) prior to hot filling and stored up to one year. Periodical evaluations of treated and untreated juices were made at time intervals with the finding that the addition of ascorbic acid had a favorable effect on flavor retention.

Some fruit juices tend to undergo a flavor change on pasteurization, their magnitude depending on the juice and the process. BIRCH et al [55] in examining this phenomenon found the flavor change related to the processed fructose and glucose components. They did not elucidate the responsible mechanism but found oxygen necessary to be present for the off-flavor development

Tab. X: Reducing sugars and required ascorbic acid levels in juices; according to BIRCH et al [55]

Juice	Reducing sugars, %	Ascorbic acid, mg/100 g	Ascorbic acid, mg/100 g
Apple	8.3	64.0	5
Grapefruit	3.2	23.5	35
Lemon	1.4	10.5	50
Orange	5.1	38.5	50
Pineapple	4.2	32.0	8
Tomato	3.4	26.0	16

(Table X) and that deaeration and addition of ascorbic acid decreased the «processed flavor». From the knowledge of the reducing sugar content of a given juice, it is possible to predict the amount of ascorbic acid required (Table XI) to prevent the off-flavor development. The following amounts of ascorbic acid were suggested for the following juices: apple, 64 mg/100 g; pineapple, 32; and tomato, 26. The citrus juices do not require additional amounts. Care must be taken to maximize the retention of desired levels of vitamin C content of juices [114].

Tab. XI: Ascorbic acid losses and ranking scores on processing pineapple juice; according to Birch et al [55]

Treatment	Ascorbic acid before processing, mg/100 g	Ascorbic acid after processing, mg/100 g	Loss of ascorbic acid, mg	Ranking score
Aerated	3.4	1.9	1.5	22
Deoxygenated	3.2	1.8	1.4	16
Aerated and AA added	82.7	81.0	1.7	14
Deoxygenated and AA added	82.5	80.8	1.7	8

Discoloration of canned, strained carrots, occurring as a brownish tinge diffused throughout the contents of the jar and as a localized gray-brown off-color in the top layer is apparently due to oxidation. It can be prevented by high vacuum. Low vacuum plus 0.01–0.1 % ascorbic acid also prevents discoloration and improves the color of the product throughout the jar [56, 57]. Other vegetable products processed with ascorbic acid are sliced beets [58, 59], cauliflower [60], and coleslaw [61].

Over the last half century mushroom cultivation has expanded greatly with various brands of canned mushrooms on the market. Concern has been shown in the glass and can packing of mushrooms on the development of a muddy grayness in the product. Sorted fresh mushrooms [62] were steam-blanched, filled into glass and tin containers (4 oz) and followed by hot water, salt and citric acid. Some had ascorbic acid added (150 mg), others were without. The containers were sealed and processed (20–23 min at 115–120° C). Observations were made on color, flavor and vitamin C content following canning and months of storage (Table XII). Flavor of the ascorbic acid treated, processed mushrooms [62] was more characteristic of freshly cooked mushroom. In the nontreated, the flavor was flat and oxidized. Flavor could be correlated with muddy-gray color. Improvement was also noted in canned mushroom soup [62] were ascorbic acid addition was made prior to sealing (Table XIII).

Ascorbic acid treatment of mushrooms in dilute brine packed in tin and glass containers was also studied by Andreotti and Ambanelli [63]. The ad-

Tab. XII: Glass-packed mushroom buttons-color and flavor improvement by ascorbic acid; according to BAUERNFEIND *et al* [62]

Sample	Ingredients added	pH	Ascorbic acid, mg/jar	Total vitamin C, mg/jar	Weight of contents, g	Color[1]	Flavor[2]
						After processing	
A-1	salt, 40 g	–	3	3	214.7	Dark; muddy gray	oxidized
2	salt, citric acid, 1.6 g	–	–	–	–	slightly dark; gray	slightly oxidized
3	salt, citric acid, 150 mg	–	–	–	211.5	good; tan	good flavor
3a	ascorbic acid	–	1-3	1-3	214.2	good; tan	good flavor
4	salt, citric acid, 300 mg	–	234	247	211.0	good; tan	good flavor
4a	ascorbic acid	–	244	248	208.9	good; tan	good flavor
5	salt, 150 mg ascorbic	–	120	126	213.1	fairly good; tan-gray	good flavor
5a	acid	–	129	137	211.1	fairly good; tan-gray	good flavor
6	salt, 300 mg ascorbic	–	241	252	218.3	good; tan	good flavor
6a	acid	–	294	294	212.9	good; tan	good flavor
7	salt, 450 mg ascorbic	–	393	411	213.0	good; tan	good flavor
7a	acid	–	282	400	206.6	good; tan	good flavor
						After storage for 3 months	
A-1		6.28	–	–	–	very dark, very muddy gray	oxidized, flat, old
2		5.77	–	–	–	dark; muddy gray	less oxidized, off-flavor
3	(same as list above)	5.50	90	101	217.6	fairly good; tan	fairly good
4		5.41	221	236	215.4	good; yellowish tan or light tan	good canned mushroom flavor
5		6.01	115	123	216.8	fairly good; tan-gray	fairly good
6		5.69	235	244	215.5	good; tan	good canned mushroom flavor
7		5.35	373	387	213.4	good; yellowish tan or light tan	good canned mushroom flavor

1 All color ratings were made on mushrooms only; there were no significant texture differences.
2 All flavor opinions were based on mushrooms and liquid.

dition of ascorbic acid (140 mg) and citric acid (250 mg) was judged the most effective treatment. Other reports [64–66] attest to the favorable action of ascorbic acid on mushrooms.

Maintenance of the keeping quality of pasteurized milk and other dairy products may be improved by the addition of ascorbic acid [67]. It has been reported that ascorbic acid addition to whole milk in the presence of tocopherols has an antioxygenic effect [68] on the milk lipids and lipoproteins. The chief function of increasing the ascorbic acid content is in the prevention or retardation of oxidized flavors frequently described as "tallowy or cardboardy".

The natural α-tocopherol content of cow's milk [69] varies with season and feeding practices, ranging from 4–30 μg/g fat. Freshly extracted cow's milk may contain as much as 30 mg ascorbic acid/l, but handling, processing, shipment or delivery practices can destroy the major portion of its natural content. Hence both tocopherol and ascorbic acid should be considered equally important in dairy product flavor stabilization. The earlier ascorbic acid papers on dairy products have been reviewed in past publications [70]. The development of oxidized flavor in milk involves multi-phase factors, namely ration of the cow, light exposure of milk, time and temperature of pasteurization, homogenization, copper level, oxygen content, oxidase activity, etc. [71–73].

It would appear that if the cow's ration provided an ample tocopherol level in the milk, avoiding undue exposure of the milk to light, proper pasteurization and homogenization, using non-copper processing equipment, low dissolved oxygen level and ample ascorbic acid levels (50 mg/l) that nutritious milk with a pleasant taste can be produced. Deaeration and ascorbic acid ad-

Tab. XIII: Flavor of mushroom soup improved by ascorbic acid; according to BAUERNFEIND et al [62]

Sample	Ingredients	Ascorbic acid content, mg per 11 oz can			
		after processing	after storage at		
			40°C	22.5°C	22.5°C
1	control pack	5.5	–	–	–[1]
2	ascorbic acid, 100 mg	79[2]	74	75	77[1]
3	control pack	5.5	–	5.6	5.8
4	ascorbic acid, 93 mg	67	63	62	61

Note: Taste panel evaluations on coded samples after processing demonstrated ascorbic acid treated product to taste more like freshly cooked product. Tests after 500 h and 12 months storage: sample 2 was superior to 1, and sample 4 was superior to 3 in flavor. At end of 12 months, non-treated samples also possessed a darker color than treated ones.

[1] pH of control, 6.10; pH of treated, 6.05.
[2] A second can opened, its contents diluted with water and heated, to serve, demonstrated an ascorbic acid content of 66 mg.

dition (50–100 mg/l) to concentrated sweetened cream [74] stabilized flavor for months of storage (6 months at 4°C) in one investigation. In another [75] ascorbic acid and tocopherol were observed to control oxidized flavor in high-fat cream. A more recent observation is the finding that ascorbic acid delays folate degradation in processed dairy and other heat treated foods [76,77].

Frozen Foods

Plant tissues which brown readily when exposed to air as a result of losing their peel, such as apples and bananas, have relatively low concentrations of ascorbic acid and highly reactive phenolases [78]. As a result of the unrestrained action of phenolase on an orthophenolic or flavonoid substrate in the presence of oxygen, colored orthoquinone compounds are produced. In the presence of adequate ascorbic acid, the orthoquinones are reversibly reduced to orthophenolic forms, and browning does not occur. The reduction products of ascorbic acid, dehydroascorbic acid and diketogulonic acid, are not browning inhibitors. When ascorbic acid is exhausted, the orthoquinones are no longer the intermediates in a reversible reaction; polymerization occurs and the browning process is irreversible [70]. Since added synthetic orthoquinone does not affect quinone formation, possibly a semiquinone forms which inhibits the enzyme reaction and which is reducible by ascorbic acid [79]. The phenolic structure varies in different fruits and vegetables, the dominant forms being chlorogenic acid, catechin, epicatechin, esculetin, dihydroquercetin, etc. [80–82].

Most varieties of peaches, apricots, pears, plums, nectarines, bananas and apples, which are generally low in natural vitamin C content, readily discolor when thawed from the frozen state with the concomitant development of off-flavor. The enzymatic oxidation responsible for discoloration can be retarded by ascorbic acid dissolved in the sugar syrup in the packaged cut-fruit prior to freezing. Some fruit varieties having intermediate levels of natural vitamin C such as strawberries, cherries and pineapple also benefit flavor or colorwise from ascorbic acid addition. Other additives [2,70] such as sulfur dioxide, cysteine, citric acid and calcium or sodium chloride [83] have been used with ascorbic acid to delay browning but may impart flavor changes, if not carefully controlled. The value of added ascorbic acid in delaying fruit browning has been known since 1938 [70]. In the preparation of frozen fruit packs, ascorbic acid is added to the sugar or sugar syrup at levels ranging from 150 to 350 mg/lb (454 g) finished product. It is important that porous or oxygen containing fruits such as apples be either thinly sliced or that the thicker slices be subjected to vacuum treatment to insure that the ascorbic acid penetrates the fruit tissue. A continuously frozen state (−20°C or below) must be maintained during storage, transportation and marketing to minimize destruction of the ascorbic acid and maintain product quality. Advantages [2] of the ascorbic acid treatment are: (a) no introduction of a foreign substance or unnatural flavors; (b) is not detected by appearance, smell or taste; (c) is easily detected by applying recognized chemical and biological tests; (d) usually increases significantly the vitamin C value of the food products; and (e) is practical from a viewpoint of cost and quality improvement.

Fish fillets, steaks and some shell fish having a fatty component undergoing oxidative rancidity in frozen storage may be benefitted by ascorbic acid application [1,2,84]. Ascorbic acid may be applied by either a dipping or spraying technique (0.5–3.0 % ascorbic acid solution). In order to assure a more even and a sufficiently thick coating, thickening agents may be added to the solution. By the ascorbic acid treatment the frozen storage shelf life of the fish may be extended several months.

ATAGIRI and NISHIMORI [85] have proposed two ascorbic acid dipping formulations for preventing loss of quality in stored fresh seafoods. Sea Rich F–A contained ascorbic acid, sodium glutamate, nicotinamide and phosphates intended for use with red fleshed fish and molluscs while Sea Rich F–D containing nicotinamide, ascorbic acid, phosphates and tocopherol is intended for oily fish. Dips were also applied to fish for frozen storage. Ascorbic acid (2 %), sodium tripolyphosphate (0.2 %), monosodium glutamate (0.2 %) and salt (7 %) have been employed as additive to prevent spoilage in frozen fillets of seer for 10 months (−20°C) compared to untreated controls only lasting 3 months (86). Shell fish also benefit from ascorbic acid treatment [87,88].

Cured Foods

The pigment heme is the basis for the color of *fresh* meat muscle. The porphyrin ring of heme combines with a globulin-like protein to form myohemoglobin, which contains bivalent iron and exhibits a bluish-red color. It changes to a bright cherry-red as heme exposed to air accumulates oxygen with the formation of oxymyoglobin wherein iron is still bivalent. The cherry-red color is unstable and the continuous exposure to air oxidation gradually (several days at 4°C) results in the formation of the more stable metmyoglobin, a compound having trivalent iron, which imparts a brownish appearance to meat. The formation of metmyoglobin is accelerated by heat, freezing, salt, some chemicals, mineral and ultraviolet light. Metmyoglobin, oxymyoglobin and myoglobin may exist simultaneously as can be seen when a ball of refrigerated ground meat is cut through so that the brownish surface, the cherry-red layer underneath, and the bluish-red interior are exhibited.

The addition of ascorbic acid (about 200 mg/kg) to *fresh* ground meat through a reducing action retards [89] the conversion of oxymyoglobin to met-myoglobin by a day or so. It does not overcome or delay meat spoilage. Treatment of fresh meat with ascorbic acid is permitted in a limited number of countries and if treatment is contemplated, current regulations should be checked. HARBERS [90] dipped bovine muscle cuts in ascorbic acid solutions (0.5–5.0 %), then wrapped, exposed to radiant energy and stored. Retardation of pigment and lipid oxidation were reported by the treatment. Preslaughter intravenous injection of sodium ascorbate has been observed to inhibit met-myoglobin formation and extend color appearance in the meat [1].

The *curing* of meat involves the addition of a nitrite salt which evolves nitric oxide gas combining with myoglobin to form the ferrous pigment, nitric-oxide-myoglobin also called nitrosomyoglobin. Heat-denaturation causes this compound to be converted to nitric-oxide-hemochromogen (nitrosomyo-chrome), a pink-red pigment. As with fresh meat, progressive oxidation produces metmyoglobin which causes the product to have a brown or gray discoloration.

Addition of ascorbate salts to the *curing* brine reduces the curing time, contributes to a better and more uniform color and improves flavor [91]. It speeds the curing action by reacting with the nitrite to give a controlled positive release of nitric oxide for ready combination with myoglobin, thus supplementing naturally occurring reducing substances in meat such as the sulfhydryls. Sodium ascorbate is capable of (a) regenerating the nitro-somyoglobin on the surface of slightly faded meat provided residual nitrite is present, (b) catalyzing the production of nitric-oxide-hemoglobin and (c) protecting the surface of cured meat from oxidation. Ascorbate treatment lowers the residual nitrite content of cured meats. More recently greater interest in the use of ascorbate in meat curing has been exhibited as a nitrosation preventive [1] either alone or in combination with α-tocopherol.

Sodium ascorbate reacts much more slowly with nitrite and is always used with nitrite in the curing pickle for pumping, injecting or covering solid pieces of milk. In comminuted meat either ascorbic acid or sodium ascorbate may be used following prescribed procedures [1,2]. The color of cured meat pigment is stabilized and initiation of fat deterioration is delayed by the presence of added ascorbate, the latter action assisted by the presence of tocopherols naturally present in meat. Ascorbyl palmitate at a level of 0.3 ppm in British sausage controls an oxidative change in the meat pigments known as «white spot», chalky white patches formed on the sausage surface [89].

Fermented or Cultured Foods

PEDERSON observed a relation between the natural ascorbic acid content and the quality of sauerkraut as reflected in its flavor, color, and texture. With this earlier observation in mind, PEDERSON and BEATTIE [92] packed sauerkraut containing lactic acid (1.5 %) and salt (2.25 %) in pint (473 ml) glass jars. Jars were also packed containing added ascorbic acid (75, 100, and 160 mg/jar). Samples were stored and examined periodically. After storage (9 months) at varying temperatures (7 and 20°C), there were no differences in color. At higher temperatures (37 and 45°C) the samples to which higher levels (160 mg) were added were rated highest in color in the majority of cases. The authors therefore find that added ascorbic acid has some effect in inhibiting color changes. Non-heat sterilized kraut, if treated with ascorbic acid (150–250 mg/lb) can be marketed for limited periods of time in heat sealed plastic bags if kept under refrigeration (4°C) [93].

Experimental packs have indicated that the application of ascorbic acid to brine-packed Spanish olives and artichoke hearts delays the development of undesirable color during shelf life. In the fermentation and preservation of green olives ascorbic acid was found beneficial by BARRET and BIDAN [94]. Olives may loose their attractive green color in the usual processing operations with alkali, the subsequent lactic acid fermentation and subsequent pickling in brine. This oxidative loss of color can be delayed or prevented by combined ascorbic acid (50–100 mg) and citric acid (200 mg/kg olives). Subsequent additions of ascorbic acid may be needed at other time intervals, in some cases.

Ascorbic acid favorably affects taste, flavor and clearness of wine and helps to stabilize its oxidation-reduction value in quantities of 25–100 mg/l. Variables inherent in wine making, such as growing region, type of grape, kind of wine and degree of maturity of the wine determine whether or not ascorbic acid should be used and in what quantity [2].

The phenolic constituents of wine tend to react with oxygen to form quinones which can cause changes in flavor and color. The reducing substances, ascorbic acid and sulfur dioxide, react with quinones and reconvert it into the original polyphenols. A higher ratio of reduced substances is an advantageous influence on wine stability and aroma. In the case of wines having a high iron content, where there is a tendency to form the cloud-producing ferri-phosphate, the presence of added ascorbic acid prevents precipitate formation by reducing the iron to the bivalent form.

Most enologists recommend ascorbic acid to be used in conjunction [95–97] with sulfur dioxide. Sulfur dioxide has antiseptic, fungicidal, antidiastase, and antioxidant properties. Ascorbic acid has a synergistic effect on sulfur dioxide and is said to be of value in resisting undesirable oxidative changes in the color and flavor of wine and to enable minimal use of sulfur dioxide, a desired objective. Utility for adding ascorbic acid in champagne and sparkling wine [98] production has been reported.

Beer has been, in increasing amounts, packaged in cans and bottles. If beer so packaged is stored for long periods, it is subject to oxidation by oxygen, as evidenced by the development of an undesirable bitter, stale flavor, loss of aroma, and haze formation [99]. Natural reducing substances in beer include reductones, melanoidins, tannins, and the SH-groups of nitrogenous compounds. A finished beer of good flavor and clarity ready for bottling should posses high reducing capacity and should be packaged with a minimum amount of dissolved air and headspace air for maximum shelf life.

Ascorbic acid is an effective antioxidant during the manufacture of beer to lessen the undesirable effects of the oxidation of beer by molecular oxygen. Ascorbic acid addition was first suggested about 1935 by GRAY and STONE [100] as a means of providing an oxygen acceptor for beer and it was subsequently demonstrated that chill and oxidation haze were reduced considerably by its addition, thereby extending shelf life. Treatment of beer with ascorbic acid depends on (a) oxidation status of the brew, as judged by ITT values; (b) mechanical devices, equipment, and handling methods; (c) amount of dissolved and container headspace oxygen (3.5 mg ascorbic acid or 4.0 g sodium salt/ml air); (d) residual ascorbate level desired after packaging; and (e) marketing practices, holding time and stability required. Amounts used vary from 1–4 g/100 l or 1.2–4.8 g/barrel.

The reactions involving ascorbic acid in beer have not been fully elucidated, but it is known that it behaves as a reductant and thereby reduces the oxidation-reduction potential (rH) which may be measured potentiometrically or colorimetrically with various redox indicators. The behavior of ascorbic acid during brewing and storage of bottled beer continues to be of interest [101]. More recently merit has been cited [102] for adding ascorbic acid to hops powder before pelleting to prevent oxidation of hops, an ingredient used in brewing.

The value of L-ascorbic acid as a fermented dough improver has been known since 1935 and is now in current commercial use in various countries [1,103–105]. The overall practical advantages of adding L-ascorbic acid to freshly milled flour for bread making are as follows: (a) enhances loaf texture and volume; (b) gives greater elasticity and gas retention to the dough; (c) improves water absorption; (d) protects fatty acids, (e) eliminates danger of over-improvement or over-treatment; (f) reduces power or minimal time or lowered consistency in continuous dough making; and (g) eliminates storage period of unimproved flour. Freshly milled flour plus ascorbic acid can be used in place of time-matured (no improver added); hence storage space is reduced. Ascorbic acid treatment of flour contributes to standardization of products for the large volume industrial baker employing complex automatic bread making equipment. Oxidation of polyunsaturated free fatty acids in flour/water slurries in the presence of and absence of ascorbic acid were investigated by Grant and Sood [106]. While added ascorbic acid (120–240 ppm) did retard oxidization of linoleic and linolenic acids, they did so over a relatively short time interval.

Durum and other wheat granular flours (semolina) require retention of their natural yellow carotenoid content for the manufacture of pasta products which have been observed to be stabilized [1] by added L-ascorbic acid.

Carbonated Foods

Some carbonated or sterilized soft drinks are prone to light induced oxidation of the flavor constituents, particularly orange and grapefruit products. These changes are due to unsaturated terpenes which are highly reactive, and which produce the characteristic rancid, oily off-notes. The addition of ascorbic acid (5–15 mg/fl oz), depending on whether the product is ready-to-drink or requiring dilution, respectively, can exert a marked stabilizing effect [107] on the flavor constituents. The mode of action is not clear but it is likely that the ascorbic acid utilizes dissolved and headspace oxygen. Another ascorbic acid action is the undesirable bleaching effect on certain added artificial colors in the beverages. It is necessary to strike an optimal balance between improved flavor stability and reduced color stability to suit the particular needs of each beverage. It is wise to establish this balance in a series of tests under the appropriate conditions [107]. Synthetic carotenoids as color additives are quite stable in soft drinks containing added ascorbic acid [3,14,108].

Apple juice concentrate (82 % total solids) diluted (15 % solids) with carbonated water, ascorbic acid added (40 mg/100 ml) was subjected to taste panel evaluation by Bright and Potter [109]. The treated carbonated juice was preferred over noncarbonated apple juice.

Tab. XIV: Effect of ascorbic acid on iron pick-up in soft drinks; according to JOHNSON *et al* [110]

Air in the can, cm^3	Added ascorbic acid, mg	Iron pick-up, ppm	
		3 months	6 months
9.7	0	1.5	2.9
2.4	0	1.1	1.9
10.2	36	1.0	1.2
2.0	36	0.8	1.0

[1] Packed in flat top 12 oz cans.
[2] Months at 25°C.

Another effect of air in carbonated drinks is the increase in internal pressure in the container and increases the ability of the product to pick up iron. Ascorbic acid (36 mg/250 ml can) added as an antioxidant reduces the amount of iron pick up (Table XIV) in the product and prolongs the shelf life of canned carbonated beverages [110].

Nutrified Foods

The availability of vitamin C from dietary sources is variable due to fluctuations in natural foods and losses incurred during harvesting, processing, storage, and pre-consumptive preparation [111]. Therefore, ascorbic acid has a different role and may be added not as an antioxidant but as a nutrient to (a) fortify natural foods having little or no vitamin C, (b) to restore losses, (c) to produce food products having a standardized quantity, and (d) to endow synthetic foods with nutritional value.

References

1 BAUERNFEIND, J C: Ascorbic acid technology in agricultural, pharmaceutical, food and industrial applications. In: SEIB and TOLBERT (eds) "Ascorbic acid: chemistry, metabolism and uses", pp 395–497. Adv Chem Ser No *200,* American Chemical Society, Washington, 1982.

2 BAUERNFEIND, J C, PINKERT, D M: Food processing with added ascorbic acid. Adv Food Res *18,* 219–315, 1970.

3 KLÄUI, H: The functional (technical) uses of vitamins. In: STEIN (ed) "University of Nottingham seminar on vitamins", pp 110–145. Churchill Livingstone, London, 1970.

4 BRIN, M: Marginal vitamin C deficiency and human health. In: COUNSELL and HORNIG (eds) "Vitamin C (ascorbic acid)", pp 359–376. Applied Science, London, 1981.

5 BAUERNFEIND, J C, CORT, W M: Tocopherols. In: JOHNSON and PETERSON (eds) "The encyclopedia of food technology", pp 891–899. AVI, Westport, 1974.

6 Johnson, F C: The antioxidant vitamins. CRC Crit Rev Food Sci Nutr *11*, 217–309, 1979.

7 Packer, J E *et al:* Direct observations of a free radical interaction between α-tocopherol and L-ascorbic acid. Nature *278*, 737–738, 1979.

8 Bayes, A L: Investigations on the use of nitrogen for the stabilization of perishable food products. Food Technol *4*, 151–158, 1950.

9 Cort, W M: Antioxidant properties of ascorbic acid in foods. In: Seib and Tolbert (eds) "Ascorbic acid: chemistry, metabolism and uses", pp 533–550. Adv Chem Ser No 200. American Chemical Society, Washington, 1982.

10 Bodannes, R S, Chan, P C: Ascorbic acid as a scavenger of singlet oxygen. FEBS Lett *105*, 195–196, 1979.

11 Lillard, D A: Effect of processing on chemical and nutritional changes in food lipids. J Food Protect *46*, 61–67, 1983.

12 Logani, M K, Davies, R E: Lipid oxidation: biological effects and antioxidants. Lipids *15*, 485–495, 1980.

13 Berger, K: Catalysis and inhibition of oxidation processes: use of antioxidants in foods. Chem Ind *5*, 194–199, 1975.

14 Kläui, H: Tocopherol, carotene and ascorbyl palmitate. Flavours, July/August, 1976.

15 Riemenschneider, R W: Oxidative rancidity and antioxidants. In: Blanck (ed) "Handbook of food and agriculture", pp 237–278. Reinhold, New York, 1955.

16 Mohler, H: Ascorbic acid as an antioxidant or synergist. Wiss Veröffentl Deut Ges Ernähr *14*, 279–295, 1965.

17 Privett, O S, Quackenbush, R W: The relation of synergist to antioxidant in fats. J Am Oil Chem Soc *31*, 321–323, 1954.

18 Pongracz, G: Antioxidant mixtures for use in food. Int J Vit Nutr Res *43*, 517–525, 1973.

19 Ambrose, A M, De Ecls, F: Biological availability of L-ascorbyl palmitate. Arch Biochem *12*, 375–379, 1947.

20 De Ritter, E *et al:* Physiological availability of dehydro-L-ascorbic acid and palmitoyl-L-ascorbate. Science *113*, 628–631, 1951.

21 Kläui, H, Pongracz, G: Ascorbic acid and derivatives as antioxidants in oils and fats. In: Counsell and Hornig (eds) "Vitamin C (ascorbic acid)", pp 139–166. Applied Science, London, 1981.

22 Cort, W M: Antioxidant activity of tocopherols, ascorbyl palmitate and ascorbic acid and their mode of action. J Am Oil Chem Soc *51*, 321–325, 1974.

23 Battna, J *et al:* Fat and vitamin A stability in the presence of Ronoxan A and other antioxidants. Int J Nutr Res *52*, 241–247, 1982.

24 Bourgeois, C F, Czornomarz, A M: Stabilization of lard by ascorbyl palmitate, α-tocopherol and phospholipids. Rev Franç Corps Gras *29*, 111–116, 1982.

25 Mattil, K F *et al:* A study of the antioxidant effectiveness of several compounds on vegetable fats and oils. Oil Soap *21*, 160–161, 1944.

26 Siegfried, B, Schneider, R: Preservation of fats and oils. Pharm Acta Helv *28*, 131–139, 1953.

27 Popovici, M *et al:* Preservation of corn oil extracted from corn germs. Ind Aliment *16*, 248–250, 1965.

28 Vitagliano, M, Vodret, A: Possible improvements in olive oil production. Olearia *14*, 137–141, 1960.

29 Herisset, A: The effect of ascorbic acid and its derivatives on the auto-oxidation of lipids. Vegetable oils: butter. Trav lab matières méd pharmacol, No 1, pp 1-4, No 2, pp 1-4. Ecole méd pharm Angers, Angers, 1954.

30 Cerutti, G: Preservation of oils: stabilizing action of an ester of ascorbic acid (ascorbyl palmitate). Olearia *10*, 39–41, 130–132, 1956.

31 Somogyi, J C, Kündig-Hegedues, H: Stabilization of oils rich in polyunsaturated fatty acids and of other dietary fats. Mitt Geb Lebensm Hyg *52*, 104–115, 1961.

32 Cerutti, G: Maintaining the freshness of some dairy products: butter stabilization. Latte *30*, 267–268, 1956.

33 Koops, J: Antioxidant activity of ascorbyl palmitate in cold stored butter. Neth Milk Dairy J *18*, 38–51, 1964.

34 Antila, V *et al:* The keeping quality of butterfat when stored dry. Finn J Dairy Sci *25*, 21–30, 1965.

35 Alifax, R: Influence of the unsaponifiable fraction on the stability of butter. Protection of butter by ascorbic acid. Ann Technol Agric *18*, 167–185, 1969.

36 US Patent 2-500-543, 1950.

37 Cerutti, G: L-ascorbic acid as antioxidant of cocoa butter. Oleagineux *13*, 95–97, 1958.

38 Sedacek, B A J: Use of antioxidants in storage of shortenings. Fette Seifen Anstrichm *70*, 795–801, 929–932, 1968.

39 Pyszniak, S: Antioxidants for lard preservation. Prace Inst Przemyslu miesnego *1*, 163–172, 1957.

40 Brown, W D *et al:* Progress on studies concerning mechanism of oxidation of oil in fish tissues. Com Fisheries Rev *19*, 27–31, 1957.

41 Tappel, A L *et al:* Unsaturated lipid peroxidation catalyzed by hematin compounds and its inhibition by vitamin E. J Am Oil Chem Soc *38*, 5–9, 1961.

42 Yamauchi, R *et al:* Reaction of 8α-hydroperoxy tocopherones with ascorbic acid. Agric Biol Chem *45*, 2855–2861, 1981.

43 Reinton, R, Rogstad, A: Antioxidant activity of tocopherols and ascorbic acid. J Food Sci *46*, 970–971, 1981.

44 Kläui, H: Use of vitamins C and E as antioxidants in food technology. In: Hallo and Hallo (eds) Nat Synth Zusatzstoffe Nahr Menschen. 14th Int Symp, 1972, pp 62–84. Steinkopff, Darmstadt, 1974.

45 Kelly, G, Watts, B M: Effect of copper chelating agents on the pro-oxidant activity of scorbic acid with unsaturated fats. Food Res *22*, 308–315, 1957.

46 Watts, B M, Faulkner, M: Antioxidant effect of liquid smokes. Food Technol *8*, 158–161, 1954.

47 Bauernfeind, J C *et al:* Home canning of fruits with L-ascorbic acid. Glass Packer *26*, (4) 268, (5) 358, 1947.

48 Wood, T: Home canning of fruits and vegetables. Cornell Extension Bulletin 792. Cornell University, Ithaca, 1956.

49 Kunz, C E, Robinson, W B: Cherry filling keeps longer. Food Packer, September, 1955.

50 Ciupercescu, V, Marinescu, I: Improving the quality of fruit in syrup by adding ascorbic acid. Lucr Inst Cercet Aliment *5*, 179–186, 1961.

51 Hope, G W: The use of antioxidants in canning apple halves. Food Technol *15*, 548–550, 1961.

52 Bauernfeind, J C: Role of ascorbic acid in the browning phenomenon of fruit juice. Symp Fruchtsaft-Konzentrate, Bristol, pp 159–185. Juris, Zurich, 1958.

53 Montgomery, M W, Petropakis, H J: Inactivation of bartlett pear polyphenol oxidase with heat in the presence of ascorbic acid. J Food Sci *45*, 1090–1091, 1980.

54 Esselen, W B *et al:* The fortification of fruit juices with ascorbic acid. Fruit Prod *26*, 11–14/29, 1946.

55 Birch, G G *et al:* Quality changes related to vitamin C in fruit juices and vegetable processing. In: Birch and Parker (eds) "Vitamin C: recent aspects of its physiological and technological importance", pp 40–67. Wiley, New York, 1974.

56 Yourga, F J: How to prevent off-color in glassed carrots. Food Indust *20*, 47, 1948.

57 Gstirner, F, Saad, S N: Keeping quality of carrots canned in glass. Z LebensmUnter-Forschung *110*, 9–14, 1959.

58 Clark, W L, Moyer, J C: Surface darkening of sliced beets. Food Technol *9*, 308–313, 1955.

59 Lusas, E W *et al:* Changes in the color of canning beets. Wisc Agr Expt Stat Res Bull *218*, 1–32, 1960.

60 CHANDLER, D R, SOOD, V K: Discoloration in processed cauliflower. Food Preserv Quart 24, 11–14, 1964.

61 CHEN, L M, PENG, A C: Effect of dip on shelf life of coleslaw. J Food Sci 45, 1556–1558, 1980.

62 BAUERNFEIND, J C et al: Better color, better flavor in processed mushrooms by adding ascorbic acid. Food Engineering 24, 88–92, 1952.

63 ANDREOTTI, R, GAMBANELLI, G: The protective action of ascorbic acid on preserved mushrooms. Industria Conserve 30, 12–15, 1955.

64 Japanese patent No 42503/72, 1972.

65 VAROQUAUX, P et al: Action of antioxidants and heat on O-diphenoloxidase of the cultivated mushroom (Agaricus bisporus). Ann Technol Agric 26, 473–486, 1977.

66 BANO, Z, SINGH, N S: Steeping preservation of an edible mushroom. J Food Sci Technol 9, 13–15, 1972.

67 CERUTTI, G: Oxidized flavor in market milk and its prevention. Proc 16th Internat Dairy Congr (Copenhagen) Section A: 663–668, 1963.

68 NAKANISHI, T, ADACHI, S: Antioxygenic action of vitamin C on dried milk. Tohoku J Agric Res 3, 271–276, 1953.

69 BAUERNFEIND, J C: Tocopherols in food. In: MACHLIN (ed.) "Vitamin E: a comprehensive treatise", pp 99–167. Dekker, New York, 1980.

70 BAUERNFEIND, J C: Use of ascorbic acid in processing food. Adv Food Res 4, 359–431, 1953.

71 DUNKLEY, W L et al: Influence of homogenization, copper and ascorbic acid on light-activated flavor in milk. J Dairy Sci 45, 1040–1044, 1962.

72 AURAND, L W et al: Some factors involved in the development of oxidized flavor in milk. J Dairy Sci 42, 961–968, 1959.

73 KING, R L: Oxidation of milk fat globule membrane material: relation of ascorbic acid and membrane concentration. J Dairy Sci 46, 267–274, 1963.

74 BELL, R W et al: Effect of L-ascorbic acid on the flavor stability of concentrated sweetened cream. J Dairy Sci 45, 1019–1020, 1962.

75 WILSON, H K, HERREID, E O: Controlling oxidized flavors in high-fat sterilized creams. J Dairy Sci 52, 1229, 1969.

76 FORD, J E et al: Influence of added ascorbic acid on the stability of folic acid and vitamin B_{12} in milk during UHT-processing and subsequent storage. Proc 19th Internat Dairy Congr, pp 567–569, 1974.

77 RUDDICK, J E: A study on the measurement and degradation of folic acid. Dissert Abstr Internat B39, 5823, 1979.

78 HENSHALL, J D: Vitamin C in canning and freezing. In: BIRCH and PARKER (eds) "Vitamin C: recent aspects of its physiological and technological importance", pp 104–120. Wiley, New York, 1974.

79 PONTING, J D: Reversible inactivation of polyphenol oxidase. J Am Chem Soc 76, 662–664, 1954.

80 BATE-SMITH, E C: Flavanoid compounds in foods. Adv Food Res 5, 262–300, 1954.

81 TANNER, H, RENTSCHLER, H: Polyphenols of stone fruits and grape juice: Occurrence and determination of chlorogenic, caffeic and quinic acid. Fruchtsaft Indust 1, 231–245, 1956.

82 SHANNON, C T, PRATT, D E: Apple polyphenol oxidase activity in relation to various phenolic compounds. J Food Sci 32, 479–483, 1967.

83 POIX, A et al: Combined action of chlorides and ascorbic acid on inhibition of enzymic browning in apple puree. Lebensm Wissens Technol 13, 105–110, 1980.

84 FREEMAN, T: Watersoluble antioxidants for seafood products. Refrigeration Sci Technol 1981, 183–188, 1981.

85 ATAGIRI, K, NISHIMORI, K: Use of vitamin C additives in sea-foods. New Food Indust 23, 58–62, 1981.

86 Himemath, G G, Sreenivasan, N: Studies on prevention of quality loss in frozen seer fillets during storage by use of additives. Mysore J Agric Sci *13*, 88–92, 1979.

87 Tsuchiya, Y *et al:* Prevention of yellow discoloration of shellfish, especially frozen scallop ligament. Reito *36*, 1011–1017, 1962.

88 Schwartz, M G, Watts, B M: Ascorbic acid as an antioxidant for frozen oysters and effects of copper-chelating ability of oyster tissue on ascorbic acid oxidation. Comm Fisheries Rev *21*, 1–6, 1959.

89 Ranken, M D: The use of ascorbic acid in meat processing. In: Counsell and Hornig (eds) "Vitamin C (ascorbic acid)", pp 105–122. Applied Science, London, 1981.

90 Harbers, C A Z: Ascorbic effects on bovine muscle pigments in the presence of radiant energy. Dissert Abstr Internat *B40*, 3684, 1981; J Food Sci *46*, 7–12, 1981.

91 Grau, R: Ascorbic acid in the treatment of meat. Wiss Veröffentl Deut Ges Ernähr *14*, 262–270, 1965.

92 Pederson, C S, Beattie, H G: Effect of processing and storage on the quality and ascorbic acid content of sauerkraut. Food Packer *27*, (7) 44–46, 1946.

93 Sedky, A *et al:* Factors affecting color and flavor of sauerkraut packaged in pliofilm bags. Food Technol *6*, 377–380, 1952.

94 Barret, A, Bidan, P: Quelques recherches recentes et leur application a la preparation des olives vertes de table. Inform Oleicoles Intern, New Ser *25*, 53–63, 1964.

95 Brown, M S: Wine from frozen grapes. Am J Enol Vitic *26*, 103–104, 1975.

96 Hernandez, M R: Study of musty flavour in various wines. Sem Vitioinic *28*, 167, 169, 171, 1973.

97 Schmitt, A: Effects of O_2 on mash and must, with special reference to the reducing agents SO_2 and ascorbic acid. Bayer Landwirtschaftl Jahrb Sonderh *58*, 70–76, 1981.

98 Merzhanian, A A *et al:* Deoxygenation of young wine for production of sparkling wine. Izvestiya Vysshikh Uchebnykh Zavedenii Pishchevaya Teknologiya *6*, 70–72, 1981.

99 Knorr, F: Significance of ascorbic acid in the brewing process. Wiss Veröffentl Deut Ges Ernähr *14*, 271–278, 1965.

100 Gray, P P, Stone, I: Oxidation in beers: oxidation stability of finished beers. J Inst Brewing *45*, 443–452, 1939.

101 Rubach, K *et al:* Behavior of ascorbic acid during storage of bottled beer. Monatschr Brauerei *33*, 163–164, 166, 1980.

102 UK patent application No GB2085027A, 1982.

103 Menger, A: Ascorbic acid in the treatment of flour. Wiss Veröffentl Deut Ges Ernähr *14*, 239–247, 1965.

104 Thewis, B N: Vitamin C in breadmaking. In: Birch and Parker (eds) "Vitamin C: recent aspects of its physiological and technological importance", pp 150–160. Wiley, New York, 1974.

105 Chamberlain, N: Use of ascorbic acid in breadmaking. In: Counsell and Hornig (eds) "Vitamin C (ascorbic acid)", pp 87–104. Applied Science, London, 1981.

106 Grant, D R, Sood, V K: Note on the antioxidant effect of ascorbic acid on flour free fatty acids. Cereal Chem *57*, 231–232, 1980.

107 Gresswell, D M: Vitamin C in soft drinks and fruit juices. In: Birch and Parker (eds) "Vitamin C: recent aspects of its physiological and technological importance", pp 136–149. Wiley, New York, 1974.

108 Mathe, L *et al:* Compositional changes in orange-containing soft drinks during storage. Szeszipar *28*, 51–53, 1980.

109 Bright, R A, Potter, N N: Acceptability and properties of carbonated apple juice. Food Prod Develop *13*, (4) 34–36, 1979.

110 Johnson, H T *et al:* Some aspects of canning soft drinks. Food Technol *9*, 643–647, 1958.

111 Erdman, J W, Klein, B P: Harversting, processing and cooking influences on vitamin C in foods. In: Seib and Tolbert (eds) "Ascorbic acid: chemistry, metabolism and uses", pp 501–532. Adv Chem Ser No *200*. American Chemical Society, Washington, 1982.

112 Reio, L: L-ascorbic acid: vitamin C a widely-used additive. Var Foeda *34*, 232–266, 1982.

113 Kläui, H: Technical uses of vitamin C. In: Birch and Parker (eds) "Vitamin C: recent aspects of its physiological and technological importance", pp 16–30. Wiley, New York, 1974.

114 Henshall, J D: Ascorbic acid in fruit juices and beverages. In: Counsell and Hornig (eds) "Vitamin C (ascorbic acid)", pp 123–137. Applied Science, London, 1981.

J. Christopher Bauernfeind, MS, PhD, 3664 NW 12th Avenue, Gainesville, Florida 32605, USA

Ascorbic Acid as a Flour and Bread Improver

H. Kläui

Food Technology Consultant, Basle, Switzerland

Key Words: Ascorbic acid · Flour improvement · Iron absorption · Bread gluten structure

Abstract: Ascorbic acid enjoys a preferential legislative status as a flour improver in many countries worldwide. Its specific properties make it a unique and ideal flour improver. As a reducing agent it exerts a protective effect on lipids against oxidation by directly reacting with lipid peroxides, and by reducing pro-oxidant metals. Ascorbic acid also improves the iron absorption, and thus helps to preserve the full nutritional value of bread. While exerting these beneficial effects, ascorbic acid is converted into dehydroascorbic acid. Dehydroascorbic acid oxidizes sulfhydryl groups to disulfides and thus strengthens the gluten structure. The reducing effect of ascorbic acid is selective: it will not split disulfides and therefore will not interfere with the gluten strengthening effect.

Introduction

Ascorbic acid is an effective flour and bread improver. It increases output in continuous and in modern batch dough-making processes. It strengthens the gluten of weak wheat flours. This is of particular importance in view of the increasing dependence on low protein wheats. Its nutritional acceptability and safety has led to the worldwide legal acceptance and use of this versatile baking aid.

Of all the technological applications, its use as flour and bread improver represents the third largest field of application - following use in meat and beverages. Large-scale manufacture, coupled with high standards of purity and economy, have led to the possibility of reducing the number or quantity of non-physiological additives normally not occurring in man's food.

The chemical properties of ascorbic acid as a powerful reducing agent have made this compound useful as an antioxidant and stabilizer. Most technological applications are in fact based on this electron-donating capacity.

Oxidation Improves the Baking Quality of Flour

However, the common flour and bread improvers are oxidizing agents (or electron acceptors). Use of the oxidation process for flour improvement has been made since the production of bread as we know and like it today. The miller had to age or «mature» the flour after milling by storing it, usually for at least 4 to 8 weeks, since freshly milled or «green» flour produced «young» dough and poor bread. Although the beneficial changes obtained by storage continue for about one year, they cannot be realized in practice for many reasons, but mainly because the period of optimum maturation varies from flour to flour, and the cost of storage would be too high.

The Development of Industrial Bread-Making and Introduction of Oxidizing Agents as Flour Improver

It was found that the uncontrolled oxidation induced by milling and storage could be replaced by chemical oxidizing agents added either to the flour or to the dough. The improvement in dough handling properties and the resulting bread quality obtained by this intentional and controlled oxidation served as a basis for the development of industrial bakeries, where the baker can no longer give individual attention to the dough. The improvement also permitted the standardization of the baking quality of the flours used, a prerequisite for the introduction of advanced rationalization, mechanization and automation, including the processes based on high intensity energy input, such as the British Chorleywood Bread Process. In such processes the time needed for the ripening or development step is drastically reduced from 3 hours to about 3 minutes, and where batches are being produced every 4 to 6 minutes (Fig.1). Moreover it is possible to produce better bread from a weak flour, a great advantage in view of the marked present trend towards weak wheats and flours with a lower protein content. Another modern process is the accelerated - or activated - dough development (ADD) procedure, where it is possible to completely omit the bulk dough fermentation time by using a proper balance of various additives - including L-cysteine.

The oxidizing agents mostly used world-wide today are ascorbic acid and potassium bromate. In the majority of the European as well as in various Latin American countries, ascorbic acid is the only permitted flour improver. This preferential status in legislation is based on its natural occurrence and its lack of any risks for health or safety, and - of course - on its efficacy.

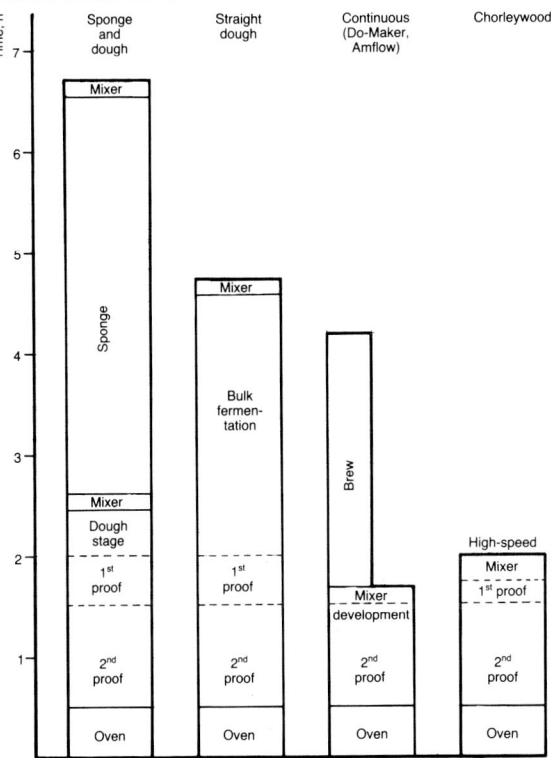

Fig. 1: Comparison of processing stages and times for bread-making systems. According to
Pyler [12].

The Discovery of the Beneficial Effects of Ascorbic Acid as Flour and Bread Improver

When the flour improving effect of ascorbic acid was discovered by Jørgensen in 1935 this finding was surprising and not easily explicable. It created some difficulties regarding the mode of action: ascorbic acid was a typical reducing agent, and not an oxidizing substance, as the other dough improvers.

The flour improvers which had been in use for some 20 years at that time were assumed to act by oxidizing proteolytic enzymes in flour. This inactivation would avoid weakening of the protein structure and thus maintain the visco-elastic and gas-retaining properties of the dough. Jørgensen assumed that the unexpected activity of ascorbic acid was due to its ability to first absorb oxygen and then release it; and the oxygen would then inhibit proteolysis.

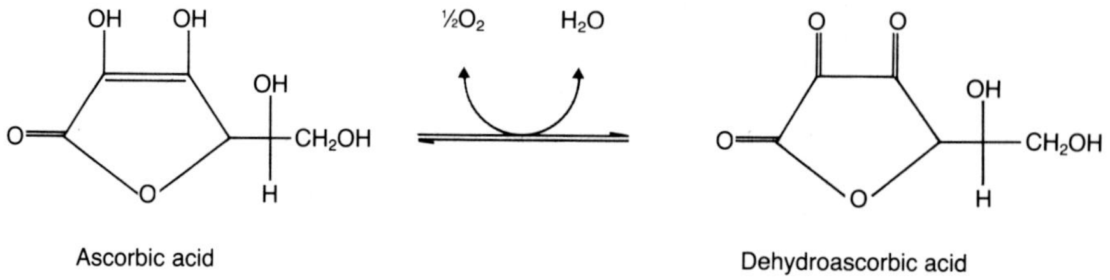

Ascorbic acid $\frac{1}{2}O_2$ H_2O Dehydroascorbic acid

Fig. 2: Oxidation of ascorbic acid.

When dehydroascorbic acid was recognized as the reversible oxidizing agent, ascorbic acid was included in all investigations regarding the mode of action of oxidizing agents as flour and bread improvers (Fig. 2).

Proposed Mode of Action

A great number of workers have studied in dough rheological, baking and other tests the reaction mechanism of dough improvers. On the basis of their results TSEN [1] supported the hypothesis of MALTHA [2] according to which the improving action of dehydroascorbic acid is due to its effect on sulfhydryl-disulfide exchange reactions: during mixing, ascorbic acid is rapidly oxidized by air to dehydroascorbic acid which, in turn, promotes the oxidation of thiol groups to disulfide links in the dough (Fig. 3).

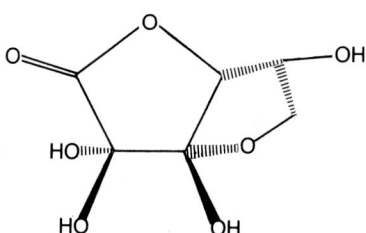

Fig. 3: Dehydroascorbic acid; according to HVOSLEF and PEDERSEN [13].

For chemically developed doughs it was suggested [3, 4] that ascorbic acid changed the water binding properties of gluten by affecting hydrogen bonds. The antioxidant effect of ascorbic acid protecting lipid components in the dough has also been considered [5].

Studies regarding the fate of added ascorbic acid support the first hypothesis, i.e. oxidation to dehydroascorbic acid and reaction with thiol compounds, whereby the dehydroascorbic acid is reduced to ascorbic acid and the thiol groups oxidized to disulfide compounds (Fig. 4). The reaction is catalyzed enzymatically, as was proven for the case of glutathione as SH compound and its oxidation by identification of the corresponding enzyme glutathione dehydrogenase (glutathione – dehydroascorbic acid oxidoreductase). The reaction is represented in figure 5.

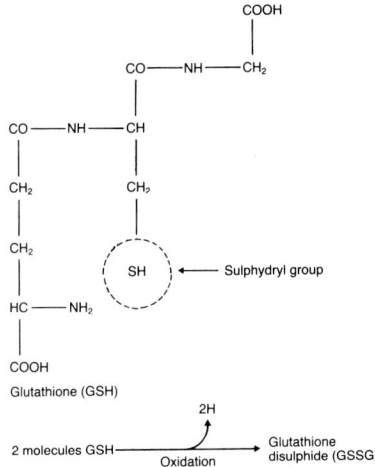

Fig. 4: Glutathione and glutathione disulphide. According to GROSCH et al [14].

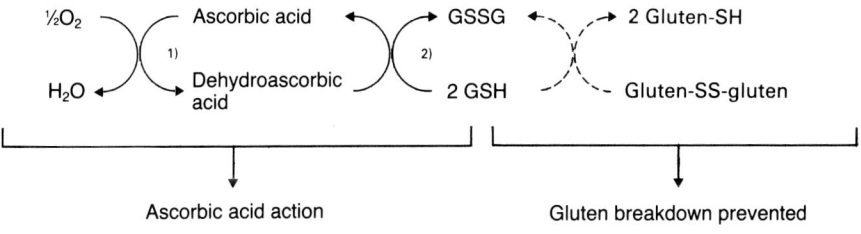

¹ Reaction catalyzed by ascorbic acid oxidase.
² Reaction catalyzed by glutathione dehydrogenase.

Fig. 5: Reaction of ascorbic acid with glutathione in dough. According to MAIR and GROSCH [6].

According to this mechanism ascorbic acid acts as a flour and dough improver by avoiding the degradation of the gluten structure induced by a sulphhydryl-disulfide interchange which, in the case of glutathione, would lead to lower molecular proteins, i.e. to weaker gluten, and this would reduce

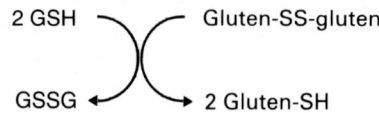

Fig. 6: Reduction of gluten structure by glutathione (sulphydryl-disulphide interchange). According to GROSCH *et al* [6].

the gas retention capacity (Fig. 6). Comments on this mechanism, particularly considering the chemical properties of ascorbic acid are given below.

The Action of Dehydroascorbic Acid

Conversion of ascorbic acid to dehydroascorbic acid. The oxidation of glutathione in the dough starts with the beginning of the mixing and kneading: it reaches 45–75 % after 1 minute, and is complete after 3 to 10 minutes [6]. This is very fast, considering that – according to the hypothesis – the oxidation of ascorbic acid to dehydroascorbic acid must precede the glutathione oxidation (Fig. 7).

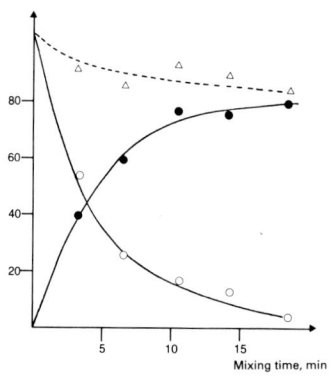

Fig. 7: Kinetics of ascorbic acid; according to NICOLAS *et al* [15]. ○ = Disappearance, dehydroascorbic acid. ● = Formation and total vitamin. △ = Loss during mixing of dough.

The mechanisms put forward for the oxidation of the ascorbic acid by oxygen in the air include the enzyme catalyzed oxidation (by L-ascorbic acid oxidase, isolated and characterised by PFEILSTICKER and ROEUNG [7]) and the heavy metal – particularly copper and iron – catalyzed oxidation. In addition to these reactions, a further possibility is discussed: lipid hydroperoxides – as the primary products of autoxidation – are strong oxidizing agents. The rapid decrease of the tocopherols present in the grain, their loss during milling, and the high content of polyunsaturated and easily oxidizable fatty acids in the wheat lipids coupled with the presence of lipoxidases may serve as an indication that the flour itself already contains powerful oxidizing agents. Ascorbic acid, as a potent H-donor, will be oxidized immediately by the hydroperoxides and by ferri- and cupri-compounds present. Since the particular step of oxigenation of lipid peroxy radicals is reversible, their reaction with ascorbic acid may even have a positive nutritional aspect, a unique feature which is not possible with any of the other oxidizing flour improvers.

The possible presence of an oxidant in dough has been mentioned in the literature [8] in connection with the observation that some ascorbic acid was converted to dehydroascorbic acid even when the doughs were mixed with nitrogen, i. e. when oxygen was excluded. These authors also refer to the fact that doughs are fully oxidized by as little as approximately 15 ppm of added dehydroascorbic acid, an amount which results easily as a sum of peroxide induced oxidation of added ascorbic acid.

The maturation period required in earlier times for flour can also be interpreted – at least partly – as a lipid oxidation process: the hydroperoxides first need some time to develop and are then inactivated slowly during further storage.

No risk of over-treating with ascorbic acid. One of the eminent practical advantages of ascorbic acid as flour improver is the impossibility of overtreating with ascorbic acid. An explanation for this behaviour refers to thiol groups in dough that are not accessible to dehydroascorbic acid, or, in other words, dehydroascorbic acid is by its nature a very mild oxidation agent and is relatively instable: it is easily reconverted to ascorbic acid, or further oxidized to 2,3-diketogulonic acid, L-threonic acid and CO_2. All these products are free of any oxidizing and thus over-treating capacity (Fig. 8).

Immediate and time-dependent effect of ascorbic acid. ELKASSABANY and HOSENEY [9] confirmed the observation of MEREDITH [10] that ascorbic acid displays an immediate and time-dependent effect. Considering the properties of ascorbic acid and the complexity of the reactions occurring in dough, it is believed that the immediate effect is due to an active oxidation of ascorbic acid by peroxides and other oxidizing agents, such as Fe (III) and Cu (II) in the presence of sufficient oxygen, and that the time-dependent reaction corresponds to the slow oxidation of ascorbic acid occurring normally in a system with very limited availability of air and where the pro-oxidant catalysts have already been – at least partly – reduced in activity.

The fact that in the absence of air, e. g. in continuous dough-making processes, some ascorbic acid remains unchanged in the dough can result in a very

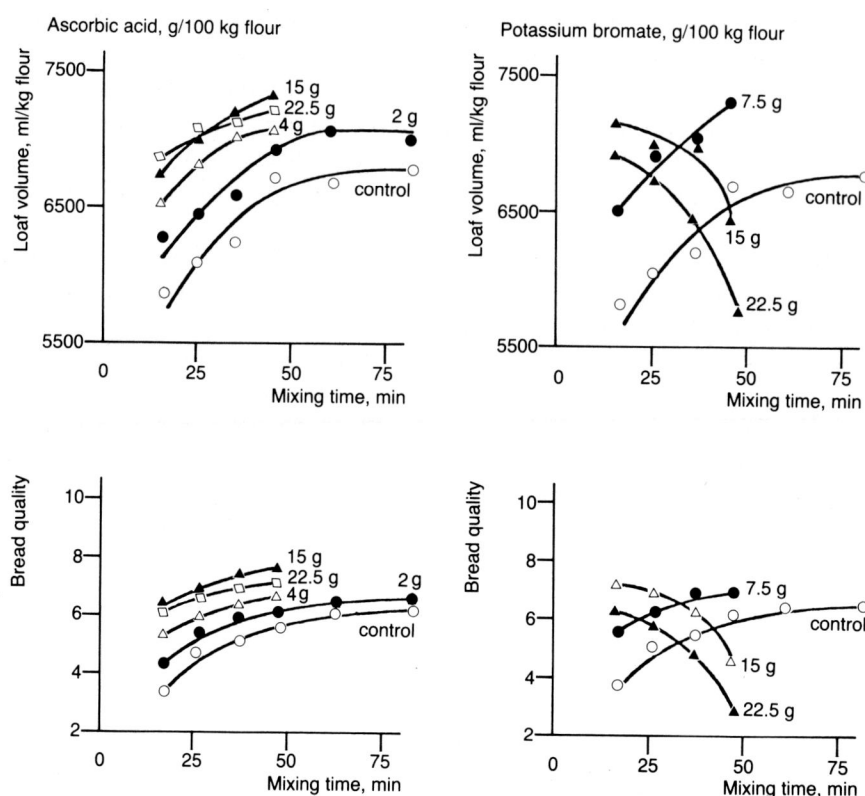

Fig. 8: Effect of various amounts of ascorbic acid and potassium bromate on bread volume and bread quality, and the effect of mixing time. (Bread quality is given on a scale of ten points.) According to DE RUITER [16].

positive effect: ascorbic acid and other reducing agents, such as L-cysteine, have a softening effect on the gluten of the flour; they therefore reduce mixing and fermentation times and thus save energy and increase capacity. The amount of unchanged ascorbic acid, however, is very small and negligible as a source of vitamin C. For enrichment purposes it has been proposed to use sodium palmitoyl ascorbate, which was found by HPLC to show a 81 % retention in baked bread [11].

Conclusion

The reducing effect of ascorbic acid is selective. Ascorbic acid does not split -S-S-bonds and therefore does not induce – undesirable – -SH, -SS-interactions. The specific properties of ascorbic acid, and particularly the beneficial effects it exerts during the oxidation to dehydroascorbic acid by reacting with lipid peroxides and by reducing pro-oxidant metals, make it a unique and ideal flour improver.

References

1 TSEN, C C: The improving mechanism of ascorbic acid. Cereal Chem 42, 86–97, 1965.
2 MALTHA, P R A: Über den Einfluss von L-Ascorbinsäure und Verbindungen mit verwandter Struktur auf die Backfähigkeit des Mehles. Getreide und Mehl 3, 65–69, 1953.
3 ZENTNER, H: Effect of ascorbic acid on wheat gluten. J Sci Food Agric 19, 464–467, 1968.
4 JOHNSTON, W R, MAUSETH, R E: The interrelations of oxidants and reductants in dough development. Baker's Digest 46, 20–22, 1972.
5 DAHLE, L K, MURTHY, P R: Some effects of antioxidants in dough systems. Cereal Chem 47, 296–303, 1970.
6 MAIR, G, GROSCH, W: Changes in glutathione content (reduced and oxidised form) and the effect of ascorbic acid and potassium bromate on glutathione oxidation during dough mixing. J Sci Food Agric 30, 914–920, 1979.
7 PFEILSTICKER, K, ROEUNG, S: Characterisation of L-ascorbic acid oxidase from wheat flour. Z Lebensm Unters Forsch 174, 306–308, 1982.
8 LILLARD, D W et al: Isomeric ascorbic acids and derivatives of L-ascorbic acid: their effect on the flow of dough. Cereal Chem 59, 291–296, 1982.
9 ELKASSABANY, M et al: Ascorbic acid as an oxidant in wheat flour dough. I. Conversion to dehydroascorbic acid. Cereal Chem 57, 85–87, 1980.
10 MEREDITH, P: The oxidation of ascorbic acid and its improver effect in bread doughs. J Sci Food Agric 16, 474–480, 1965.
11 HOSENEY, R C et al: Use of salts of 6-acyl esters of L-ascorbic and D-isoascorbic acids in breadmaking. Cereal Chem 54, 1062–1069, 1977.
12 PYLER, E J: Comparison of different bread-making systems. Baker's Digest 56, (4), 22–26, 1982.
13 HVOSLEF, J, PEDERSEN, B: Structure of dehydroascorbic acid in solution. Acta Chem Scand B 33, 503–511, 1979.
14 GROSCH, W et al: Vorkommen von Glutathion in Weizenmehl und -teig. Getreide Mehl Brot 32, 175–177, 1978.
15 NICOLAS, J et al: Effects of some parameters on the kinetics of ascorbic acid destruction and dehydroascorbic acid formation in wheat flour doughs. Lebensmittel-Wiss Technol 13, 308–313, 1980.
16 DE RUITER, D: Some observations on the effects of different breadmaking systems. Baker's Digest 42, (10), 24–33, 1968.

Dr. Heinrich Kläui, Kilchgrundstrasse 77, CH-4125 Riehen, Switzerland

The Use of L-Ascorbic Acid in Improving the Quality of Pasta

L. Milatović

Institute of Food Technology and Biochemistry, Faculty of Agriculture – Zemun, University of Belgrade, Belgrade, Yugoslavia

Key Words: L-Ascorbic acid · Dehydroascorbic acid · Pasta processing · Spaghetti · Soft wheat flour · Semolina · Redox reaction · Lutein · Carotenoids and colour · Lipoxigenase · Gluten · High temperature drying · Cooking properties of pasta

Abstract: The effect of L-ascorbic acid (AA) on the commercial and cooking qualities of pasta were compared in products with different basic ingredients using controls. Tests covered such aspects as colour, texture, and taste. These criteria were improved by the addition of AA during processing, particularly in pasta made from common flour instead of the traditional semolina. This is important for the production of pasta in countries where durum wheat is not grown. Analyses showed that the addition of AA also reduced loss of solid matter and protein in the cooked product. Among the most important production parameters at the three manufacturing sites were the temperatures of the water used and those employed in drying. Lower temperatures gave better results in AA assays on the final product.

Pasta products are important items in the staple diet of many countries, particularly so in Italy, Argentina, France, Greece, Switzerland, Germany and Turkey. The yearly per capita consumption of pasta for the whole of Italy is 33 kg, but in the south (with some 28 million inhabitants) it attains over 60 kg. In Argentina it is about 24 kg, in Switzerland 12 kg, in France and Greece 9 kg, in West Germany 8 kg, and in Yugoslavia 5 kg. Pasta owes its increasing popularity to easy preparation and good storage properties. It is also inexpensive.

Background Information

Pasta products constitute a preserved foodstuff made from flour or semolina and water, with or without added ingredients. Such products are available pressed, shaped, dried and packed. The raw material used in pasta processing includes semolina made from a species of wheat known as *Triticum durum,* flour milled from *Triticum aestivum,* and flour from corn or rice. In Italy the main constituent is semolina with an added maximum of 10 % wheat flour. A distinction is moreover made in Italy between two types of semolina, namely *semola* and *semolato,* which must conform to official standards.

In some countries, *durum* wheat is not grown, so the harder and vitreous varieties of wheat milled from *Triticum aestivum* are employed. Often the resultant pasta is however of inferior quality, with regard to colour, surface and cooking properties. Compromises have been made, and the proportion of semolina to soft wheat flour in pasta varies from country to country. In yet other countries, particularly European, the harder varieties of *Triticum aestivum* are almost unobtainable, and our experiments were mainly conducted using the softer varieties.

A means is obviously required of improving the quality of pasta made either entirely or partly of common wheat flour. The addition of dry gluten [1], sugar esters or monoglycerides of fatty acids or other emulsifying agents has been proposed. But according to several authors [2–8] L-ascorbic acid (AA) has been employed most successfully, both for reducing loss of colour as well as for improving cooking properties. The explanation for the former effect is that AA is a strong reducing agent and inhibits the oxidation of pigments. The formula [20] in Figure 1 shows how AA takes part in redox reactions.

During mixing AA is rapidly oxidized by air, by ferric and cupric compounds present in flour, or by hydroperoxides, to dehydroascorbic acid, which in turn promotes oxidation of thiol groups to disulfide links in the dough. Moreover, it has been shown that the addition of 20–150 ppm AA to water, semolina, or flour used for macaroni dough, considerably inhibits the destruction of pigments [2]. An actual increase in yellow colour has been claimed, particularly for long-cut products such as spaghetti. The greatest improvement in colour was achieved in pasta products made from the traditional semolina produced from varieties of durum wheat that have high lipoxygenase activity [3]. The quantity of AA mentioned above was however used in the old system of pasta processing, where low drying temperatures, as well as longer mixing and drying times, were used for the dough [7]. L-AA was shown here to be a fully competitive lipoxygenase inhibitor. In pasta, lipoxygenase activity is connected with the oxidation of carotenoids (lutein). Some authors [2, 7, 15]

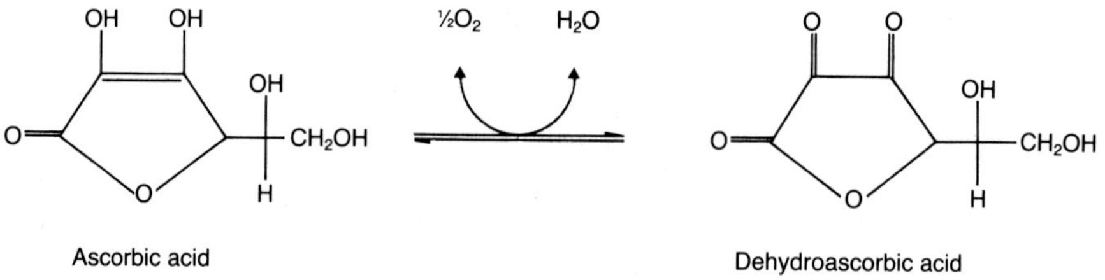

Ascorbic acid   Dehydroascorbic acid

Fig. 1: Oxidation of ascorbic acid.

stress that AA inhibits this activity when the vacuum system is used for dough processing.

High Temperature Drying and other Processing Aspects

Between 1975 and 1977, macaroni processing was greatly improved by the following innovations:
a) Drying at temperatures over 60° C
b) High capacity plant and Rototherm predryers
c) Shorter processing times
d) Sterilization during drying

These advances improved the quality of pasta in all respects [16], particularly where soft wheat flour was used. But between 1980 and 1983 it became apparent that there were two approaches to obtain the optimum benefit from high temperature (HT) drying.

The first was its application during the initial phase but after the first phase of predrying, when pasta has about 17.5–18.5% moisture content (in the Rototherm). This was followed by drying cycles at decreasing temperatures.

The second was to use high temperatures during the final drying phase, after predrying at conventional temperatures.

Both systems have the advantage of greatly reducing overall drying time and keeping the product relatively sterile. The Pavan system corresponds to the first approach [21], while the second is recommended by some American authors [29, 30].

The temperature of the water used in making dough is also important. Guidelines at present observed in the pasta industry are:
a) between 36 and 45° C for cold dough making;
b) between 45 and 65° C for the warm system using HT drying;
c) between 75 and 80° C for very warm processing (15).

Most industrial plants use the warm system, since the temperature range of 45–65° C is suitable for both long-cut pasta and bulkier shapes [16].

When egg is added, the water temperature should not exceed 50°C, i.e. the temperature of the dough must remain about 40°C since albumen plays the most important role in the product's flexibility and coagulates at 49°C. When AA is added the temperature of the water used should not exceed 55°C, otherwise degradation of the additive will be accelerated [17]. For small shapes of cut pasta and hollow macaroni, the water temperature should be between 36 and 45°C. If *semolato* or low grade wheat flour with less than 28% of wet gluten is used, the cold system with temperatures of 36–45°C is preferable [17].

The flour employed should not have more than 10 % of its particles smaller than 150 μm or larger than 340 μm. Particles exceeding the latter size impede the activity of the various enzymes and ions in the dough. This reduces the desired effect of AA.

In the warm processing system, dough preparation is shorter owing to the quicker hydration of gluten. This causes the starch to swell rapidly, which is desirable in dough making. Such conditions also improve the possibility of retaining the yellow colour of pasta products.

The very warm system is restricted to pasta produced from semolina or flour with over 32 % wet gluten content. Water between 75 and 80°C produces the most rapid hydration of gluten and gelatinization starch, but AA decomposes at this temperature and thus has no beneficial effect on the product.

That AA does improve the commercial quality of pasta products when added under the right conditions has been confirmed by our 1983 studies, which were the first of their kind[1]. The improvements were observed in both colour and cooking properties. The quantities of the additive used in our experiments finally ranged from 200 to 400 ppm. The best results in Yugoslavia were obtained with 300 ppm for long-cut pasta made from soft wheat flour milled from *Triticum aestivum*. The product also contained egg, and AA was first dissolved in the water used for making the dough.

Materials and Methods

The raw materials employed varied according to location. At the Mapimpianti semi-industrial pilot a mixture of equal quantities of *semola* and wheat flour was used, while pure *semola* only was employed at the Del Verde industrial high-capacity plant. At a similar plant, Danubius in Yugoslavia, soft wheat flour only was used.

AA was supplied by its leading producer F. Hoffmann-La Roche, Basle [22,23]. Other ingredients were local tap water and commercial fresh eggs or melange. All raw materials conformed to local standards.

The three principal raw materials were subjected to organoleptic and rheological tests, as well as to chemical analyses. Further information on materials and methods is contained in an upcoming paper by this author.

---

[1] *Studies were conducted at the following locations:*
Mapimpianti. Galliera-Veneta, Padua, Italy; a semi-industrial pilot plant with HT drying. Del Verde. Fara San Martino, Abruzzo, Italy; does not use HT drying. Danubius. Novi Sad, Yugoslavia; HT drying.

Tab. I: Chemical characteristics of the raw materials (semola, mixture, and soft wheat flour)

Properties	Del Verde semola	Mapimpianti mixture (semola + flour)	Danubius soft wheat flour
Moisture, %	15.8	15.0	14.9
Ash, %	0.83	0.67 (0.50)[1]	0.39
Lipids, %[2]	–	–	1.56
Proteins, %[2]	11.7	11.0	10.5
Acidity	–	–	1.56
Gluten[3]			
Wet (0), %	34.9	29.3	24.0
Wet (30), %	37.7	30.4	–
Dry, %	13.3	9.0 (7)[1]	7.0
Quellzahl of gluten[4]			
First (0)	5	8	–
Second (30)	1	10.5	–
Value of sediment	–	–	13
Pigments as lutein equivalents, ppm	3.9	2.5	–

[1] Values in brackets correspond to the standards for Italian white wheat flour (from *Tr. aestivum).*

[2] Lipids were analyzed by the Soxhlet and proteins by the Kjeldahl method ($N \times 5.7$).

[3] The quantity of wet gluten was analyzed immediately after washing and again after 30 min.

[4] The Quellzahl was analyzed immediately after washing the gluten and again after 30 min.

Tab. II: Comparison of the granulation of Italian commercial semola and experimental flour and semola

Sieve aperture (DIN 4188), μm	US Standard sieves (ASTME 11–70); sieve No.	Material remaining on sieve, %		
		Italian commercial semola (18)	experimental semola (Del Verde)	experimental flour and semola (Mapimpianti)
630	approx. 22–25	0	0	0
500	35	1.2	5	0.3
400	approx. 40–45	14.6	30	1.4
315	approx. 45–50	30.7	30	12.8
200	approx. 70–80	32.4	26	28.5
Through 200		21.1	9	56.3
Total		100.0	100	99.3

Processing Parameters and Plant at the Three Sites

Mapimpianti

This semi-industrial pilot plant was equipped with an F-20 extruder former, a TM 20 shaker predryer, a CD 20 continuous dryer with 3 selections, and a vacuum pump.

The formula for the pasta produced during the experiment was: 30 l warm water per 100 kg of a mixture of equal parts of Italian *semola* and white wheat flour, with or without 200/400 ppm of AA. Each experiment was performed twice, 300 kg pasta being produced per run. In this case AA was added to the flour. The final product was a short type of hollow macaroni. Prior to the experimental work, exclusively *semola* had been used as raw material. This provided useful data for comparison.

It is obvious from Table II that the granulation [18] of the Mapimpianti mixture was too fine, most particles being smaller than 200 μm. This quality is adequate for baking bread but not for processing pasta. The *semola* was also finer than the usual commercial varieties used in Italy [22].

The following processing parameters were kept constant during the experiment:

Temperature of tap water added to raw material	63°C
Moisture content of pressed dough	31.5 %
Mixing time	8 min
Vacuum pressure during mixing	$8.3 \cdot 10^{-2}$ bar
Shaping pressure	110 bar
Transport time of pasta through shaker	45 sec
Temperature of air entering predryer or shaker	70°C
Temperature of cut pasta immediately after predrying	45°C
Moisture content of pasta before HT drying	28.5 %
Relative humidity in first section of dryer	71.6 %
Temperature of hot air at entrance to dryer	74°C
Moisture content of pasta at end of first section	20.5 %
Temperature of pasta at exit of first dryer section	60°C
Temperature of air at entrance to second dryer section	58°C
Relative humidity in second section	82.4
(The two ensuing sections have lower drying temperatures).	
Moisture content at end of drying and stabilization	12.2 %
Total drying time	8 h 45 min

Experiments were made continuously, the dryer being kept full in order to obtain constant, optimum hydrothermic conditions. This is an essential feature for work on this type of plant.

Del Verde

This industrial high-capacity plant was equipped throughout with units supplied by «Pavan».

The formula for the pasta was 30 l water per 160 kg of best quality *semola* (for granulation see Table II). 200/400 ppm AA were dissolved in the water, the temperature being 50°C. The final products were nested fettuccini pasta, some 300 kg being processed. The experimental work was performed during the normal course of production.

The processing parameters at Del Verde were as follows:

Water temperature	50°C
Dough mixing time	15 min
Vacuum pressure	$8.3 \cdot 10^{-2}$ bar
Moisture content of dough	29.5 %
Pressure of extruder	120 bar
Air temperature during predrying (Incartatore)	48°C
Duration of predrying	3–5 min
Subsequent moisture content	24.5–25 %

The pasta then entered the main dryer sections, final data of which are given in Table III.

Tab. III: The hydrothermic conditions in drying nested fettuccini

Dryer section	Dry thermometer, °C	Relative humidity, %	Drying time, min	Moisture content in final product, %
I	47	68.8		17.5[1]
II	45	77.7	55	14.8
III	45	88.5	55	13.0
IV	45	70.5	55	12.4
V	40	–	55	12.0
VI	30	–	55	11.7
VII	30	–	55	11.0
VIII	30	–	55	10.5
IX	30	–	55	9.8

[1] End of predrying.

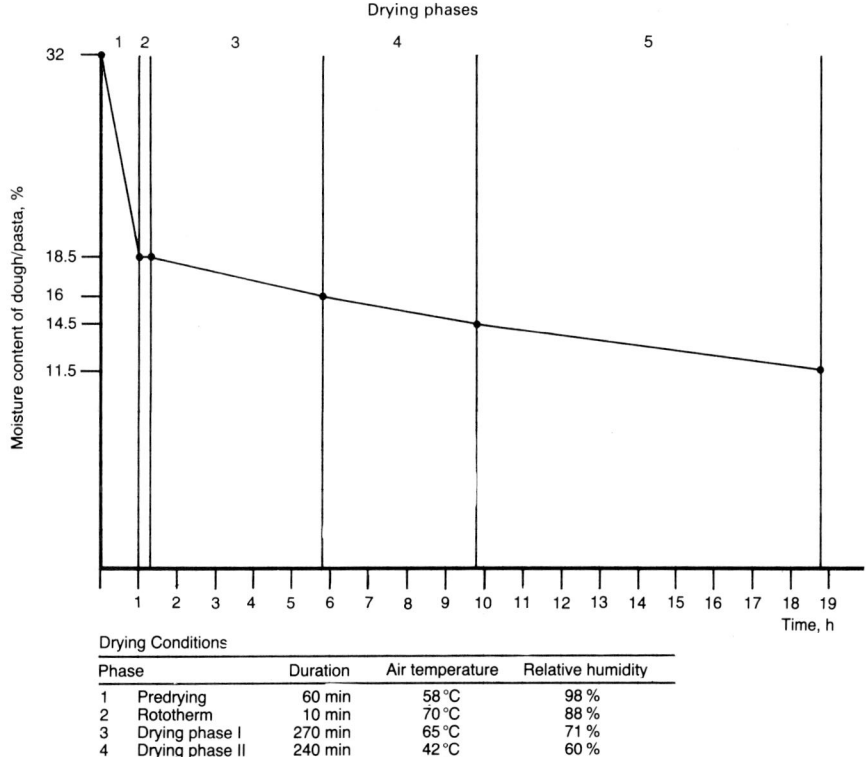

Drying Conditions

Phase		Duration	Air temperature	Relative humidity
1	Predrying	60 min	58 °C	98 %
2	Rototherm	10 min	70 °C	88 %
3	Drying phase I	270 min	65 °C	71 %
4	Drying phase II	240 min	42 °C	60 %
5	Drying phase III	540 min	29 °C	–

Fig. 2: Drying data for HT processing of pasta at the Danubius plant.

Danubius

This plant is equipped with modern Pavan machinery and employs HT drying. The high temperature, however, is applied here during the initial phase with the Rototherm system [21]. See Figure 2.

The formula was as follows: 77 kg soft wheat flour milled from *Triticum aestivum:* 19–20 l warm water; 3 kg egg powder or 10 kg fresh egg (melange); and 300 ppm AA dissolved in the water. The finished product was long cut spaghetti.

The water used at Danubius contains 0.1 to 0.3 mg/l of Fe^{3+}. Since this acts as a catalyst in the degradation of AA, the quantity of the additive was increased to 300 ppm.

Table IV shows the granulation of the flour. About 12 % of it had particle sizes of less than 195 μm and about 6 % were over 350 μm. This proportion is optimum when using HT drying.

Higher amounts of fine particles are unfavourable since the warm water added causes a too rapid dough formation and difficulties are incurred in the mixing and pressing stages.

The processing parameters at Danubius were as follows:

Water temperature	50°C
Mixing time	15 min
Vacuum pressure during dough mixing	$7.3 \cdot 10^{-2}$ bar
Moisture content of dough	32°C
Extruder pressure for spaghetti	110 bar
Temperature of dough immediately after shaping	34°C

Tab. IV: Granulation of Yugoslavian soft wheat flour

Sieve aperture, μm	US Standard sieves; sieve No.	Flour remaining on sieve, %
450	approx. 35–40	0
350	approx. 45	5.6
250	60	49.4
220	approx. 70	26.9
195	approx. 75	6.4
146	approx. 100	4.6
125	120	3.5
Through 125		3.5
Total		100.0

Drying data are shown in Figure 2. As in the case of «Del Verde», the experimental work was conducted in the course of normal production, and since the final product was intended for export, the moisture content was less than that laid down by local standards.

Methods of Adding Ascorbic Acid

The stability of AA is affected by the presence of oxygen, heavy metals and enzymes, as well as by the temperature of water in which it has been dissolved. The time it is exposed to these factors is also very important [26].

AA may be added to any of the ingredients used in making dough, such as to the basic semolina or flour. Alternately, it may be dissolved previously in the water, or mixed with other additives such as powdered egg, dry gluten, or starch, dry soya protein and emulsifiers. Each method has its particular advantages and disadvantages.

Tab. V: The characteristics of commercial raw pasta with and without AA

Pasta product	Colour (assessed visually)		Strength		Aroma and taste		Appearance
	with AA	without AA (control)	with AA	without AA (control)	with AA	without AA (control)	
Short, cut (Mapimpianti)	pale yellow less «greyish»	greyish, less yellow (pale)	normal	normal	normal	normal	no remarks
Fettuccini or nidi (Del Verde)	slightly more yellow	yellow	normal	normal	normal	normal	no remarks
Spaghetti (Danubius)	intense yellow (some samples slightly brownish)	less yellow	flexible	less flexible	normal	normal	Much more friable without AA than with it. Presence of white points on both samples. No fissure. Brighter with AA than without it. Slightly smoother with AA.

If AA is added to the semolina or flour it must be well mixed and attention paid to accurate weighing, as well as to the time the mixture is stored. This procedure is advisable in well equipped plants only.

One problem involved in adding AA to the water used for dough making is constituted by the direct employment of the main supply in production; large, intermediate water storage tanks are thus needed for dissolving the additive. Once AA has been added, moreover, the water must be kept at prescribed temperatures and for short periods only. Another problem is that tap water may contain traces of zinc, iron, and copper ions [26, 27]. Since they act as catalysts in the oxidation of AA it may be necessary to eliminate them, thus incurring extra production costs.

No particular problems are involved in adding L-AA to other powdered additives. If, however, it is added to emulsifiers or anti-foaming agents, special equipment is necessary [15].

Criteria for Tests

Attention was mainly directed to measuring three objective criteria, namely:
1) solid matter in the cooked product
2) the yield per 100 g of raw product
3) the solid matter left in the water used for cooking and rinsing

The final test for the acceptability of a pasta product is its cooking quality. Cooked pasta must be firm, resilient, and certainly not sticky [29]. In our research we used visual methods and a panel of professional tasters.

Results

The colour of pasta is one of the most important features for its commercial acceptance. In recent years, three major methods have been developed for predicting the product's final colour and evaluating its suitability [6, 25]:

1) visual comparisons with standard samples

2) chemical pigment extraction

3) light reflectance measurements

The relationships between these different methods have been widely discussed.

The results on colour given in Table V represent visual comparisons and show clearly that all the samples treated with AA had more intense colour than the controls. An improvement in texture is also apparent in the pasta made from soft wheat flour at «Danubius», the Yugoslavian plant.

The spectrophotometric readings obtained by measuring ground pasta samples [28] given in Table VI show little difference between colour values on samples treated with AA and on controls. All they have done is to reveal differences in dominant wavelengths, purity of colour, and relative brightness in all samples. Yet it should be stressed that there are distinctly visible differences in colour. The pasta made by adding about 200 ppm of AA had a more intense yellow colour.

Tab. VI: Spectrophotometre readings

Measurement	Pasta products with and without AA						
	Mapimpianti; from mixture		Del Verde; from semola			Danubius; from flour	
	AA 200 ppm	no AA	AA 400 ppm	AA 200 ppm	no AA	AA 300 ppm	no AA
Dominant wavelength, nm	574.8	574.1	575.7	575.9	576.4	574.8	575.9
Purity of colour	0.197	0.192	0.314	0.304	0.321	0.183	0.191
Relative brightness	69.7	69.6	67.4	67.9	67.6	70.3	70.1

An additional attempt was made to objectify the results by another method. The colouring matter was measured by the extraction and purification of carotenoids, i. e. an assay of total carotenoids was made calculated as their lutein equivalent at a wavelength of 445 nm. The results are summarized in Tables VII and VIII. The data indicate that slightly less carotenoids were pre-

Tab. VII: Content of total carotenoids (as lutein equivalent) in pasta products (ppm) [22]

Samples	Short-cut pasta (Mapimpianti)	Fettuccini or nidi (Del Verde)	Spaghetti (Danubius)
Control without added AA	2.7	3.5	2.0
With 200 ppm AA	2.3	3.4	–
With 300 ppm AA	–	–	1.5
With 400 ppm AA	2.3	3.3	–
Raw material: semola	–	3.9	–

Tab. VIII: Content of total carotenoids (as lutein equivalent) after 3 and 6 months in fettuccini («Del Verde») [22]

Samples	After 3 months, ppm	After 6 months, ppm	Remarks
Controls	3.5	3.3	No significant changes
200 AA added	3.1	3.4	in total carotenoids
400 AA added	3.6	3.6	after storing the pasta 3 and 6 months under normal atmospheric conditions.

sent after the addition of AA. Visually however, the contrary would appear to be the case, for the samples treated with AA have improved colouring.

The various types of pasta produced for the experiments were tested for their cooking properties at all of the three locations mentioned and in the laboratories of Hoffmann-La Roche in Basle, Switzerland. Local tap water was used in all cases. The results are recorded in Table IX.

With respect to taste, texture and flavour, no great difference was evident between cooked Mapimpianti pasta treated with AA and the controls. It will be recalled that the pasta at this plant was made from a mixture of equal parts of semolina and flour. The colour was nevertheless the desired yellowish hue in samples to which AA had been added, whereas the controls were greyish. There was likewise an increase in yellow colouring in Del Verde products that

Tab. IX: The results of cooking Mapimpianti. Del Verde and Danubius varieties of pasta made from mixture (semolina plus flour), pure semolina, and pure flour respectively [22]

Origin of sample	Solid matter of raw product[1], %	Yield from 100 g of pasta[2], g	Solid matter of cooked pasta[3], %	Solid matter[4] in cooked and rinsing water, g	Solid matter[4] in rinsing water, %
Mapimpianti					
No AA	88.6	321	26.4	11.58	1.38
AA added (400 ppm)	88.8	330	26.3	9.79	1.24
Del Verde					
No AA	91.8	371	25.0	4.32	0.55
AA added (200 ppm)	91.6	348	25.0	4.49	0.57
AA added (400 ppm)	91.8	350	26.0	3.83	0.49
Danubius					
No AA	90.0	337	28.3	6.17	–
AA added (300 ppm)	90.2	361	25.5	6.78	–

[1] Dried at 100°C to obtain constant weight.
[2] Cooked 15 min, in 1000 ml of water with 2 g NaCl added. Rinsed with 250 ml of water and allowed to drip for 2 min.
[3] Dried at 100°C to constant weight.
[4] Including NaCl.

had received 200 to 400 ppm AA. The same can be said of the spaghetti produced at Danubius, with the added observation that the product made with 300 ppm AA expanded more on cooking than the controls.

Very little difference existed in the analyses carried out in the SOUR-Mlinpred laboratory in Novi Sad [24] from those performed on identical samples in Basle. The Yugoslavian results given in Table X clearly indicate that spaghetti made from soft wheat flour is improved with respect to cooking properties by the addition of 300 ppm AA. The additive also caused the spaghetti to retain its yellow colour and brightness. Water absorption was slightly increased and the quantity of dried residue reduced. Far less flaked sediment was noted in the water used for cooking after allowing it to settle for 24 hours.

The effect of AA on protein loss after cooking was also determined. The Kjeldahl method of analysis revealed differences in the residue contained in the cooking water. 100 g samples of Danubius spaghetti were used. The results are given below.

Spaghetti processed without AA:
Weight of total dried residue, of which 0.56 g was pure
protein, in cooking water.   9.8 g/100 g

Spaghetti processed with AA:
Weight of total dried residue, of which 0.50 g was pure
protein, in cooking water.   9.1 g/100 g

Tab. X: The characteristics of cooked Danubius spaghetti (made from soft wheat flour) [24]

	Sample without AA		Sample with 300 ppm AA	
Cooking time, min	12[1]	15	13[1]	15
Absorption of water, %	206.5	225	228	243
Quantity of dried residue, %	6.9	7.1	5.9	7.0
Appearance of cooked pasta	normal	overcooked	normal	overcooked
Colour (visible)	yellowish	yellowish	yellow	yellow
Taste (organoleptic)	pleasant	pleasant	slightly resistent, pleasant	pleasant
Brightness (visible)	surface bright	bright	very bright	bright
Turbidity of cooked water	very turbid	very turbid	visibly less turbid	very turbid
Height of sediment from residue after 24 hours	29.1	29.7	25.5	27.3
Height of flaked sediment after 24 hours	1.9	2.7	1.5	2.3

[1] Time of cooking fixed according to the moment at which the starch nucleus in spaghetti disappeared.

Identical analyses were carried out in Novi Sad and Basle without any significant difference in results.

It should be stressed at this juncture that the structure of protein is destroyed in pasta at temperatures approaching 80°C [30]. It was in fact recently reported [29] that this already took place at temperatures exceeding 72°C.

Analysis of AA in the Final Product

To conclude our tests, the amount of AA was determined in all samples of pasta by potentiometric titration [23]. The results are given in Table XI.

Tab. XI: The AA content of final uncooked pasta products used in the study

Sample	AA, mg/kg product
Mapimpianti (raw material)	
Mixture with AA	400
Mixture without extra AA	17[1]
Mapimpianti (pasta)	
Mixture with 400 ppm AA	265
Mixture without extra AA	10[1]
Del Verde (fettuccini)	
Semola with 400 ppm AA	290
Semola with 200 ppm AA	155
Semola without extra AA	15
Danubius (spaghetti)	
Flour with 300 ppm AA	0[2]
Flour without extra AA	0

[1] AA was probably added to the wheat flour to improve baking quality.
[2] AA completely destroyed during processing in Rototherm at 70°C.

Discussion

Dough used for making pasta has moisture contents ranging from 29 to 31 %. Under such conditions AA has less effect than in dough used for baking [9], where the moisture content is about 65 %. Hence, more AA must be added in pasta processing than in baking bread. The actual amount depends on many factors, including the granulation of the semolina or flour used, the water temperature, the mixing time, the temperature of the dough before drying and that used in the drying process [19, 30]. Moreover, the time taken for mixing the various ingredients of pasta is merely 12–16 minutes, so that more additive is again required in order to achieve its optimum effect in such a short period [10–14].

The amount of AA added may be reduced in pasta processing employing low or medium temperature ranges, but our work has shown that it should not be below 220 ppm. The method of adding AA, e.g. whether to the basic raw material, the water, or to other additives, may also have some influence on the redox reaction [31–33].

The temperature of the water in which AA has been dissolved ought not to exceed 55°C, and that of the dough containing the additive and egg should be below 48°C before pressing. Large amounts of AA were found in finished pasta products processed without HT drying, e.g. in those produced at Del Verde and Mapimpianti. No trace of the additive remained in the pasta produced by Danubius on account of the HT predrying and Rototherm units employing a temperature of 70°C.

It was established that AA had a positive influence on the commercial and culinary qualities of pasta. The colour of the dried product was a bright yellow, much of which remained even after cooking. Compared with the controls, there was marked improvement in many respects. The loss of solid matter in the cooking water, for example, was also reduced after preparing spaghetti made at «Danubius». The dried product was moreover less friable after being processed with AA.

The addition of AA is recommended for the production of pasta made from soft wheat flour or from a mixture of equal parts of semolina and flour. Low grade wheat flour with a wet gluten content of less than 25% requires a minimum addition of 200 ppm AA.

A predrying air temperature exceeding 72°C and a relative humidity of less than 80% is not recommended.

This sector of nutrition employing AA requires further research with respect to the following items:
a) The influence of HT drying on enzyme lipoxygenase activity
b) The action of AA in dough after mixing, pressing, shaping, and predrying
c) The combined effect of AA and emulsifiers on the commercial and cooking qualities of pasta
d) The optimal method of adding substances such as AA in modern processing plants

e) The measurement of visible colour in pasta products (neither spectro-photometric techniques nor lutein assay really correspond to visual results)

It is highly probable that once this field of research has been completed, fresh impetus will be given to producing a staple food on an even larger scale.

Acknowledgements: Information on plants, processing aspects and technical assistance were obtained from G. Pavan, Dr. G. Papotto and G. Didone, as well as from other specialists in Pavan, Del Verde and Mapimpianti in Italy.

Assistance on technical points was also supplied by Lj. Obradović, G. Bejarović, M. Franciskovic and Dr. M. Zeželj of OOUR-Danubius and SOUR-Mlinpred in Yugoslavia.

Acknowledgement is also made of the support afforded by F. Hoffmann-La Roche & Co. Ltd., Switzerland, particularly by Dr. F. Leuenberger and P. Schuler of the Vitamin and Fine Chemicals Division.

References

1 Spunger, J, Matthews, R H: Nutrient content of pasta products. Cereal Foods Wld 27, 558-561, 1982.

2 Milatovic, L: La vitamina C nella tecnologia dei cereali. Chiriotti, Pinerolo, 1967.

3 Walsh, D E et al: Inhibition of durum wheat lipoxidase with L-ascorbic acid. Cereal Chem 47, 119-125, 1970.

4 Grant, R D: Studies of the role of ascorbic acid in chemical dough development. I. Reaction of ascorbic acid with flour-water suspensions. Cereal Chem 51, 684-692, 1974.

5 Grant, R D, Sood, K V: Note on the antioxidant effect of ascorbic acid on flour free fatty acids. Cereal Chem 57, 231-232, 1980.

6 Elkassabany, M et al: Ascorbic acid as an oxidant in wheat flour dough. II. Rheological effects. Cereal Chem 57, 85-87, 1980

7 Milatovic, L, Martinek, M: Kemija u ind (Zagreb) 16, 461, 1967.

8 Nicolas, J: Effets de différents paramètres sur la destruction des pigments caroténoides de la farine de blé tendre au cours du pétrissage. Ann Technol Agric 27, 695-713, 1977.

9 Schuler, P: Ascorbic acid as a flour improver. Technical Information, Hoffmann-La Roche, Basel, 1982.

10 Goodwin, W T, Mercer, I E: Introduction to plant biochemistry, pp 198-199. Pergamon Press, Oxford, 1972.

11 Stepchkov, K A et al: USSR Patent No 275000 (1970).

12 Globe, F E et al: US Patent No 50-18058 (1970).

13 Glicksman, M: Utilization of natural polysaccharide gums in the food industry. Adv Food Res 11, 109-200, 1962.

14 Ukiti, M: Japanese Patent No 50-18058 (1975).

15 Nazarov, I N: Technologia makaronik izdellii. Pishc prom Mosca, pp 61-62, 1978.

16 Dexter, J E et al: High temperature drying: effect on spaghetti properties. Food Sci 46, 1741-1746, 1981.

17 Milatovic, L: The technology of pasta products. Unpublished lecture. Faculty of Agriculture, University of Belgrade-Zemun, 1981/1982.

18 Sollberger, H: Bühler Diagram No 53. Uzwil, 1972.

19 Matsuo, R R, Irvine, G N: Rheology of durum wheat products. Cereal Chem 52, 131r-135r, 1975.

20 Roche Technical Bulletin, Hoffmann-La Roche Basel, 1982.

21 Pavan, G: High temperature drying process and pasta quality. Report of Officine Meccaniche Pavan, Galliera, 1979.

22 Schuler, P: Private communication.
23 Pongracz, G: Neue potentiometrische Bestimmungsmethode für Ascorbinsäure und deren Verbindungen. Z Anal Chem *253,* 271–274, 1971.
24 Research laboratory methods of SOUR-MLINPRED. Factory for macaroni production Danubius, Novi Sad, 1983.
25 Alary, R *et al:* Tecnica molitoria: 776–783, 1980.
26 Menger, A: Tecnica molitoria: 23–32, 1982.
27 Johnston, R A *et al:* Note on comparison of pigment extraction and reflectance colorimeter methods for evaluating semolina color. Cereal Chem *57,* 447–448, 1980.
28 AACC Method 14–21, pp 1–2, 1961.
29 Dexter, J E *et al:* Grain research laboratory. Compression tester: instrumental measurement of cooked spaghetti stickiness. Cereal Chem *60,* 139–142, 1983.
30 Manser, J: Optimale Parameter für die Teigwarenherstellung am Beispiel von Langwaren. Getreide Mehl Brot *35,* 75–83, 1981.
31 Dexter, J E *et al:* High temperature drying: effect on spaghetti properties. Food Sci *46,* 1741–1746, 1981.
32 Tsen, C C: The improving mechanism of ascorbic acid. Cereal Chem *42,* 86–97, 1965.
33 Maltha, P R A: Über den Einfluss von L-Ascorbinsäure und Verbindungen mit verwandter Struktur auf die Backfähigkeit des Mehles. Getreide Mehl *3,* 65–69, 1953.
34 Mair, G, Grosch, W: Changes in glutathione content (reduced and oxidised form) and the effect of ascorbic acid and potassium bromate on glutathione oxidation during dough mixing. J Sci Food Agric *30,* 914–920, 1979.

Prof. Dr. Ljubomir Milatovic, Barutanski Jarak 5, Pancićeva, 41000 Zagreb, Yugoslavia

Vitamin C – A Modulator of Host Defense Mechanism

An Overview

K. Schmidt and U. Moser

Department of Surgery, University of Tübingen, Tübingen, West-Germany, and Department of Vitamin and Nutrition Research, F. Hoffmann-La Roche & Co Ltd, Basle, Switzerland

Key Words: Vitamin C/Ascorbic acid · Content in phagocytes · Transport into phagocytes · Inhibition of transport · Stimulation of transport · Immunomodulation by ascorbic acid

Abstract: The ascorbic acid content in plasma and leucocytes is decreased under different conditions such as various diseases and marginal nutrition. It is well known that ascorbate stimulates chemotactic migration and a positive effect on phagocytosis is observed. The uptake of ascorbate in human granulocytes is mediated by an active transport mechanism which is dependent on the concentration of the substrate in the incubation medium and on temperature, the maximum being at 40 °C. Glucose is a strong and specific inhibitor of the uptake with a K_i of 3.7 mM. The similarity between the inhibition of the transport of glucose and of ascorbate by phlorizin gives rise to the assumption that there may be a common transport mechanism. Chemotactically active peptides such as N-formyl-L-methionyl-L-leucyl-L-phenylalanine stimulate the uptake of ascorbate whereas the chemotactically inactive L-methionyl-L-leucyl-L-phenylalanine remains without effect. Vitamin C may therefore act as a modulator of host defense mechanisms. Some possible interactions with the metabolism of neutrophils are discussed.

Introduction

A disturbance of homeostasis in living tissues is followed by activation of host defense reactions. These activation processes involve cellular and humoral mechanisms resulting in an acute inflammatory response. In the first line of the non specific inflammatory response polymorphonuclear leucocytes (PML) and macrophages undergo functional stimulation. In an ordered sequence of cellular events adherence, degranulation, diapedesis, chemotaxis and phagocytosis occur. Although the molecular mechanisms underlying the inflammatory response are not completely understood a few reactions have been established as being important components. Among those are ligand receptor interactions, changes in membrane transport, oxidative and hydrolytic processes, membrane fusion, changes in metabolic pathways such as the hexose monophosphate shunt, and second messenger concentration. Sophisticated mechanisms are required in order to protect host tissues during the inflammatory response against endogenous oxidative and hydrolytic agents.

Vitamin C as a biological redox reagent interferes with the oxidative processes during the inflammatory response thereby modulating specific cellular functions such as chemotaxis, degranulation etc. Furthermore it is well established that ascorbate levels are decreased in human granulocytes in various diseases associated with an impaired host defense as well as under marginal nutrition. The present paper describes various aspects of the content and transport of ascorbate in phagocytic cells in relation to chemotactic and phagocytic stimulation. In addition the significance of ascorbate in selected clinical disorders with impaired host defense is discussed.

Part of these data have been reported elsewhere [1, 2].

Method

Human blood was obtained by venipuncture from male and female volunteers. White blood cells were isolated from human blood according to the method described by BÖYUM [3] using metrizoate and polymorphonuclear granulocytes from this crude cell fraction on a Percoll gradient as described in detail by HJORTH et al [4]. Rat peritoneal macrophages were obtained by suction of the intraperitoneal fluid 5 days after i.p. injection of 0.5 ml mineral oil and purified by a two step Percoll/sucrose density gradient. Pure alveolar macrophages were obtained by repeated lavage of the lung of adult rats as described by TRUSH et al [5].

The procedure for the experiments with $(1-^{14}C)$ascorbic acid was as follows: 10 ml blood were mixed with 10 ml of an isotonic buffer, pH 7.4, containing 5.4 mM KCl, 0,8 mM $MgSO_4$, 0.8 mM NaH_2PO_4, 25 mM $NaHCO_3$, 5.5 mM glucose, 0.1 mM citric acid, 120 mM NaCl, plus 2 % dextran in order to separate the erythrocytes. Thrombocytes and lymphocytes were separated using Percoll (d = 1.076) and the remaining erythrocytes were removed by hypotonic lysis. The granulocytes were washed 3 times and finally resuspended in the buffer mentioned above which in addition contained 1.3 mM $CaCl_2$ and 4 % bovine serum albumin. 5 x 10^6 cells were incubated in a total volume of 1.0 ml in a shaking water bath for 45 minutes at 37° with 2 x 10^5 - 5 x 10^5 dpm $(1-^{14}C)$ascorbic acid, stopped on ice and washed. (^{14}C)activity was counted in INSTA-GEL after disruption of the cells in 1 N NaOH.

Ascorbic acid has been determined using the method of ZANNONI et al [6], partly with modifications according to OKAMURA [7] and to BEUTLER and BEINSTINGL [8].

Results and Discussion

Ascorbate content of unstimulated phagocytes

According to the different determination methods for ascorbic acid a wide variety of normal values of intracellular ascorbate concentration can be extracted from the literature. The mean values of ascorbate measured in peripheral blood granulocytes from healthy subjects are in the range of 10 to 40 $\mu g/10^8$ cells as determined by 6 different authors (Table I). In addition attention has to be paid to artifacts due to the methods used for isolation of the cells [9]. Macrophages for example can easily be stimulated during the purification process and in experiments with granulocytes the purity of the cell population is often not assessed [10]. The principal methodological difficulties of intracellular ascorbate measurement are discussed in detail elsewhere [11].

Tab I: Ascorbic acid content in PML

Source	Ascorbate content, $\mu g/10^8$	Citation
30 children (6 months–14 years)	25.4 ± 4.6	Bingöl et al [52]
18 men	9.9 ± 2.5	Attwood *et al* [53]
20 men	9.3 ± 3.0	Evans *et al* [24]
21 women	9.5 ± 2.1	Evans *et al* [24]
26 women	13.9 ± 5.1	Attwood *et al* [53]
31 women	39.0 ± 28.0	Briggs and Briggs [54]
25 persons	35.0 (21–53)	Denson and Bowers [55]
50 elderly persons	13.4 (2–36)	Denson and Bowers [55]
14 persons	20.5 ± 8.4	Schmidt and Moser this publication
7 women	7.8 ± 1.9	Schmidt and Moser this publication
6 men	8.2 ± 1.4	Schmidt and Moser this publication

Similar variations have been found in granulocytes from a single blood sample by only using two different isolation procedures and two different determination methods for intracellular ascorbate concentration (Table II). Table III shows ascorbate concentrations in alveolar as well as peritoneal macrophages. The 4.5-fold higher values of the latter may be explained by interference with the mineral oil used for collection of the cells in the peritoneal cavity. Besides these discrepancies the findings demonstrate that the ratio of the intra- to extracellular concentrations of ascorbate is larger than 10. Hence, granulocytes as well as macrophages have to maintain an ascorbate gradient across the membrane.

Transport of ascorbic acid into unstimulated PML

Ascorbic acid is accumulated in several tissues by an active transport mechanism as it is shown by an extensive pharmacokinetic study of

Tab II: Methodical effects on the apparent ascorbic acid content in PML

Isolation	Assay	Ascorbic acid found, $\mu g/10^8$
Pure granulocytes	α,α'-bipyridyl	9.5
(dextran/Percoll)	DNPH	9.5
Buffy layer	α,α'-bipyridyl	22.6
(methylcellulose)	DNPH	34.2

Tab III: Ascorbic acid content in macrophages

Source		Ascorbate content, $\mu g/10^8$	Citation
14	rabbits (alveolar)	54.7 (38.0–82.1)	De Chatelet et al [56]
6	rats (alveolar)	42.4 ± 13.5	Castranova et al [57]
5	rats (peritoneal)	183 ± 65	Schmidt and Moser this publication

(1–^{14}C)ascorbic acid in guinea pigs [12]. It is not the topic of this paper to review the literature concerning ascorbate transport but some relevant references shall be given below.

Most endocrine glands accumulate ascorbic acid like the adrenals [13–15], which also secrete the newly taken up ascorbic acid after stimulation [16,17]. Organs like brain [18], placenta [19], kidney [20], lung [21] have an active transport mechanism as well as leucocytes [22].

(1–^{14}C)ascorbic acid is accumulated in isolated human PML as a function of the concentration of ascorbic acid in the incubation medium. Assuming a volume of 320 fl per cell, the concentration of ascorbic acid can be calculated to be 10–15 times higher inside the cells than in the medium if the addition does not exceed the physiological range. At concentrations over 1 mM, the ratio ascorbic acid inside/outside reaches the value 1 (Fig. 1). The calculation is only based on the uptake of labelled ascorbic acid during the incubation period; therefore, the concentration inside the cell is rather underestimated. All of the (1–^{14}C)ascorbic acid can be found in the reduced form inside the cell as it is shown by thin-layer-chromatography (Fig. 2).

Incubating the cells in presence of 0.26 mM ascorbate shows that the uptake is completely suppressed at 4°C. The slight decrease of the rate of uptake at 37° and 40°C is probably due to the decrease of the ascorbate concentration since ascorbic acid is unstable in aqueous solutions [23] (Fig. 3). The uptake is fastest in the temperature range of 37–40°C; beyond this temperature cells

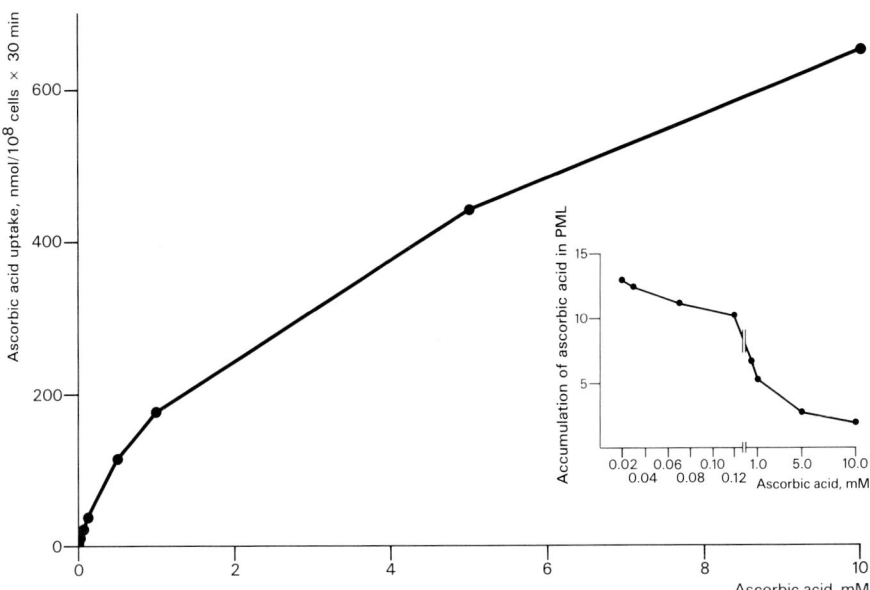

Fig. 1: Variation of ascorbic acid uptake with substrate concentration. The accumulation (inset) is calculated from $(1-^{14}C)AA$ found in the cells assuming a volume of $32\mu l/10^8$ cells. The ratio AA «in» (mM) / AA «out» versus AA «out» is plotted.

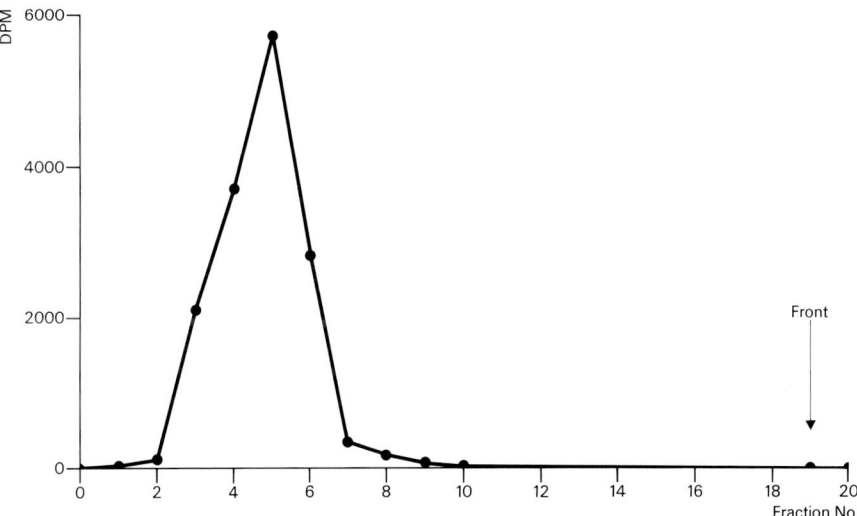

Fig. 2: TL chromatogram of $(1-^{14}C)$ascorbic acid. Granulocytes are incubated for 45 min as described under 'method'. Cells are washed and disrupted by sonification. Cold AA is added to avoid degradation of the active AA and a sample applied on a silica gel plate. Solvent: chloroform: methanol: H_2O: acetic acid 65 : 50 : 15 : 1 (by volume).

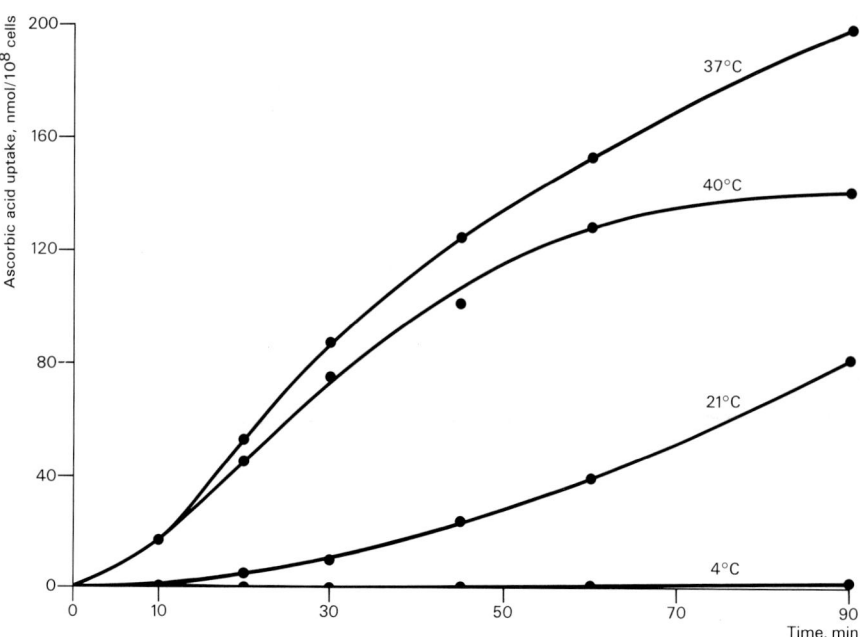

Fig. 3: Uptake of ascorbic acid with respect of time. 6 x 10^6 granulocytes are incubated with 0.26 mM (1-^{14}C)AA at different temperatures. No activity can be found in the cells at 4°C. During the incubation, AA is rapidly degraded in the medium. So far, a saturation could not be achieved.

start to leak (Fig. 4). From the Arrhenius plot (Fig. 4, inset) an activation energy of the transport of 25.0 kcal/M can be estimated.

These results confirm earlier observations by Evans *et al* [24] about an active transport mechanism for ascorbic acid in PML. Passive diffusion becomes apparent only above physiological concentrations in the medium.

Evans *et al* [24] as well as Loh and Wilson [25] found a positive correlation between plasma ascorbic acid and ascorbic acid content in PML, the slope of the linear regression analysis being 0.0039 ± 0.0009 1/10^9. From Figure 1 regarding the range between 0.018 and 0.12 mM ascorbate, a linear correlation between uptake and concentration of ascorbic acid in the medium with a slope of 0.0032 1/10^9 is obtained. This implies an identical dependence of the ascorbate content in PML on the outside concentration under either *in vivo* or *in vitro* conditions.

Ascorbate content of stimulated phagocytes

Evidence on the immunostimulatory effects of ascorbate has been successively accumulated during the last couple of years. Enhanced random

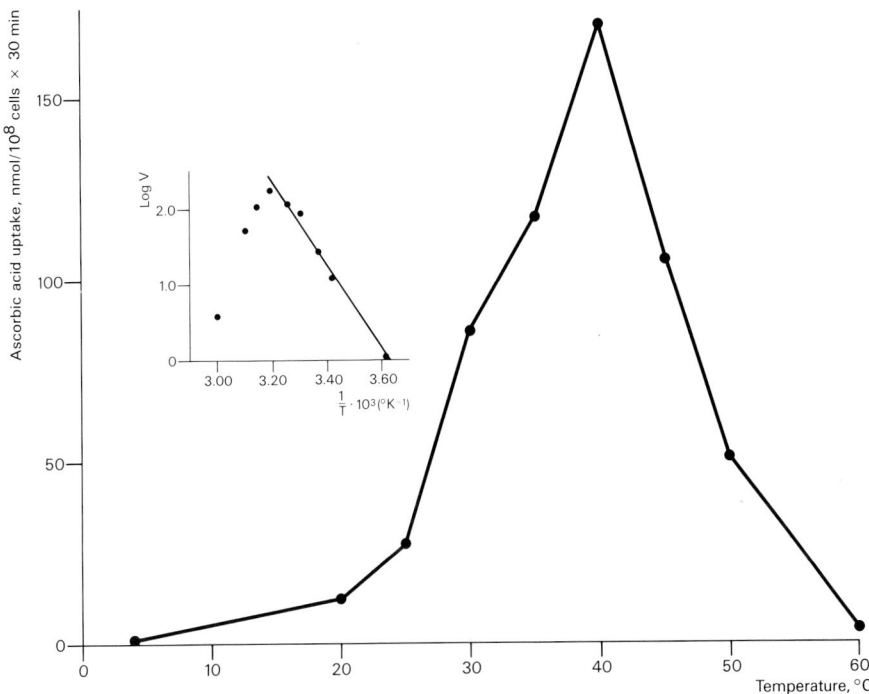

Fig. 4: The uptake of ascorbic acid as a function of temperature. 5 x 10⁶ granulocytes are incubated with 0.29 mM (1–¹⁴C)AA at the different temperatures indicated. The cells start to leak at temperatures over 40°C and are completely destroyed at 60°C. The activation energy can be estimated from the Arrhenius plot (inset) to be 25.0 kcal/mol.

migration and chemotactic response of human granulocytes by ascorbate was reported by Goetzl *et al* [26]. Similar findings were published by Anderson [27], Dallegri *et al* [28], and Sandler *et al* [29]. Greendyke *et al* [30] reported enhanced phagocytic activity of human neutrophils in the presence of ascorbate in vitro. There is, however, a considerable controversy regarding the significance of extra- versus intracellular ascorbate levels in host defense reactions. On the other hand, the available data on intracellular ascorbate concentrations of stimulated phagocytes are very limited. We have therefore re-examined in the present study the effects of functional stimulation of polymorphonuclear neutrophils from human peripheral blood as well as of peritoneal and alveolar macrophages of the rat on intracellular ascorbate levels. For phagocytic stimulation in vitro two different experimental systems, opsonized zymosan and 12-O-tetradecanoylphorbol-13-acetate were used.

Tab IV: Intracellular ascorbate concentrations of phagocytes before and after stimulation by zymosan or PMA ($\mu g/10^8$cells)

Cell population	Unstimulated	Stimulated (zymosan)	Stimulated (PMA)
White blood cells	33 ± 14 [18]	29 ± 19 [5]	
Polymorphonuclear blood cells	22 ± 8 [34]	23 ± 6 [7]	
Mononuclear blood cells	53 ± 15 [8]	44 ± 15 [7]	
Peritoneal macrophages	183 ± 65 [5]	105 ± 53 [5]	
Alveolar macrophages	167 ± 54 [10]	94 ± 10 [5]	106 ± 27 [5]

The effect of phagocytic stimulation of the different cell populations on the intracellular ascorbate levels is given in Table IV. It is evident that only macrophages loose half their ascorbate content into the medium during stimulation by zymosan or phorbolmyristate acetate (PMA). It has to be emphasized that the incubation medium does not contain ascorbic acid; therefore only an outflow can be recognized, but not a possible increase of the uptake. White blood cells (polymorphonuclear as well as mononuclear) seem to conserve the ascorbate inside the cells by restricting the transport through the cell wall in the direction of uptake.

Transport of ascorbic acid into stimulated PML

Phagocytic cells such as PML and macrophages migrate toward attractants like bacteria after chemotactic stimulation. A large number of di- and tripeptides containing formylmethionine which resemble bacterial chemotactic factors [31] have been synthesized [32,33]. Their ability to induce chemotactic activity correlates with the release of lysosomal enzymes, whereas the unformylated peptides are ineffective regarding both activities [33]. Specific receptor sites for N-formylmethionyl peptides have been identified on human PML [34]. The number of binding sites is approximately 2000 which is in the same range as the number of receptors per cell for several hormones.

PML exposed to formylmethionyl peptides increase the uptake of ascorbate up to 2.5 fold compared to the unstimulated control (Fig. 5). f-Met-Leu-Tyr, f-Met-Leu-Phe (FMLP) and f-Met-Phe are the most effective, f-Met-Val and f-Met-Try stimulate to a lesser extent whereas Met-Leu-Phe is inactive.

The functional importance of the striking parallelism between chemotactic activation and ascorbate uptake remains to be elucidated.

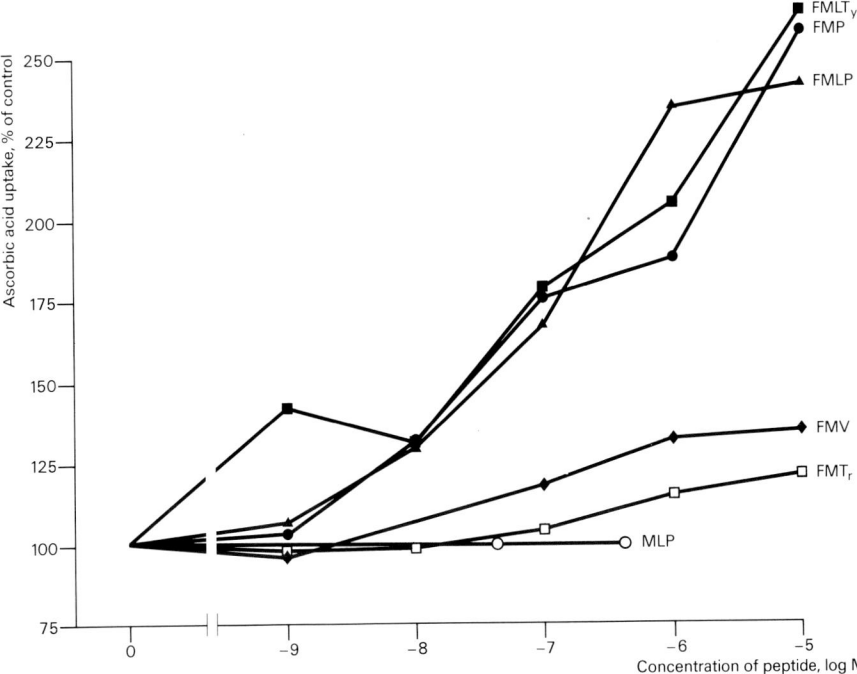

Fig. 5: Effect of chemotactic peptides on ascorbate uptake. Granulocytes are incubated as described under method except that the concentration of bovine serum albumin is 0.5 %. This concentration is just sufficient in order to avoid cell clumping and does not inhibit the action of the peptides. FMLTy = N-Formyl-methionyl-leucyl-tyrosine. FMP = N-Formyl-methionyl-phenylalanine. FMLP = N-Formyl-methionyl-leucyl-phenylalanine. FMV = N-Formyl-methionyl-valine. FMTr = N-Formyl-methionyl-tryptophan. MLP = Methionyl-leucyl-phenylalanine.

Inhibition of the ascorbate uptake

2-Deoxyglucose and 3-O-methylglucose competitively inhibit dehydroascorbate uptake. The K_m for DHA uptake is in the range of 2.4–3.2 mM and the K_i of the inhibition by the glucose analogues between 2.9 and 3.2 mM. The authors conclude that DHA transport is mediated by glucose transport systems [35].

Incubation of isolated PML in presence of $(1-^{14}C)$ascorbate with increasing amounts of glucose leads to a similar inhibition of the ascorbate uptake (Fig. 6). From the Hill plot a K_i of 3.7 mM can be calculated and the slope of 0.9 indicates the stoichiometry of ascorbate/glucose binding to be 1.

Phlorizin, a potent inhibitor of glucose transport in small intestinal brush border membrane and renal cortex vesicles [36] inhibits ascorbate as well as

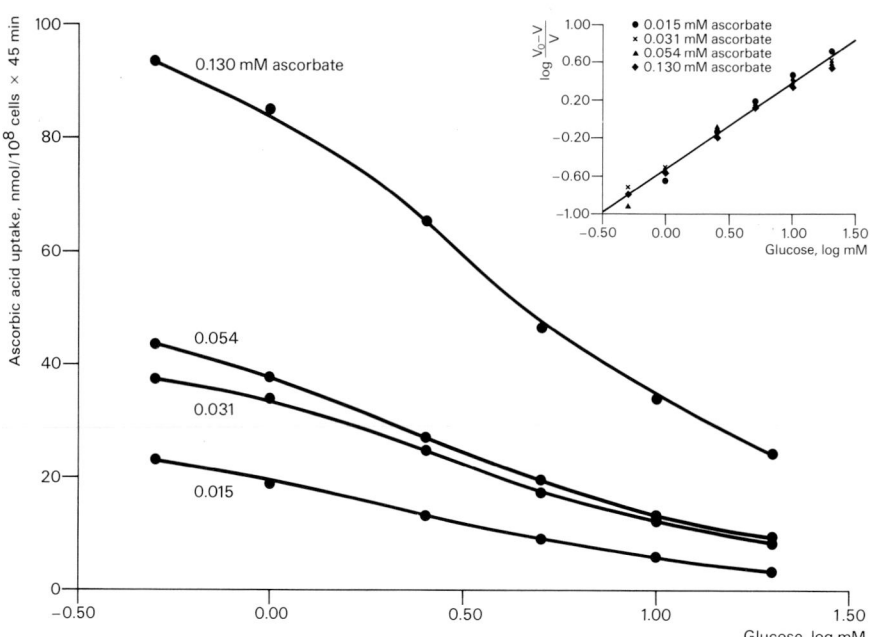

Fig. 6: Inhibition of the ascorbic acid uptake in granulocytes by glucose. 3–6 x 10^6 granulocytes are incubated with 0.015 mM, 0.031 mM, 0.054 mM or 0.13 mM (1–^{14}C)ascorbic acid plus 0–20 mM glucose. From the Hill plot (inset) the K_i = 3.7 mM and the slope = 0.91 can be estimated.

glucose uptake in PML (Fig. 7). Again, this suggests a similar transport mechanism for both substrates. Phlorizin (10 mM) not only inhibits the unstimulated but also the FMLP-stimulated ascorbate uptake by the same extent, the figures being 61.4 % and 64.4 %, respectively. Whereas SH-reagents like cysteine and DTT are without effect, 1.0 mM KCN blocks the uptake by about 70 % (Fig. 8) which means that the process requires energy. Furthermore, the inhibition by glucose seems to be specific since neither fructose nor galactose interfere with ascorbate uptake (Table V).

Tab. V: Inhibition of the ascorbic acid uptake in granulocytes by hexoses

Addition, mM	Ascorbic acid uptake, nmol/10^8 cells × 45 min		
	glucose	galactose	fructose
0	104.9	104.9	104.9
2.5	61.9	101.5	104.1
5.0	45.2	92.2	107.9
10.0	31.9	83.3	109.6

5.2 × 10^6 cells are incubated as described under Method with 0.05 mM (1–^{14}C) ascorbic acid (460 000 dpm).

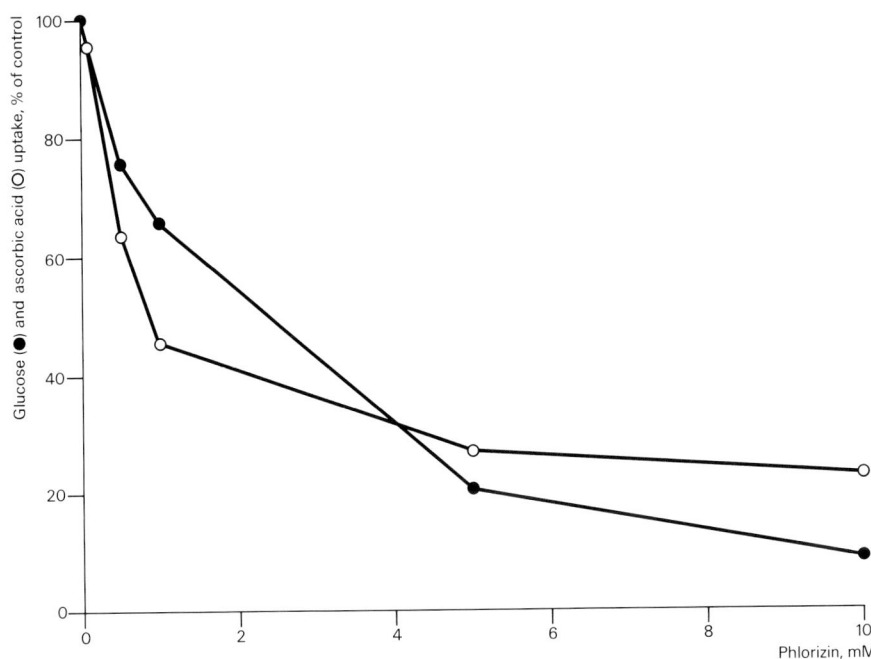

Fig. 7: Inhibition of the ascorbic acid uptake by phlorizin. 4.9 x 10^6 cells are incubated either with 0.02 mM (1–^{14}C)AA or with 0.02 mM U–^{14}C-glucose. 100% of the glucose uptake is 4263 dpm/10^8 cells x 45 min and of the AA uptake 18533 dpm/10^8 cells x 45 min.

In order to distinguish whether only the uptake of ascorbate is affected by glucose or also its release, PML are loaded with (1–^{14}C) ascorbate for 45 min. After removal of the extracellular ascorbate, the PML are reincubated in presence of different amounts of glucose. Only about 4% of the total activity inside the cells are released during the 45 min of incubation which is considered to be within the experimental error (Fig. 9). Hence glucose does not provoke a release of ascorbate out of the cells. Ascorbate seems to be kept very firmly inside the cells since up to now a release could not be observed under any circumstances *in vitro*.

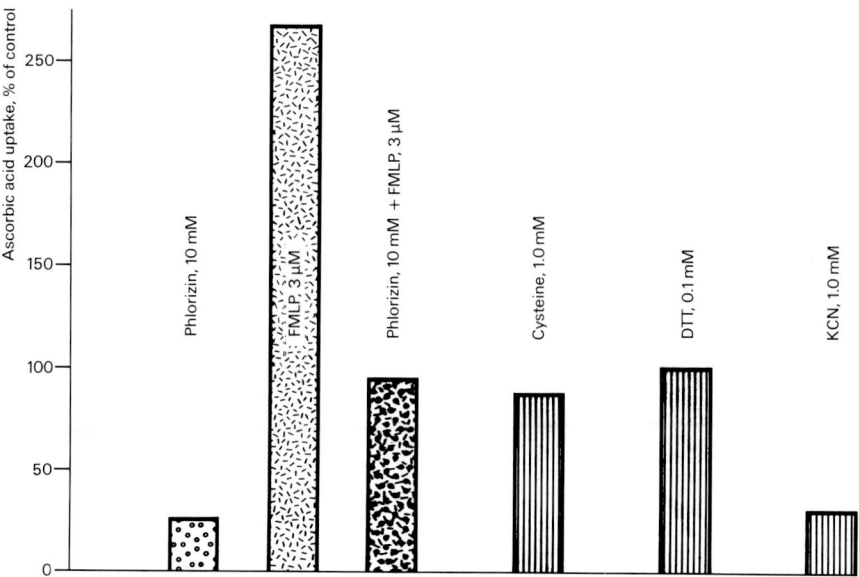

Fig. 8: Effect of formyl-methionyl-leucyl-phenylalanine (FMLP), cysteine, dithiothreitol (DTT) and KCN on the uptake of ascorbic acid. $5.1–6.2 \times 10^6$ cells are incubated as described under Method. 0.5 g/100 ml albumin is added in experiments with FMLP (bars 1-3) and 0.11 mM $(1-^{14}C)$ AA is present in all experiments. FMLP and phlorizin are dissolved in DMSO which has no effect on the AA uptake. The control rates (100 %) are as follows: Bars 1-3 = 25.9 nmol/10^8 cells $\times$ 45 min. Bars 4-5 = 90.4 nmol/10^8 cells $\times$ 45 min. Bar 6 = 82.9 nmol/10^8 cells $\times$ 45 min. 10 mM phlorizin inhibits the uptake by 61.4 % and the FMLP-stimulated uptake by 64.4 %.

Conclusion

Polymorphonuclear leucocytes accumulate ascorbic acid in order to maintain a concentration inside the cell which exceeds by far the plasma concentration.

However, a clear correlation between ascorbate content and functional behaviour of neutrophils could only be found in chronic granulomatous disease (CGD) and Chediak-Higashi syndrome. Anderson [37] treated three children with CGD by adding a daily dose of 1 g ascorbate to the standard regimen. In all patients there was an improvement in neutrophil motility as well as a slight increase in the hexose monophosphate shunt which is in agreement with an investigation by De Chatelet et al [38].

Impaired PML motility of an 11-month-old child due to Chediak-Higashi syndrome could be restored with 200 mg ascorbate daily. The improved chemotactic activity was associated with an increased antimicrobial activity

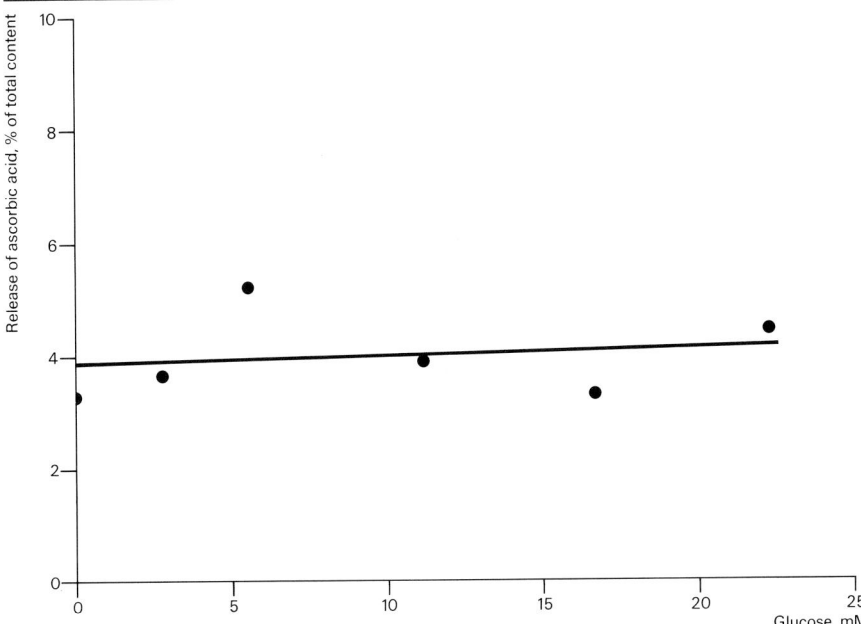

Fig. 9: Effect of glucose on the release of ascorbic acid. 5×10^6 granulocytes are incubated with 0.12 mM (1–^{14}C) AA for 45 min. The accumulated 87.1 nmol/10^8 cells represent 100 % total content. The cells are reincubated without AA for additional 45 min in presence of glucose and the remaining AA measured in the cells.

[39]. Several population groups are described in the literature with a significantly decreased ascorbic acid level in the plasma and hence also in leucocytes. These include chronic hemodialysis patients [40–42], psychogeriatric patients [43], institutionalized patients [44], elderly persons [44], etc. Whether the diminished ascorbate content is important for a general risk of impaired neutrophil function is not clear; many other factors may be involved as well. Since ascorbate seems to utilize the same transport system as glucose, diabetic persons might need more ascorbic acid in order to maintain an adequate level in the cells.

The fact that chemotactic peptides stimulate the uptake of ascorbic acid strengthens the speculation that ascorbate is acting as a modulator of immune functions. Redox reactions are very important not only during the respiratory burst but also in activating and desactivating PML collagenase by disulfide/thiol interchange [45]. The regulation of the activity of these proteases, which include also elastase and cathepsin-G, determines whether inflammation will damage connective tissue. α_1-Proteinase inhibition can be inactivated by oxidation of methionine residues in or near the active site [58].

Furthermore, ascorbic acid increases cyclic GMP in human monocytes, but not in PML [29]. Since chemotaxis is stimulated in both cell types the question arises whether the changes in cyclic GMP were too small to be detectable or, alternatively, ascorbate may be acting through other second messengers.

Microtubules have been implicated in phagocyte chemotactic responses. There is experimental evidence suggesting a functional link between chemotactic activation as well as degranulation of phagocytes and post-translational fixation of tyrosine into the alpha-chain of tubulin catalyzed by tubulin tyrosine ligase [46,47]. Tubulin tyrosinolation is abnormally increased in patients with Chediak-Higashi syndrome which can be related to the increased oxidative metabolism in these cells. Ascorbate, like other reducing agents such as GSH, cysteine, or DTT, restores the activity to a normal level [48]. Moreover ascorbate has been shown to promote microtubule assembly [49].

Another issue related to ascorbate as a modulator of immune functions stems from the fact that it may act as a coupling factor between peripheral blood or tissue phagocytic stimulation and granulocyte differentiation and maturation in the bone marrow. Functional stimulation of phagocytes increases the production of metabolites of ascorbic acid in the extracellular space. Dehydroascorbate is taken up by granulocyte progenitor cells in the bone marrow thereby activating a dehydroascorbate reductase (EC 1.8.5.1) [50]. This process is parallelled by differentiation of granulocyte progenitors to mature granulocytes [51]. At the moment, it is not clear whether this effect is a consequence of an interaction with prostaglandin E_2-mediated inhibition of granulocyte maturation or of a stimulated cytoskeletal rearrangement by ascorbate (Fig. 10).

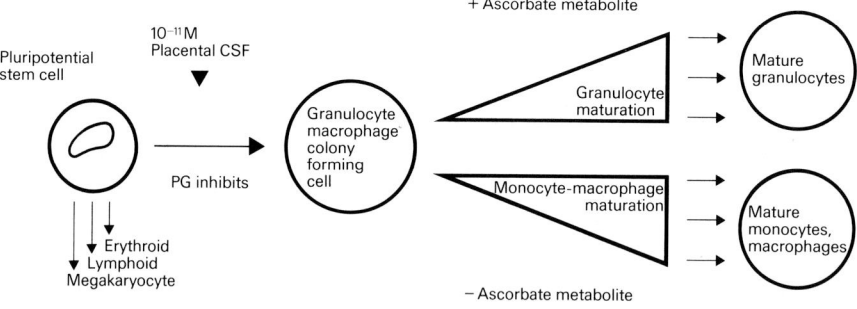

Fig. 10: Possible involvement of ascorbic acid in cell differentiation. CFS = Cell stimulating factor. PG = Prostaglandin.

References

1   Moser, U, Weber, F: Uptake of ascorbic acid by human granulocytes. 15th FEBS Meeting, Brussels, Symposium S-03, abstract 35, 1983.

2   Moser, U, Weber, F: Uptake of ascorbic acid by human granulocytes. Int J Vit Nutr Res 54, 47–53, 1984.

3   Böyum, A: Isolation of mononuclear cells and granulocytes from human blood. Scand J Clin Lab Invest 21, suppl 97, pp 77–89, 1968.

4   Hjorth, R et al: A rapid method for purification of human granulocytes using percoll. A comparison with dextran sedimentation. J Immunol Methods 43, 95–101, 1981.

5   Trush, MA et al: The generation of chemiluminescence by phagocytic cells. In: De Luca (ed) "Methods in enzymology", vol 57, pp 462–494. Academic Press, New York, 1978.

6   Zannoni, V et al: A rapid micromethod for the determination of ascorbic acid in plasma and tissue. Biochem Med 11, 41–48, 1974.

7   Okamura, M: An improved method for determination of L-ascorbic acid and L-dehydroascorbic acid in blood plasma. Clin Chim Acta 103, 259–268, 1980.

8   Beutler, HO, Beinstingl, G: Bestimmung von L-Ascorbinsäure in Lebensmitteln. Dtsch Lebensm-Rdsch 76, 69–75, 1980.

9   Evans, RM et al: Effect of platelets on apparent leucocyte ascorbic acid content. Ann Clin Biochem 17, 252–255, 1980.

10 Adams, DO: Macrophages. In: Jakoby and Pastan (eds) "Methods in enzymology", vol. 58, pp 494–506. Academic Press, New York, 1979.

11 Cooke, JR, Moxon, RED: The detection and measurement of vitamin C. In: Counsell, JN, Hornig, DH (eds) "Vitamin C (ascorbic acid)", pp 167–198. Applied Science, London, 1981.

12 Hornig, D, Hartmann, D: Kinetic behaviour of ascorbic acid in guinea pigs. In: Seib and Tolbert (eds) "Ascorbic acid: chemistry, metabolism, and uses", pp 293–316. Advances in Chemistry Series No 200. American Chemical Society, Washington, 1982.

13 Clayman, M et al: Specificity of action of adrenocorticotrophin in vitro on ascorbate transport in rat adrenal glands. Biochem J 118, 283–289, 1970.

14 de Nicola, AF et al: Hormonal control of ascorbic acid in rat adrenal glands. Endocrinology 82, 436–446, 1968.

15 de Nicola, AF et al: In vitro uptake of ascorbic acid 1–^{14}C by adrenal glands of different species. Gen Comp Endocrinology 11, 332–337, 1968.

16 Finn, FM, Johns, PA: Ascorbic acid transport by isolated bovine adrenal cortical cells. Endocrinology 106, 811–817, 1980.

17 Daniels, AJ et al: Secretion of newly taken-up ascorbic acid by adrenomedullary chromaffin cells. Science 216, 737–739, 1982.

18 Sharma, SK et al: Active transport of ascorbic acid in adrenal cortex and brain cortex in vitro and the effects of ACTH and steroids. Can J Biochem Physiol 41, 597–604, 1963.

19 Streeter, ML, Rosso, P: Transport mechanism for ascorbic acid in the human placenta. Am J Clin Nutr 34, 1706–1711, 1981.

20 Toggenburger, G et al: Na$^+$-dependent, potential-sensitive L-ascorbate transport across brush border membrane vesicles from kidney cortex. Biochim Biophys Acta 646, 433–443, 1981.

21 Wright, JR et al: Ascorbate uptake by isolated rat lung cells. J Appl Physiol 51, 1477–1483, 1981.

22 Bigley, R, Stankova, L: Uptake of oxidized and reduced ascorbate by human leucocytes. J Exp Med 139, 1084–1092, 1974.

23 Hornig, DH, Moser, U: The safety of high vitamin C intakes in man. In: Counsell and Hornig (eds) "Vitamin C (ascorbic acid)", pp 225–248. Applied Science, London, 1981.

24 Evans, RM et al: The distribution of ascorbic acid between various cellular components of blood, in normal individuals, and its relation to the plasma concentration. Br J Nutr 47, 473–482, 1982.

25 Loh, HS, Wilson, CWM: Relationship between leucocyte and plasma ascorbic acid concentrations. Br Med J 3, 733–735, 1971.

26 Goetzl, EJ et al: Enhancement of random migration and chemotactic response of human leucocytes by ascorbic acid. J Clin Invest 53, 813–818, 1974.

27 Anderson, R: Ascorbic acid and immune functions: mechanism of immunostimulation. In: Counsell and Hornig (eds) "Vitamin C (ascorbic acid)", pp 249–272. Applied Science, London 1981.

28 Dallegri, F et al: Effects of ascorbic acid on neutrophil locomotion. Int Archs Allergy Appl Immun 61, 40–45, 1980.

29 Sandler, JA et al: Effects of serotonin, carbamylcholine, and ascorbic acid on leukocyte cyclic GMP and chemotaxis. J Cell Biol 67, 480–484, 1975.

30 Greendyke, RM et al: In vitro studies on erythrophagocytosis. II. Effects of incubating leukocytes with selected cell metabolites. J Lab Clin Med 63, 1016–1026, 1964.

31 Schiffmann, E et al: The isolation, and partial characterization of neutrophil chemotactic factors from Escherichia coli. J Immunol 114, 1831–1837, 1975.

32 Schiffmann, E et al: N-formylmethionyl peptides as chemoattractants for leucocytes. Proc Natl Acad Sci USA 72, 1059–1062, 1975.

33 Showell, HJ et al: The structure-activity relations of synthetic peptides as chemotactic factors and inducers of lysosomal enzyme secretion for neutrophils. J Exp Med 143, 1154–1169, 1976.

34 Williams, LT et al: Specific receptor sites for chemotactic peptides on human polymorphonuclear leucocytes. Proc Natl Acad Sci USA 74, 1204–1208, 1977.

35 Bigley, R et al: Interaction between glucose and dehydroascorbate transport in human neutrophils and fibroblasts. Diabetes 32, 545–548, 1983.

36 Toggenburger, G et al: Phlorizin as a probe of the small-intestinal Na^+, D-glucose cotransporter. A model. Biochim Biophys Acta 688, 557–571, 1982.

37 Anderson R: Assessment of oral ascorbate in three children with chronic granulomatous disease and defective neutrophil motility over a 2-year period. Clin Exp Immunol 43, 180–188, 1981.

38 De Chatelet, LR et al: Stimulation of the hexose monophosphate shunt in human neutrophils by ascorbic acid: mechanism of action. Antimicrob Agents Chemother 1, 12–16, 1972.

39 Boxer, LA et al: Correction of leucocyte function in Chediak-Higashi syndrome by ascorbate. New Engl J Med 295, 1041–1045, 1976.

40 Sullivan, JF, Eisenstein, AB: Ascorbic acid depletion in patients undergoing chronic hemodialysis. Am J Clin Nutr 23, 1339–1346, 1970.

41 Sullivan, JF, Eisenstein, AB: Ascorbic acid depletion during hemodialysis. J Am Med Ass 222, 1697–1699, 1972.

42 Pönkä, A, Kuhlbäck, B: Serum ascorbic acid in patients undergoing chronic hemodialysis. Acta Med Scand 213, 305–307, 1983.

43 Hontely, S et al: Serum level of vitamins A, C, E, folate, and iron in female psychogeriatric patients in comparison with their controls. Nutr Rep Int 27, 1101–1111, 1983.

44 Schorah, CJ: Vitamin C status in population groups. In: Counsell and Hornig (eds) "Vitamin C (ascorbic acid)", pp 23–47. Applied Science, London, 1981.

45 Macartney, HW, Tschesche, H: Characterisation of β_1-anticollagenase from human plasma and its reaction with polymorphonuclear leucocyte collagenase by disulfide/thiol interchange. Eur J Biochem 130, 85–92, 1983.

46 Kobaysahi, T, Flavin, M: Tubulin-tyrosine ligase: purification and application to studies of tubulin structure and assembly. J Cell Biol 75, 285, 1977.

47 Hoffstein, S et al: Role of microtubule assembly in lysosomal enzyme secretion from human polymorphonuclear leukocytes. J Cell Biol 73, 242–256, 1977.

48 Nath, J et al: Tubulin tyrosinolation in human polymorphonuclear leucocytes: studies in normal subjects and in patients with the Chediak-Higashi syndrome. J Cell Biol 95, 519–526, 1982.

49 Boxer, LA et al: Enhancement of chemotactic response and microtubule assembly in human leucocytes by ascorbic acid. J Cell Physiol 100, 119–126, 1979.

50 Bigley, RH et al: Human cell dehydroascorbate reductase, kinetic and functional properties. Biochim Biophys Acta 659, 15–22, 1981.

51 Anderson, R et al: Dehydroascorbate uptake as an in vitro biochemical marker of granulocyte differentiation. Cancer Res 43, 4696–4698, 1983.

52 Bingöl, A et al: Plasma erythrocyte, and leukocyte ascorbic acid concentrations in children with iron deficiency anemia. J Pediatr 86, 902–904, 1975.

53 Attwood, EC et al: Determination of platelet and leucocyte vitamin C and the levels found in normal subjects. Clin Chim Acta 54, 95–105, 1974.

54 Briggs, M, Briggs, M: Vitamin C requirements and oral contraceptives. Nature 238: 277, 1972.

55 Denson, KW, Bowers, EF: The determination of ascorbic acid in white blood cells. A comparison of W.B.C. ascorbic acid and phenolic acid excretion in elderly patients. Clin Sci 21, 157–162, 1961.

56 De Chatelet, LR et al: Ascorbic acid levels in phagocytic cells. Proc Soc Exp Biol Med 145, 1170–1173, 1974.

57 Castranova, V et al: Ascorbate uptake by isolated rat alveolar macrophages and type II cells. J Appl Physiol Respirat Environ Exercise Physiol 54, 208–214, 1983.

58 Carp, H, Janoff, A: Potential mediator of inflammation. Phagocyte-derived oxidants suppress the elastase-inhibitory capacity of alpha$_1$-proteinase inhibitor in vitro. J Clin Invest 66, 987–995, 1980.

K.H. Schmidt, MD, PhD, Department of Surgery, University of Tübingen, D–7400 Tübingen, West Germany

Causes of Gastric and Esophageal Cancer. Possible Approach to Prevention by Vitamin C

J.H. WEISBURGER

American Health Foundation,
Naylor Dana Institute for Disease Prevention,
Valhalla, New York, USA

Key Words: Vitamin C · Gastric cancer · Esophageal cancer · Colon cancer · Nitrosamines · Nitrite · Nitrate

Abstract: In the US gastric cancer was one of the main types of cancer decades ago, but in the last fifty years has declined sharply. However, it is still an important disease in Japan, Central America, parts of South America west of the Andes, and in Eastern and Northern Europe.

Recently, research has shown that treatment of certain foods, such as fish or beans with nitrite, mimicking pickling or smoking, yields a powerful direct acting mutagen with properties similar to that of the synthetic mutagen N-methyl-N'-nitro-N-nitrosoguanidine (MNNG), which is also an effective carcinogen for the glandular stomach in rats. The mutagen from nitrite-treated pickled fish has not yet been identified, but we have shown that it can cause glandular stomach cancer in rats.

Vitamin C is an antagonist to nitrite and therefore an inhibitor of the formation of this mutagen. Epidemiological studies also show that migrants from high risk regions for stomach cancer to low risk regions tend to acquire the habit of eating more foods containing vitamin C.

Cancer of the esophagus in the Western world is seen in individuals who smoke cigarettes and drink alcohol excessively. This disease occurs also in other populations without these risk factors, but living in areas like Eastern Iran, Southern Soviet Union, parts of China and South Africa. The specific risk factor has not been identified, but epidemiological studies note that people at high risk customarily do not have access to foods rich in vitamin C. It is suspected that this plays a role and that the active carcinogen may be of the nitrosamine type.

It is clear that prevention of these important cancer types in parts of the world is feasible by lowering the intake of pickled, salted and smoked foods (that will be useful also in lowering the risk for hypertension and stroke) and

increasing the daily presence from childhood onward of an adequate supply of foods with vitamin C and probably vitamin E, or to make available to such populations these vitamins at moderate dosages with each meal.

Introduction

Worldwide epidemiological studies on the incidence and mortality rates of diverse cancers and consideration of how these rates change in migrant populations from an area of high risk to low risk or vice versa indicate that life style elements, especially tobacco smoking or chewing and nutritional factors, play a major role in the occurrence of many of the principal forms of cancer [1–4]. Additional data on the same point consist in the observation that time

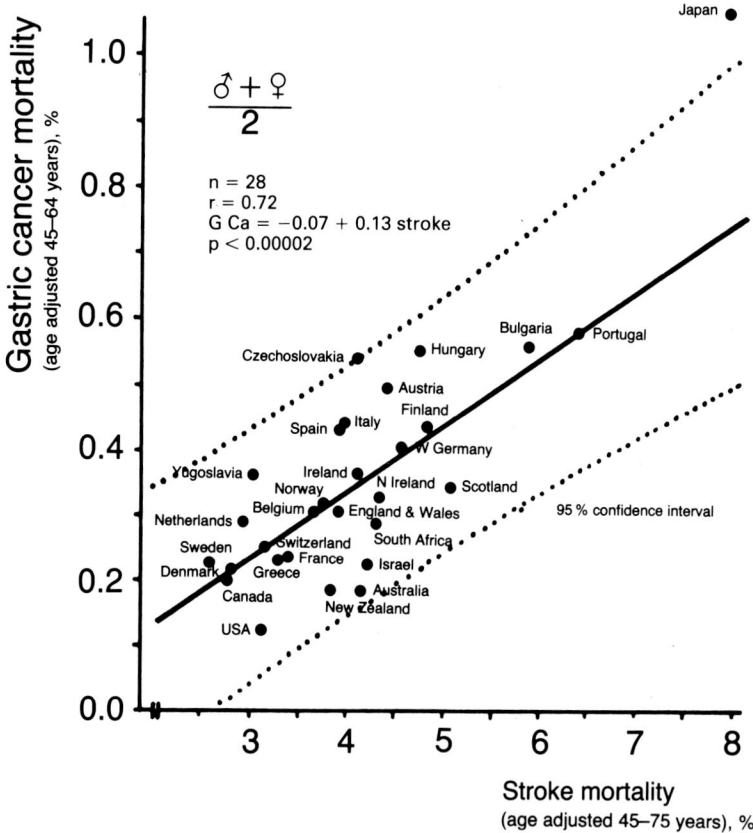

Fig. 1: The geographic relationship between stroke and gastric cancer mortality for the average of both sexes, 1965–1970. Japan was excluded from the calculation of the regression line [13].

trends also can be related to personal habits and life style elements. Thus, in the Western World, the main cancers associated with nutrition are those in the large bowel, breast, prostate, as well as pancreas, ovary and endometrium [5]. These same cancers are much less frequent in an equally industrialized area with an economically high standard of living, namely Japan [6, 7]. The key difference between Japanese life style and that prevalent in the West is nutrition, and specifically the fact that in traditional Japan the customary diet contained only 10–15 % of calories in fat, whereas in the Western world 40–45 % of calories are in fat [5, 8, 9].

At the same time, countries such as Japan, Central and Western South America, and also Eastern and Northern Europe exhibited a high incidence of stomach cancer, albeit, in most of these high risk areas for stomach cancer there has been a declining trend [10, 11]. The rate of decline has been more rapid in specific countries and regions than in others. Countries with a high risk for gastric cancer often have a high prevalence of hypertension, and hence, a high mortality from cerebro-vascular accidents, ascribed to a generally high intake of salt (Fig. 1) [12].

Where efforts were made to deliberately lower salt intake, as in Belgium, both gastric cancer and hypertensive diseases declined more rapidly than in other regions where no specific efforts were made to decrease salt consumption (Fig. 2) [13].

On the other hand, in many regions of the world, such as Central America, Japan, Northern and Eastern Europe, where preservation of foods through refrigeration has become progressively more common, older methods such as pickling, salting, or smoking have been used less frequently (Table I) [14, 15]. This accounts in part for the decreased incidence of hypertensive disease and a beginning decrease in the incidence of stomach cancer [13, 15].

Tab. I: Changes in Puerto Rico 1946–1966 expressed in percentage of households

	1946	1966
Appliances		
Charcoal cooker	37	1
Elec./gas cooker	4	70
Refrigerator	11	88
Animal protein		
Lunch	< 50	71
Supper	15	75
Codfish	75	75

Compiled from data in Fernandez
[16].

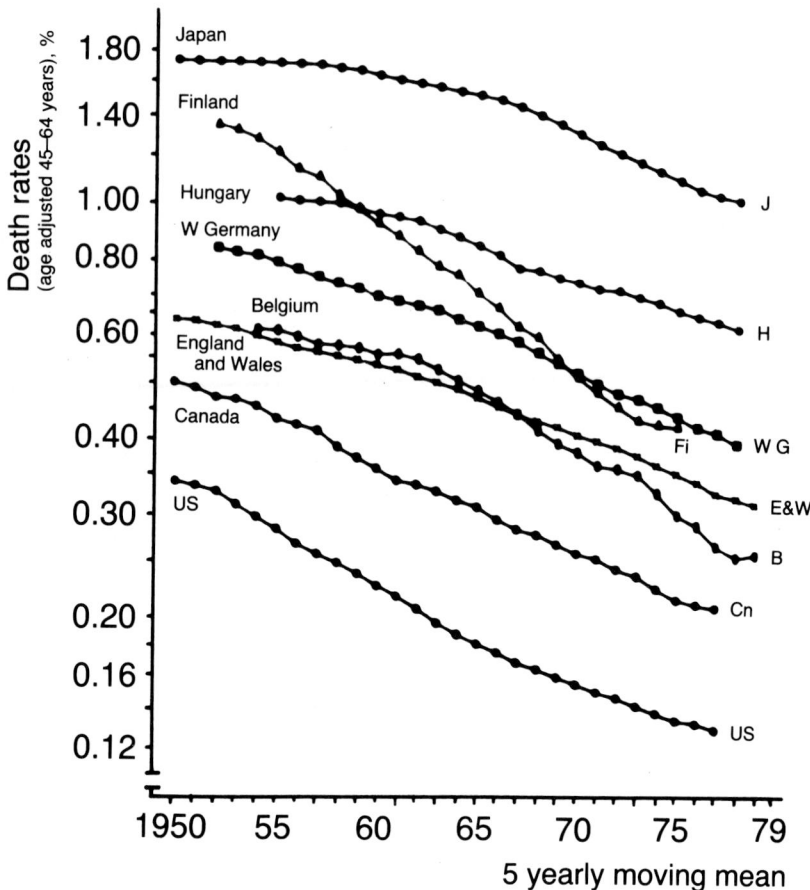

Fig. 2: Time trends in gastric cancer mortality (males). The decrease since 1968 is fastest in Finland and Belgium and slowest in Japan and Hungary [13].

In the last fifty years, more effective distribution of fresh fruits and vegetables has also contributed to improved nutrition [9, 16–20]. Historically, fresh fruits and vegetables were freely available mainly during harvest time and for a limited period thereafter. In northern areas of the world, such vitamin C containing foods were less frequently consumed in winter and early spring. The main source of vitamin C was at an ever decreasing level because of storage losses in foods such as potatoes. In areas of Northern Japan and parts of Latin America, where the main starch consumed was in the form of rice, the vitamin C intake was subject to even more severe seasonal variations.

In this report we will describe the role of vitamin C intake or the relative deficiency of vitamin C in the occurrence of gastric and esophageal cancers. There are also some suggestions that the use of vitamin C may play a role in modifying the risk for large bowel cancer, although the data for this disease are not definitive.

Esophageal Cancer: Nature of Associated Carcinogens

Cancers of the head and neck are related to heavy tobacco use in the form of cigarette smoking or by the habit of snuff inhalation or tobacco chewing in the Western world, particularly combined with a heavy consumption of alcohol [21–23]. Certain tobacco-specific nitrosamines, such as nitrosornornicotine, comprise a substantial portion of the genotoxic carcinogens in tobacco smoke, chews, and snuff [24]. The specific association of these carcinogens with cancers at sites related to the use of tobacco remains to be fully documented, but it seems that alcohol acts as a cocarcinogen [25, 26]. TUYNS [22] has noted a protective effect by vitamin C in an area, such as Calvados, France, in the occurrence of esophageal cancer presumably associated with smoking and drinking (Fig. 3)

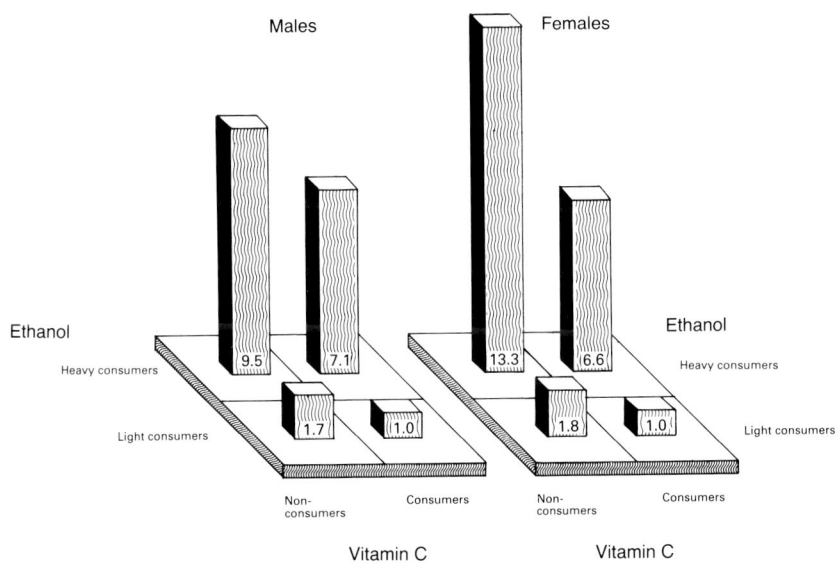

Fig. 3: Effect of vitamin C on the incidence of esophageal cancer in populations who are light or heavy consumers of alcohol and who smoke cigarettes [22].

The underlying mechanism is not clear but may relate to cell duplication rates as affected by vitamin C. The formation and properties of connective tissue may also be involved.

In areas of the world such as Eastern Iran and Central China, the high incidence of esophageal cancer does not appear to be related to heavy use of tobacco and alcohol as it is in Western countries [27–31]. In Iran, the poor quality of the diet with a low intake of fresh vegetables and fruits and the possible smoking of opium-tobacco or chewing of the resulting tar appear to be contributing factors [30]. Likewise, in the Transkei, a change in dietary habits away from sorghum to maize or wheat, and a seasonal poor intake of micronutrients has been noted to be associated with increases in the occurrence of esophageal cancer (Table II) [20, 27].

Tab. II: Nutrient intakes and risk for esophageal cancer (Iran, China, Transkei). Data from GROENEWALD et al [20]

	%
< 2/3 of RDA and inadequate intakes for	
Calcium	90
Nicotinic acid	79
Riboflavin	55
Vitamin C	50

Seasonal variation is important, especially for vitamins A and C.

Consumption of traditional preserved foods such as salted fish and pickled vegetables among the Southern Chinese people have been associated with their high incidence of nasopharyngeal and esophageal cancers [29, 31, 32]. The salted fish is commonly «pickled» in a crude salt solution of rock or sea salt containing nitrate. Significant levels of N-nitrosodimethylamine (NDMA) and other nitrosamines have been detected in salted fish. Rats fed salted fish daily produced urine that showed mutagenic activity in the Ames test [33]. Extracts from pickled vegetables, which are commonly contaminated with fungus, showed mutagenic, transforming, and promoting activity in different biological systems.

Thus, it would seem that certain specific nitrosamines are associated with the causation of cancers in the oral cavity and esophagus. In the Western world where the use of tobacco products is involved, nitrosonornicotine and related compounds, are likely candidates as the relevant carcinogens [24]. In Iran, Southern Soviet Union and Central China, the specific carcinogens are not yet known and may well be different for each area. In China, the compounds may be in the diet, or formed from dietary constituents, in which case vitamin C or vitamin E, or foods containing these micronutrients may be effective inhibitors.

Stomach Cancer: Nature of Associated Carcinogens

Cancer of the glandular stomach occurs in high incidence in Japan, Iceland, mountainous interior regions of Central and Western Latin America, and some Eastern European countries. In contrast, Western Europe, many Anglo-Saxon countries (except Wales in the United Kingdom), and the United States have a low incidence [3, 5, 10, 15]. Over the last 50 years, gastric cancer rates in the United States have steadily declined from 38 to 9/100 000 for men and 28 to 4/100 000 for women [34].

Tab. III: Vitamin C and stomach cancer, studies in Norway 1967–1978.
From BJELKE [18]

Value of vitamin C index	Case-control study			Prospective study[1]		
	relative risk	number of cases	number of controls	relative risk	number of cases	number of cases expected
< 15	1.0	76	317	1.0	46	32.8
15–21	0.7	63	348	0.6	39	46.1
> 22	0.5	88	729	0.6	31	37.1

[1] Excluding stump carcinomas.

Positive correlations with dietary risk factors in high risk populations have been made for diets with a high consumption of dried, salted fish, pickled vegetables, smoked fish, and a low vegetable intake as well as for a reduced vitamin C intake, particularly on a seasonal basis (Table III). Another correlation has been made between elevated levels of nitrate in foods and drinking water that occurs due to high levels in the soil and water supply [35–38]. The latter correlation holds only in the periodic absence of fresh vegetables as sources of vitamin C, an antagonist of nitrite [11]. When fresh vegetables and fruits are more widely available, measurement of urine nitrate alone fails to correlate with risk. When crude salt or saltpeter is used in the preservation of certain foods such as fish, this may constitute another source of nitrate [15]. Japanese migrants to Hawaii whose diet contained a higher intake of uncooked vegetables such as celery, lettuce, and tomatoes, and fresh fruit juices, correlated with a low risk of gastric cancer as compared to indigenous Japanese and first generation Japanese migrants to Hawaii [17].

Alkylnitrosoureido compounds such as N-methyl-N'-nitro-N-nitrosoguanidine (MNNG) are carcinogens that have the characteristic of inducing glandular stomach cancer in animal models [38, 39]. SANDER [40] found that such carcinogens were formed through the reaction of nitrite and suitably substituted secondary amines or amides. The reaction of the nitrosation of alkylamides such as methylurea has been studied by MIRVISH [10, 41], who also made the important discovery that ascorbic acid had an inhibitory effect on the nitrosation of methylurea and alkylamines [42].

Tab. IV: Mutagens formed by nitrosation of different types of fish.
From WEISBURGER et al [43]

		Salmonella typhimurium TA 1535, revertants/g of fish
Fresh fish		
A	Salt water	
	Shad, flounder	0
	Cod	29
	Haddock	39
	Sanma	595
	Aji	610
	Iwashi	1320
B	Fresh water	
	Catfish	0
	Bluegill	8
	Sunfish	11
Canned fish		
	Salmon	4
	Anchovies	26
	Jack mackerel (light muscle)	9
	Jack mackerel (dark muscle)	55
	Herring	63
	Sardines	72

Reaction of a homogenate of certain kinds of fish commonly eaten in Japan with nitrite at pH 3 mimicking gastric conditions yielded high levels of direct-acting mutagens (Table IV). YANO [46] discovered alkylating activity in several kinds of fish, including mackerel, treated with nitrite. We noted that formation of the mutagen was blocked by the simultaneous presence of vitamin C. A mutagenic extract from the reaction of nitrite and Sanma induced adenocarcinomas of the glandular stomach in Wistar rats (Table V) [43]. The nature of the mutagen(s) obtained from these reactions is as yet unknown, but the mode of formation and inhibition, along with the

Tab. V: Sites and incidence of tumors in rats given extract of fish treated with nitrite or fish alone. From WEISBURGER et al [43]

Group and treatment	Effective No. of rats	Forestomach		Glandular stomach			Pancreas		Small intestine: adenocarcinoma
		papilloma	squamous cell carcinoma	adenoma	adenocarcinoma	adenosquamous carcinoma	adenoma	adenocarcinoma	
I: Fish extract alone	8[a]	0	0	0	0	0	0	0	0
II: Fish extract + NaNO$_2$	12[b]	0	2[c]	2[d]	2[e]	1[f]	2	1	1[f]

a Three rats had interstitial cell adenoma of testis, 1 renal nephroblastoma, 1 rhabdomyosarcoma.
b Eight rats had at least one of tumors tabulated here. In addition the following miscellaneous tumors were noted: 1 rat had cortical adenoma of adrenal gland, 1 had follicular adenoma of thyroid gland, and 1 had pulmonary adenoma.
c One rat also had a pancreatic adenoma, and the other had an adenocarcinoma.
d One rat had only an adenoma, but the other also had an adenocarcinoma.
e One rat also had an adenocortical adenoma, and the other had a gastric adenoma and a thyroid adenoma.
f The only tumor in 1 rat.

mutagenicity/carcinogenicity results suggest a possible alkylnitrosoureido compound. We have observed that the precursor found in fish is a rather polar compound, most likely with a carboxyl group, and of course, a nitrosatable amino group to yield the reactive, direct-acting mutagen. Under similar conditions treatment of beans as eaten in Latin America also yielded mutagenic activity with properties somewhat similar but not identical to that found in nitrite-treated fish [47].

Furthermore, reaction of soy sauce and select other Japanese foods with nitrite under gastric conditions yielded a mutagenic product [48]. Attempts to isolate the precursors in soy sauce met with success for they yielded 1-methyl-1,2,3,4-tetrahydro-β-carboline-3-carboxylic acid, a synthetically prepared nitroso derivative that is not mutagenic. The chemistry involved in the production of a mutagen from this precursor is not yet completely known. In any case, it is quite apparent that nitrite reacting under conditions of pickling with salt and vinegar or under conditions prevailing in the stomach with foods eaten in high gastric cancer regions yielded chemicals with the property consistent with that of a gastric carcinogen. Glutathione may play a role in the release of reactive products in the glandular stomach [49, 50].

Nitrite is essential for the formation of such gastric carcinogens. The available nitrite load can be measured by estimating the urinary nitroso-amino-acid products [51]. Nitrate in foods is converted to nitrite during storage at room temperature for 24 hours, a reaction inhibited by cold storage or refrigeration [43]. Also, nitrate can be reduced efficiently to nitrite by the oral bacterial flora.

All of these different lines of evidence lead to the conclusion that the human consumption of salted and pickled foods may result in gastric cancer through the action of an active agent (or agents) that has the properties of alkylnitrosoureido compounds formed from nitrite and undefined substrates. The fact that the formation of such carcinogens may be blocked by vitamin C or by vitamin E is most important. It provides an effective tool for the avoidance of such carcinogens and thus of gastric and esophageal cancer caused by these agents.

Colon Cancer: Effect of Vitamin C

We have discussed above the protective effects of vitamin C for cancer of the esophagus and cancer of the stomach. There was a satisfactory mechanistic explanation of the role of vitamin C in the prevention of these forms of cancer. In this respect, an effect in carcinogenesis of the large bowel is somewhat unexpected and currently a proven mechanism is not at hand. It is possible that vitamin C affects cell duplication rates and connective tissue integrity and patency. REDDY et al [52] found that under some conditions, specifically the induction of colon cancer by 1,2-dimethylhydrazine, ascorbic acid displayed a protective effect. This was true only when the carcinogen was given as a single dose but not when given as multiple treatments. This suggests that the protective effect is rather weak. In addition, no effect was found with the direct-acting carcinogen N-methyl-N-nitrosourea injected intrarectally, which suggests that the effect with dimethylhydrazine depends on a modification of the metabolism of this agent.

BRUCE et al [53] discovered that the stools of certain individuals on a Western diet contained mutagenic activity, a finding that was confirmed by WILKENS et al [54], MOWER et al [55], VENITT et al [56], KÜNLEIN et al [57] and REDDY et al [58]. Mutagenic activity was found only in individuals on a Western diet, and populations on a vegetarian diet, which might involve a higher intake of fiber as well as vitamins, had no mutagens. When BRUCE et al [53] first discovered mutagens in the stools of individuals, it was thought that these mutagens were nitrosamines, and it seemed logical that their formation should be inhibited by vitamins C and E [59]. The finding of lower mutagenic activity when vitamins C and E were added was actually made. It is now known, however, that one of these fecal mutagens is in the form of a fecapentaene, a highly unsaturated aliphatic compound produced by specific bacteria [60, 61]. Thus, at this time it is less clear why vitamin C lowers mutagenic activity, although vitamin C and vitamin E may help stabilize the membranes in the bacteria that are the source for these fecal mutagens. In addition, feces of individuals on a Western diet may also contain metabolites of mutagens found in fried food [62, 63], and it is not yet clear how vitamin C affects the production of these metabolites.

DECOSSE [64] noted from a small sample of patients with familial polyposis that vitamin C delayed the neoplastic change typical of this genetically initiated disease. In a large scale trial, this effect was less apparent [65]. BRUCE et al [66] have underway a clinical trial of vitamin C and vitamin E to examine whether patients with polyps having undergone a polypectomy would have a lower recurrence rate.

Cancer Therapy by Vitamin C

CAMERON and PAULING reported in a preliminary note [67] the finding in a hospital in Scotland that patients with diverse types of cancer not treated with chemotherapeutic agents but given amounts of 10–15 g/day of vitamin C in divided doses appeared to have better survival than patients not so treated. A test of this interesting finding at the Mayo clinic could not confirm this effect [68]. However, the patients at Mayo had undergone conventional chemotherapy and were in late stage disease. PAULING [69] noted that the mechanism of action of vitamin C might be to stimulate or at least maintain reasonably functional the immunological competence, thus, accounting for the lack of positive response in the patients at Mayo since conventional chemotherapy is immunosuppressive. Results of a new study, just published, where the prior use of cytotoxic drugs is taken into account, again failed to demonstrate any effect of vitamin C in the treatment of colorectal cancer [69a, 69b]. It would appear that more basic research, perhaps in animal models [70], utilizing new technology to determine immunologic competence might be helpful in accounting for discrepancies in the clinical literature.

Historic Intake Patterns of Vitamin C in Foods

Vitamin C disappearance data obtained from the tabulation of diverse foods by the United States Department of Agriculture show that the nominal intake of vitamin C has not changed very much in the last 80 years [19]. Indeed, about 1903 the daily estimated disappearance was 104 mg/day, and in 1980 it was 120 mg/day (Table VI) [9].

Tab. VI: Vitamins available from 1910 to 1980.
Data from [9,19]

Year	Vitamin			
	A, IU	B_1, mg	B_2, mg	C, mg
1910	7600	1.63	1.82	107
1920	7900	1.52	1.82	104
1930	8000	1.54	1.84	103
1940	8500	1.55	1.90	115
1950	8400	1.90	2.29	105
1960	8000	1.85	2.28	108
1970	8200	1.93	2.35	114
1980	8000	2.16	2.32	123

It is important to consider the significance of the overall estimated values. It seems reasonable to assume that prior to the availability of home refrigeration in the United States [11], and even more so in other regions of the world [20], that there would have been a much greater variation in intake. One can surmise that historically there was an adequate, even high intake in the summer and early fall, and then a progressive decline during the winter and spring. In the United States and Eastern Europe, the main food in fall and winter providing such vitamin C presumably was potatoes, and it is well known that this food progressively loses vitamin C during storage. In countries such as Japan, Central and Northern China, Central or Western Latin America where the main carbohydrate is in the form of rice, particularly in the lower socioeconomic groups, the daily vitamin C intake could be expected to undergo even more sizable fluctuations between summer and winter. At this point, there are relatively few data available for vitamin C, but for vitamin A it has been noted that the lower socioeconomic groups seem to consume much less than middle and upper classes (Table VII) [16], and a like comment can be made about fluctuations in vitamin C intake [8, 10, 15, 41, 70, 71].

Tab. VII: Constituents of various 2400-calorie diets in Puerto Rico. Adapted from FERNANDEZ [16]

	Protein, g	Fat, g	Carbohydrate, g	Calcium, g	Protein, g	Vitamin A, IU
USA	55	99	321	0.35	1.29	7895
Puerto Rico						
City family	86	76	340	0.28	1.49	2419
Country family	59	62	401	0.29	0.73	1220

Specific Aspects of the Reaction of Vitamin C With Nitrite

In the previous discussion, we have indicated that population studies reveal an effect of the reaction of certain precursors in food with nitrite as being associated in specific regions of the world with gastric cancer and of distinct precursors in foods in other parts of the world with cancer of the esophagus [6, 22, 27-33]. Further, it appears that intake of foods containing vitamin C, and perhaps Vitamin E and selenium, have an antagonistic effect in the occurrence of these cancers [71-73]. There are laboratory studies to document a protective effect of vitamin C [2, 10, 11, 15, 43, 51, 71-74].

MIRVISH et al [42] discovered that the production of dimethylnitrosamine resulting from the treatment of the drug oxytetracycline, and also other secondary or tertiary amines or amides, with nitrite was blocked by vitamin C (Table VIII). This germinal experiment has been duplicated many times and depends on the previously known reaction of ascorbate with N_2O_3 or $H_2NO_2^+$.

Tab. VIII: Effect of ascorbate on the yield of *N*-nitroso compounds.
From MIRVISH *et al* [42]

Experiment No.	Base, mM	Nitrite, mM	Ascorbate, mM	pH	Time min	Yield from amine of urea, %		Blocking, %
						without ascorbate	with ascorbate	
Oxytetracycline								
1	21.6	315	475	2.8	1320	44	0	100
2	21.6	315	475	3.8	1320	63	0.045	99.9
Morpholine								
3	25	50	100	2	30	20	0.48	98
4	25	50	100	3	30	65	0	100
5	25	50	100	4	30	34	0	100
Piperazine								
6	10	10	20	1	60	35	0.58	98
7	10	10	20	2	20	44	1.2	98
8	10	10	20	3	10	56	0.33	99
9	10	10	20	4	15	54	0.24	99
N-Methylaniline								
10	2.5	2.5	5	3	5	68	27	60
11	2.5	2.5	5	4	10	16	8.8	45
Methylurea								
12	5	10	20	1	10	85	6.9	92
13	5	10	20	2	10	58	7.6	87
14	20	20	40	3	30	27	0	100
Dimethylamine								
15	500	50	100	1	60	0.042	0.076	−80
16	500	50	100	2	60	0.27	0.29	−7
17	500	50	100	3	60	0.76	0.20	74
18	500	50	100	4	60	0.92	0.03	97
19	20	300	500	2	1440	2.2	0.17	92
20	20	300	500	2.8	1380	20	1.7	91
21	20	300	500	3.8	1380	82	1.4	98

Tab. IX: Effect of ascorbic acid on the formation of methylnitrosourea in potato incubated at pH 1.5.[1]
From RAINERI and WEISBURGER [72]

μCi methyl-^{14}C-urea (100 ppm methylurea)	Nitrite (100 ppm)	[Ascorbate]: [nitrite]	Methylnitrosourea formed[2] ± SE, ppm	Inhibition, %
+	−	−	0.0 ± 0.0	−
+	+	0	19 ± 1.1	0
+	+	1	12 ± 0.8	37
+	+	2	5.0 ± 0.4	74
+	+	4	1.4 ± 0.2	93

[1] 5 g samples of homogenized boiled potato (adjusted to pH 1.5 were incubated in triplicate at 37° for 10 minutes.
[2] Recovery of methylnitrosourea was 35 %.

In our laboratory, we have noted that the formation of a powerful direct-acting mutagen that could also induce glandular stomach cancer when certain fish were reacted with salt and nitrite, could be completely blocked when vitamin C was added prior to nitrite [15, 72]. A model experiment in which the promutagen methylurea was added to potatoes containing nitrite demonstrated a progressively reduced formation of nitrosomethylurea (Table IX) as a function of the amount of vitamin C added [72].

Vitamin C and Other Micronutrients

As noted, vitamin C has a pronounced effect on reactions with nitrite. Vitamin E has a similar role and these two micronutrients in some instances have a synergistic interaction in minimizing nitrosamine formation [72,73]. One explanation is that vitamin C is water soluble and reacts mainly with precursors in the aqueous phase, whereas vitamin E is lipid soluble and favors inhibiting nitrosamine formation in the fat component in certain foods. With the potential of nitrosation of precursors in both an aqueous and lipid medium, a greater effect is seen with both vitamin C and E and other components such as sorbate [75, 77].

Vitamin C and Drug-Carcinogen Metabolism

Drugs and carcinogens are metabolized actively by several complex enzyme systems, especially the cytochrome P-450 system and prostaglandin synthetase located on the endoplasmic reticulum of cells and tissues, as well as more specialized systems such as the cytosolic, soluble xanthine oxidase. A number of essential cofactors are required for the cytochrome P-450 system. In most of the rodent laboratory animals that have the capacity to synthesize vitamin C, this micronutrient is usually present in adequate amounts in the tests for this enzyme activity without need for the exogenous vitamin. It seems that vitamin C plays a specific role in the activities of this critical set of enzymes, but the specific site where ascorbate plays such a role has not yet been definitely pinpointed [10, 35, 70, 71, 78–84]. The cytochrome P-450 system is less active in scorbutic guinea pigs. It is possible, nonetheless, that the scorbutic guinea pig, where protein synthesis is also depressed, has a general rather than a specific deficiency of enzymes. This is an area where more research is needed on the role of vitamin C in an important metabolic system that is not yet completely elucidated. Several recent papers have appeared [84a–c].

Vitamin C and Cell Transformation

Vitamin A and carotene have been studied extensively as possible chemopreventive agents [71, 85]. While not all of the mechanisms are known, vitamin A throught its membrane effects stabilizes the differentiated forms of cell systems. Benedict et al [86] discuss the use of ascorbic acid in studies of cell transformation by chemicals, particularly by polycyclic aromatic hydrocarbons. They demonstrated that ascorbic acid blocked transformation by 3-methylcholanthrene of mouse cell line C3H/10T½. Unlike retinoids, this inhibition appeared to be quite stable even when vitamin C was no longer added to the cell system in the later stages of the test. In addition, vitamin C could revert cells that had been transformed previously to a normal growth pattern. These important observations have not yet been explained as to the underlying relevant mechanism.

Vitamin C as a Mutagen

Some years ago, Stich et al [87] noted that solutions of vitamin C displayed mutagenic activity. It was realized, however, that this effect depended in large measure on the simultaneous presence of some heavy metal ions such as copper. In turn, the effect reflected the production of hydrogen peroxide from oxygen by vitamin C and copper where the hydrogen peroxide acted as the mutagen. It is known that polyhydroxylated chelating agents such as ascorbic acid or maleic acid can function in this manner, as was described in connection with the properties of the Fenton or the Udenfriend reagents. When the solutions of ascorbic acid were completely free of heavy metals, mutagenicity was not seen [88]. Schaumberger [88a] has published a critical overview.

Comment

The consideration of various lines of evidence drawn from multi-disciplinary approaches suggests that nutrition and specific nutritional components, as well as dietary habits, in various parts of the world may play an important role in the causation and development of a number of types of major human neoplasms.

The current concept of cancer causation indicates the overall carcinogenic process can be split into a number of sequential steps, all of which appear necessary before a clinically invasive cancer occurs [89]. This sequence of events has been demonstrated by numerous studies in animal models, and there is no reason to assume that it would not also hold for the initiation, development, and progression of human cancers. Mutagens, which may be initiating, genotoxic carcinogens, are found in certain salted, pickled, or smoked foods, an area that clearly needs further research in identifying those mutagens and demonstrating their relevance in human cancer causation.

Gastric cancer appears to have specific risk factors, pickled and salted fish or beans or residence in areas with geochemical or agricultural sources of nitrate intake, not balanced by the presence of vitamin C, vitamin E, or certain phenolic antioxidants and nitrite traps such as propyl gallate or tannins. In the MNNG-induced gastric cancer model, salt (sodium chloride) has a co-carcinogenic effect [see 10, 71]. This observation may also mimic the human environment, for Joossens and Geboers [12, 13] have documented a parallelism in international trends between gastric cancer and hypertension. A reduction in the use of salt would have dual benefits of lowering gastric cancer and also reduce the risk of hypertension.

The possible genotoxic carcinogen involved is postulated to be of the alkylnitrosamide type. The formation of such compounds is inhibited by vitamin C, vitamin E, and certain antioxidants. This fact can be used as a preventive approach to deliberately decrease the risk for gastric cancer. Furthermore, cancer of the oral cavity and esophagus, highly prevalent in some parts of the world, appears to depend on the presence of certain nitrosamines, the amount of which can also be lowered by anticarcinogens such as vitamins C or E (Table X).

Tab. X: Nutritional factors involved in certain human cancers

Source of genotoxic carcinogen	Enhancing factors	Inhibiting factors	Organs affected
Nitrite + specific foods (fish, beans, *not* meats)	salt	vitamin C vitamin E propyl gallate, tannins	stomach, oral cavity, esophagus

1 Mechanisms discussed in text.

If current research extends and amplifies findings that the salting, pickling, or smoking methods of food preparation yield carcinogens for certain nutritionally linked cancers, it will be possible to design approaches throught which the formation of such carcinogens can be prevented, and hence lower the risk for important types of cancer in many parts of the world. Along these lines, research on optimal levels of vitamins, minerals, antioxidants, and other micronutrients in the current diet could provide a broad basis for chemoprevention. Cancers at other target sites appear susceptible to inhibitory modulation, albeit not prevention by vitamins and other micronutrients, and especially by vitamin C [7, 51, 71, 90–92]. Because of other exogenous influences such as smoking [93, 94], the requirements for vitamins are increased. Over the last several years, new facts and perspectives have been acquired on the causes and modifiers of cancers with the highest mortality, as well as on the underlying mechanisms. Further research with emphasis on nutritional factors may provide feasible and practical means of cancer prevention.

References

1 DOLL, R, PETO, R: The causes of cancer: Quantitative estimates of avoidable risks of cancer in the United States today. J Nat Cancer Inst 66, 1196–1305, 1981.
2 BRUCE, W R et al (eds): Banbury Rpt 7. Gastrointestinal cancer: endogenous factors. Cold Spring Harbor Laboratory, Cold Spring Harbor, 1981.
3 SCHOTTENFELD, D, FRAUMENI, J F, Jr: Cancer epidemiology and prevention. Saunders, Philadelphia, 1982.
4 Surgeon General Report. The health consequences of smoking. Cancer. US Govt Pub No DHHS (PHS) 82-50179. Superintendent of documents, US Government Printing Office, Washington, 1982.
5 REDDY, B S et al: Nutrition and its relationship to cancer. Adv Cancer Res 32, 237–345, 1980.
6 HIRAYAMA, T: Diet and cancer. Nutr Cancer 1, 67–80, 1979.
7 HIRAYAMA, T: A large-scale cohort study on the relationship between diet and selected cancer of digestive organs. Banbury Rept 7, 409–430, 1981.
8 OISO, T: Incidence of stomach cancer and its relation to dietary habits and nutrition in Japan between 1900 and 1975. Cancer Res 35, 3254–3258, 1975.
9 GORTNER, W A: Nutrition in the United States, 1900–1974. Cancer Res 35, 3246–3253, 1975.
10 MIRVISH, S S: The etiology of gastric cancer. J Natl Cancer Inst 71, 631–647, 1983.
11 WEISBURGER, J H, HORN, C L: On the factors associated with esophageal and gastric cancer in man. Banbury Rpt 12, 523–528, 1982.
12 JOOSSENS, J V, GEBOERS, J: Salt and hypertension. Prev Med 12, 53–59, 1983.
13 JOOSSENS, J V, GEBOERS, J: Epidemiology of gastric cancer: A clue to etiology. In: SHERLOCK et al (eds) Precancerous lesions of the gastrointestinal tract, pp 97–114. Raven Press, New York, 1983.
14 FJELLSTRÖM, P: Diet in the nordic countries in olden times. Nordic Council Arct Med Res Rep No. 31, 7–13, 1982.
15 WEISBURGER, J H: N-Nitroso compounds: diet and cancer trends. An approach to the prevention of gastric cancer. In: SCANLAN and TANNENBAUM (eds) N-Nitroso compounds. Am Chem Soc Symp Ser 174, 305–317, 1981.
16 FERNANDEZ, N A: Nutrition in Puerto Rico. Cancer Res 35, 3272–3291, 1975.
17 KOLONEL, L N et al: Nutrient intakes in relation to cancer incidence in Hawaii. Br J Cancer 44, 332–339, 1981.
18 MAGNUS, K: Trends in cancer incidence. Causes and practical implications, p 176. Hemisphere, Washington and McGraw-Hill, London, 1982.
19 MARSTON, R M, WELSH, S O: Nutrient content of the national food supply, 1981. Natl Food Rev 21, 17–21, 1983.

20 Groenewald, G et al: Nutrient intakes among rural Transkeians at risk for oesophageal cancer. SA Med J 60, 964–967, 1981.

21 Tuyns, A J et al: Le cancer de l'oesophage en Ille et Villaine en fonction de niveaux de consommation d'alcool et de tabac. Des risques qui se multiplient. Bull Cancer 64, 45–60, 1977.

22 Tuyns, A J: Protective effect of citrus fruit on esophageal cancer. Nutr Cancer 5, 195–200, 1984.

23 Groupé, V, Salmoiraghi, G C (eds): Alcohol and cancer workshop. Cancer Res 39, 2840–2852, 1979.

24 Hecht, S S et al: Carcinogenicity and metabolic activation of tobacco specific nitrosamines: current status and future prospects. In: Proc 8th Inter Meeting on N-nitroso compounds–occurrence and biological effects. IARC Sci Publ. In press, 1984.

25 Kouros, M et al: The influence of various factors on the methylation of DNA by the oesophageal carcinogen N-nitrosomethylbenzylamine. I. The importance of alcohol. Carcinogenesis 4, 1081–1084, 1983.

26 McCoy, G D et al: Differential effect of chronic ethanol consumption on the carcinogenicity of N-nitrosopyrrolidine and N'-nitrosonornicotine in male Syrian golden hamsters. Cancer Res 41, 2849–2854, 1981.

27 Rensburg, S J van: Epidemiologic and dietary evidence for a specific nutritional predisposition to esophageal cancer. J Natl Cancer Inst 67, 243–251, 1981.

28 Day, N E: Some aspects of the epidemiology of esophageal cancer. Cancer Res 35, 3304–3307, 1975.

29 Yang, C S: Research on esophageal cancer in China: A review. Cancer Res 42, 2633–2644, 1980.

30 Joint Iran-International Agency for Research on Cancer Study Group. Esophageal cancer studies in the Caspian Littoral of Iran: results of population studies-a prodrome. J Natl Cancer Inst 59, 1127–1138, 1977.

31 Armstrong, R W et al: Salted fish and inhalants as risk factors of nasopharyngeal carcinoma in Malaysian Chinese. Cancer Res 43, 2967–2970, 1982.

32 Ho, J H et al: Salted fish and nasopharyngeal carcinoma in Southern Chinese. Lancet ii, 626, 1978.

33 Fong, L Y et al: Preserved foods as possible cancer hazards: WA rats fed salted fish have mutagenic urine. Int J Cancer 23(4), 542–46, 1979.

34 Silverberg, E: Cancer statistics. Ca-A Cancer J Clinicians 33, 15, 1983.

35 Hartman, P E: Nitrates and nitrites: Ingestion, pharmacodynamics, and toxicology. In: de Serres and Holländer (eds) Chemical mutagens, vol. 7, pp 211–294. Plenum, New York, 1982.

36 National Academy of Sciences. Nitrates: an environmental assessment. National Academy Press, Washington, 1978.

37 Hartman, P E: Overview: nitrite load in the upper gastrointestinal tract-past, present, and future. Banbury Rept 12, 415–436, 1982.

38 Jensen, O M: Nitrate in drinking water and cancer in Northern Jutland, Denmark, with special reference to stomach cancer. Ecotoxicol Environ Safety 6, 258–267, 1982.

39 Bralow, S P, Weisburger, J H: Experimental carcinogenesis in the digestive organs. Clinics Gastroenterol 5, 527–542, 1976.

40 Sander, J et al: Nitrite and nitrosable amino compounds in carcinogenesis. Gann Monogr 17, 145–160, 1975.

41 Mirvish, S S: In vivo formation of N-nitroso compounds: Formation from nitrite and nitrogen dioxide, and relation to gastric cancer. Banbury Rept 12, 227–242, 1982.

42 Mirvish, S S et al: Ascorbate-nitrite reaction: Possible means of blocking the formation of carcinogenic N-nitroso compounds. Science 177, 65–68, 1972.

43 Weisburger, J H et al: Inhibition of carcinogenesis: vitamin C and the prevention of gastric cancer. Prev Med 9, 352–361, 1980.

44 ICHINOTSUBO, D Y, MOWER, H F: Mutagens in dried/salted Hawaiian fish. J Agric Food Chem *30*, 937–939, 1982.

45 STEMMERMAN, G N, MOWER, H: Gastritis, nitrosamines, and gastric cancer. J Clin Gastroenterol *3*, suppl 2, pp 23–27, 1981.

46 YANO, K: Alkylating activity of processed fish products treated with sodium nitrite in simulated gastric juice. Gann *72*, 451–454, 1981.

47 PIACEK-LLANES, B G, TANNENBAUM, S R: Formation of an activated N-nitroso compound in nitrite-treated fava beans *(Vicia faba)*. Carcinogenesis *3*, 1379–1384, 1982.

48 WAKABAYASHI, K *et al:* Presence of 1-methyl-1,2,3,4-tetrahydro-β-carboline-3-carboxylic acid, a precursor of a mutagenic nitroso compound, in soy sauce. Proc Natl Acad Sci USA *80*, 2912–2916, 1983.

49 BOYD, S C *et al:* High concentrations of glutathione in glandular stomach: Possible implications for carcinogenesis. Science *205*, 1010–1011, 1979.

50 KLEIHUES, P, WIESTLER, O: Involvement of thiols in MNNG-induced gastric cancer: Biochemical and autoradiographic studies. IARC Sci Publ No. 57, pp 603–608. 1984.

51 MAGEE, P N (ed): Nitrosamines and human cancer. Banbury Rpt 12. Cold Spring Harbor Laboratory, Cold Spring Harbor, 1982.

52 REDDY, B S *et al:* Effect of dietary sodium ascorbate on 1,2-dimethylhydrazine- or methylnitrosourea-induced colon carcinogenesis in rats. Carcinogenesis *3*, 1097–1099, 1982.

53 BRUCE, W R *et al:* A mutagen in the feces of normal humans. In: HIATT *et al* (eds) Origins of human cancer, pp 1641–1646. Cold Spring Harbor Laboratory, Cold Spring Harbor, 1977.

54 EHRLICH, M *et al:* Mutagens in the feces of 3 South-African populations at different level of risk for colon cancer. Mutat Res *64*, 231–240, 1979.

55 MOWER, H F *et al:* Fecal mutagens in two Japanese populations with different colon cancer risks. Cancer Res *42*, 1164–1169, 1982.

56 VENITT, S, BOSWORTH, D: The development of anaerobic methods for bacterial mutation assays: aerobic and anaerobic fluctuation tests of human faecal extracts and reference mutagens. Carcinogenesis *4*, 339–345, 1983.

57 KUENLEIN, H V *et al:* The effect of short-term dietary modification on human fecal mutagenic activity. Mutat Res *113*, 1–12, 1983.

58 REDDY, B S *et al:* Metabolic epidemiology of large bowel cancer. Fecal mutagens in high- and low-risk populations for colon cancer. A preliminary report. Mutat Res *72*, 511–519, 1980.

59 DION, P W *et al:* The effect of dietary ascorbic acid and α-tocopherol on fecal mutagenicity. Mutat Res *102*, 27–37, 1982.

60 GUPTA, I *et al:* Structures of fecapentaenes, the mutagens of bacterial origin isolated from human feces. Biochem *22*, 241–245, 1983.

61 HIRAI, N *et al:* Structure elucidation of a potent mutagen from human feces. J Am Chem Soc *104*, 6149–6150, 1982.

62 BARNES, W S *et al:* Mutagens in cooked foods: possible consequences of the Maillard reaction. In: WALLER and FEATHER (eds) The Maillard reaction in foods and nutrition. Am Chem Soc Symp Ser *215*, 485–506, 1983.

63 REDDY, B S and co-workers: Unpublished data.

64 DeCOSSE, J J: Potential for chemoprevention. Cancer *50*, 2550–2553, 1982.

65 BUSSEY, H J R *et al:* A randomized trial of ascorbic acid in polyposis coli. Cancer *50*, 1434–1439, 1982.

66 BRUCE, W R *et al:* The endogenous production of nitroso compounds in the colon and cancer at that site. In: MILLER *et al* (eds) Naturally occurring carcinogens-mutagens and modulators of carcinogenesis, pp 221–228. Japan Scientific Society Press, Tokyo, and University Park Press, Baltimore, 1979.

67 CAMERON, E, PAULING, L: Supplemental ascorbate in the supportive treatment of cancer: prolongation of survival times in terminal human cancer. Proc Natl Acad Sci USA 73, 3685–3689, 1976.

68 CREAGAN, E T et al: Failure of high-dose vitamin C (ascorbic acid) therapy to benefit patients with advanced cancer. New Engl J Med 301, 687–690, 1979.

69 PAULING, L: Vitamin C therapy of advanced cancer. New Engl J Med 302, 694, 1980.

69a MORTEL, C G et al: High-dose vitamin C versus placebo in the treatment of patients with advanced cancer who have had no prior chemotherapy. New Engl J Med 312, 137–141, 1985.

69b WITTES, R E: Vitamin C and cancer. New Engl J Med. 312, 178–179, 1985.

70 KAWASAKI, H et al. Influence of oral supplementation of ascorbate upon the induction of N-methyl-N'-nitro-N-nitrosoguanidine. Cancer Lett 16, 57–63, 1982.

71 National Research Council National Academy of Sciences. Diet, nutrition and cancer. National Academy Press, Washington, 1982.

72 RAINERI, R, WEISBURGER, J H: Reduction of gastric carcinogens with ascorbic acid. Ann NY Acad Sci 258, 181–189, 1975.

73 LUBIN, B, MACHLIN, L J (eds): Vitamin E: biochemical, hematological, and clinical aspects. Ann N Y Acad Sci 393, 1–506, 1982.

74 PARK, S-C et al: A study on mutagenicity of Korean taste marine foods and mutagenic suppressive activity of ascorbate. Korean J Biochem 12(2), 45–57, 1980.

75 MERGENS, W J: Efficacy of vitamin E to prevent nitrosamine formation. Ann N Y Acad Sci 393, 61–69, 1982.

76 TANNENBAUM, S R: Reaction of nitrite with vitamins C and E. Ann N Y Acad Sci 355, 267–277, 1980.

77 MASSEY, R C et al: The effects of ascorbic acid and sorbic acid on N-nitrosamine formation in a heterogenous model system. J Sci Food Agric 33, 294–298, 1982.

78 CONNEY, A H et al: Metabolic interactions between L-ascorbic acid and drugs. Ann N Y Acad Sci 92, 115–127, 1961.

79 ZANNONI, V G, SATO, P H: Effects of ascorbic acid on microsomal drug metabolism. Ann N Y Acad Sci 258, 119–131, 1975.

80 BELVEDERE, G et al: Hydroxylation of benzo(a)pyrene and binding of (-)trans-7,8-dihydroxy-7,8-dihydrobenzo(a)pyrene metabolites to deoxyribonucleic acid catalyzed by purified forms of rabbit liver microsomal cytochrome P–450. Effect of 7,8-benzoflavone, butylated hydroxytoluene and ascorbic acid. Biochem Pharmacol 29, 1693–1702, 1980.

81 BLACK, H S, GERGUIS, J: Use of the Ames test in assessing the relation of dietary lipid and antioxidants to N-2-fluorenylacetamide activation. J Environm Pathol Toxicol 4, 131–138, 1980.

82 BOCK-HENNIG, B S et al: Activating and inactivating reactions controlling 2-naphthylamine mutagenicity. Arch Toxicol 50, 259–266, 1982.

83 DOWNGANG, F, EMEROLE, G: Metabolism of aflatoxin B_1 (AFB$_1$), aflatoxin G_1 (AFG$_1$) and vitamin C intake by guinea pig liver preparation in vitro. Biochem Pharmacol 31, 2327–2330, 1982.

84 THORGEIRSSON, S S et al: Effect of ascorbic acid on the in vitro mutagenicity and in vivo covalent binding on N-hydroxy-2-acetylaminofluorene in the rat. Mutat Res 70, 395–398, 1980.

84a SOM, S et al: Ascorbic acid: scavenger of superoxide radicals. Acta Vitaminol Enzymol 5, 324–350, 1983.

84b Review: Elucidation of the biochemical role of ascorbic acid. Nutr Rev 42, 392–394, 1984.

84c SMART, R C, ZANNONI, V G: Effect of ascorbate on covalent bindings of benzene and phenol metabolites to isolated tissue preparations. Toxicol Appl Pharmacol 77, 334–343, 1985.

85 STÄHELIN, H B et al: Vitamin A, cardiovascular risk factors, and mortality. Lancet i, 394–395, 1982.

86 Benedict, W F et al: Differences in anchorage-dependent growth and tumorigenicities between transformed C3H/10T½ cells with morphologies that are or are not reverted to a normal phenotype by ascorbic acid. Cancer Res 42, 1041–1045, 1982.

87 Stich, H F et al: Mutagenic action of ascorbic acid. Nature 260, 722–724, 1976.

88 Norkus, E P et al: Studies on the mutagenic activity of ascorbic acid in vitro and in vivo. Mutat Res 117, 183–191, 1983.

88a Schamberger R G: Genetic toxicology of acorbic acid. Mutagen Res 131, 135–159, 1984.

89 Weisburger, J H, Williams, G M: Chemical carcinogenesis. In: Doull et al (eds) Toxicology: the basic science of poisons, 2nd ed, pp 84–138. Macmillan, New York, 1980.

90 Wassertheil-Smoller, S et al: Dietary vitamin C and uterine cervical dysplasia. Am J Epidemiol 114, 714–724, 1981.

91 Dunham, W B et al: Effects of intake of L-ascorbic acid on the incidence of dermal neoplasms induced in mice by ultraviolet light. Proc Natl Acad Sci USA 79, 7532–7536, 1982.

92 Levander, O A, Cheng, L (eds): Micronutrient interactions: vitamins, minerals and hazardous elements. Ann N Y Acad Sci 355, 1–371, 1980.

93 Kallner, A B et al: On the requirements of ascorbic acid in man: steady-state turnover and body pool in smokers. Am J Clin Nutr 34, 1347–1356, 1981.

94 Hornig, D H, Glatthaar, B E: Cf this book, pp 139–155.

John H. Weisburger, PhD, MD (hc), Director, Naylor Dana Institute, American Health Foundation, Dana Road, Valhalla, NY 10595, USA

Vitamin C Deficiency in São Paulo State, Brazil

D. WILSON

Department of Nutrition, University of São Paulo School of Public Health, São Paulo, Brazil

Key Words: Vitamin C · Deficiency · Brazil · Dietary pattern Survey · Symptoms · Eating habits · Food consumption

Abstract: Faulty nutrition is the forerunner of deficiency disease. Twenty towns in São Paulo state, Brazil, were surveyed to ascertain dietary vitamin C intake. The overall consumption of nutritional foodstuffs was low, and against this background figured a low intake of dietary sources of vitamin C, i.e. vegetable and fruit. This dietary pattern is dictated by a variety of factors, chief of which are cost and cultural preferences. Fruit juices might offer a palatable and convenient source of vitamin C, although the commercial, preserved brands have a lower content per drinking portion than do freshly made juices. In a survey of the population of all towns in the state, no cases of scurvy were found, although many families had a diet with insufficient vitamin C content. A large number of symptoms indicative of, but not specific for, vitamin C deficiency were found, the most frequent of which was atrophy of lingual papillae (16.8 % of total population surveyed). The findings indicate that clinical vitamin C deficiency is not a problem in São Paulo state, but might become so in the future if the present low levels of intake are maintained.

Introduction

In many parts of Brazil, the question of vitamin C deficiency has been overshadowed by other health problems. Deficiency diseases in general have received insufficient attention owing to the difficulties in carrying out specific studies, i.e. lack of personnel and suitable equipment, and insufficient material support.

In the state of São Paulo, however our group has been fortunate in being able to carry out studies in deficiency disease. Epidemiological studies have been favoured as they offer much information that can be used for the benefit of the entire population. Clinical studies, although important in deciding immediate measures, do not supply the means for a long-term solution.

Deficiency diseases are determined by many interacting factors, in particular socio-economic influences, among which number eating habits. The latter, although of cultural origin, are subject to change by external factors such as the mass media which play a forceful role in introducing fashionable nutritional fads. This is unfortunate, as these same media could be used to engender more healthy attitudes towards nutrition.

Another important factor is the economic climate. Eating habits rely for their maintenance on food availability, which in turn depends on food production. The latter is dictated by the production priorities and the technological means to make production sufficiently cost-efficient to make food prices attractive to the majority of consumers.

Faulty nutrition, if allowed to continue, will lead to subclinical malnutrition, which will eventually result in clinical signs and symptoms, after which it is merely a matter of time before overt deficiency disease appears. In the present study, we were limited to consideration of the first and third of these three stages.

Survey of Eating Habits in São Paulo State

A survey of food consumption was performed in 20 towns in São Paulo state, selected to provide a representative distribution through all regions. Data on all types of food, including those that do not contribute to vitamin C intake, were collected.

As can be seen from Table I, meat consumption is generally low, and beef, chicken and fish dominate this category. The only type of fish to be mentioned is sardines as they are the cheapest and, therefore, most frequently consumed. In coastal towns, the daily per capita sardine consumption is 3.6 times higher than the state average, although, contrary to expectations, consumption of other types of fish on the coast was not higher than in inland areas.

The low egg consumption is related to many factors, such as the belief that too many eggs are harmful, but mainly to their high cost. Liver and mussels have been included in our list, although they are consumed only in small quantities, because they are the only types of meat to contain vitamin C (content = 0.1 %).

Fat consumption is not high, and is mainly in the form of vegetable oil. Margarine, butter and cream are eaten in small amounts; lard and coconut fat were in the past eaten in large amounts, but their consumption has now decreased, reflecting a change in habit.

Tab. I: Food consumption in 20 towns of São Paulo state, Brazil: daily per capita average

Food item	Amount, g
Meat and eggs	
Beef	40
Chicken	35
Sardines – in 20 towns	25
– in 3 coastal towns	90
Eggs	12
Liver	2
Mussels	2
Fat	
Vegetable oil	40
Margarine	4
Lard	4
Butter	2
Coconut fat	< 1
Cream	< 1
Sugar	
Sucrose	71
Paste sweets	< 1
Chocolate	< 1
Legumes	
Beans	41
Peas	10
Milk and milk products	
Fresh whole milk	70
Powdered whole milk	3
Curdled milk	1
Fresh cheese	3
Cured cheese	1
Condensed milk	1
Cereals	
Rice	153
Wheat	
Bread	60
Macaroni	11
Wheat flour	8
Biscuits	3
Maize	
Cornflour	5
Corn meal	2
"Maizena"	2

Sugar intake, especially in the form of sucrose, is high. Consumption of milk and milk products (Table I) is very low, and is virtually limited to liquid milk, powdered whole milk being consumed mainly by small children.

Of the legumes (Table I), beans are the most frequently consumed, but do not contribute to vitamin C intake, whereas peas which have a vitamin C content of 26 mg/100 g are eaten in far smaller quantities for reasons that are partly cultural and partly economic.

Table I also shows the average consumption of cereals, rice being eaten in the largest quantities, followed as a distant second by wheat products. Corn (maize), although grown in the state, does not contribute greatly to the diet. In general, cereals are of no importance with regard to vitamin C intake, but do have a bearing on general nutritional status.

As a nutritional class vegetables (Table II) are an important dietary source of vitamin C, although much of it is lost or destroyed by cooking. Only watercress, cucumber and lettuce are almost always eaten raw, although the latter are poor in vitamin C.

Tab. II: Vegetable consumption in 20 towns of São Paulo state: daily per capita average

Decreasing order of vitamin C content, mg/100 g		Decreasing order of daily consumption, g/person	
Kale	125	Tomatoes	19
Pimento[2]	114	Onions	10
Broccoli	94	Chuchu	8
Cauliflower	82	Cabbage	7
Mustard greens	62	Lettuce	6
Pumpkin sprouts	58	Kale	4
Tomato paste	49	Vegetable marrow	4
Spinach	46	Carrots	3
Watercress[1]	44	Chicory *(Chicorium intybus)*	2
Cabbage[2]	43	Cucumber	2
Okra	29	Pumpkin	2
Turnips	26	Cauliflower	1
Tomatoes[2]	23	Endive *(Chicorium endivia)*	1
Chuchu	20	Eggplant	1
Vegetable marrow	19	Palmetto	1
String beans	18	Pimentos	1
Palmetto	17	Tomato paste	1
Pumpkin	15	Broccoli	< 1
Cucumber[1]	14	Beetroot	< 1
Lettuce[1]	12	Mushrooms	< 1
Chicory	11	Mustard greens	< 1
Onions[2]	10	Pumpkin sprouts	< 1
Carrots[2]	5	Okra	< 1
Beetroot	5	Spinach	< 1
Eggplant	5	String bean	< 1
Endive *(Chicorium endivia)*	5	Turnips	< 1
Mushrooms	3	Watercress	< 1

[1] Consumed raw.
[2] Consumed both raw and cooked.

As can be seen from Table II, the vegetables that are eaten in the largest quantities are not the best sources of vitamin C. This is largely due to economic reasons, as those that are richest in vitamin C also tend to be more expensive, with the notable exception of kale. On the whole, vegetables contribute little to vitamin C intake as the best sources are consumed in smaller quantities, the content is greatly reduced by cooking, and consumption is, on the whole, low.

A potentially important dietary source of vitamin C is fruit (Table III). Guavas have by far the highest content. Lemons, although rich in vitamin C (51 mg per edible 100 g), are in reality a poor source as they are generally consumed in the form of juice which is either used in small quantities as a seasoning, or diluted with water to make lemonade with at most, 10 % lemon juice content. The high cost of other fruit reduces their role as a source of vitamin C, with the exception of oranges. Thus, it would be logical to encourage an increase in the consumption of oranges, particularly in the form of juice. The consumption of oranges is, in fact, already comparatively high, as can be seen from Table III. On the whole, consumption of fruit is low, and efforts should be made to increase it, particularly in improving availability and lowering prices.

Tab. III: Fruit consumption in 20 towns of São Paulo state: daily per capita average

Vitamin C content, mg/100 g		Daily average consumption, g/person	
Guava	218	Orange	21
Strawberry	70	Banana	7
Orange	59	Watermelon	5
Mango	53	Papaya	4
Lemon	51	Apple	2
Papaya	46	Pineapple	2
Tangerine	36	Tangerine	2
Peach	28	Avocado	1
Pineapple	27	Jaboticaba	1
Jaboticaba	23	Pear	1
Banana	11	Guava	1
Avocado	10	Lemon	1
Apple	6	Mango	1
Pear	5	Peach	1
Watermelon	5	Strawberry	1

Fruit juices. Fruit juices are prepared from a variety of fruits and, in theory, might offer a palatable and convenient means of supplementing vitamin C intake. Commercial preserved juices are available, some of which are advertised as "containing" vitamin C, and thereby suggest that they are rich sources of this nutrient. We tested some brands of fruit juice to determine their vitamin C content (Table IV). Some of these juices were concentrated (i. e. orange, tangerine and lemon) and would be diluted before drinking.

Tab. IV: Average vitamin C content in commercial preserved fruit juice in São Paulo state; according to Roncada M J *et al:*Rev Saúde públ *11,* 39–46, 1977

Fruit	Type	Container	Vitamin C content, mg/100 ml ± 2 SE
Orange	concentrated	can	158.1 ± 7.4
Tangerine	concentrated	can	56.2 ± 4.8
Lemon	concentrated	can	31.0 ± 4.0
Pineapple	whole	bottle	11.5 ± 1.1
	whole	bottle	5.3 ± 1.1
	whole	bottle	7.7 ± 1.0
Cashew *(Anacardium occidentale)*	whole	bottle	100.4 ± 8.8
	whole	bottle	93.1 ± 13.4
	whole	bottle	142.2 ± 1.6
	ready for use	can	25.7 ± 0.4
Passionfruit *(Passiflora SP)*	whole	bottle	10.3 ± 1.0
	whole	bottle	1.6 ± 2.0
	whole	bottle	7.3 ± 1.2
	ready for use	can	1.9 ± 3.2
Tamarind	whole	bottle	5.1 ± 1.8
	whole	bottle	6.1 ± 1.0
Guava *(Psidium guatava)*	whole	bottle	19.2 ± 3.0
	whole	bottle	21.5 ± 3.6

Tab. V: Vitamin C content of fresh fruit juice in São Paulo state; according to Roncada M J *et al:*Rev Saúde públ *11,* 39–46, 1977

Fruit	Vitamin C content, mg/100 ml ± 2 SE
Orange	43.6 ± 11.8
Pineapple	41.6 ± 16.7
Lemon (Tahiti)	37.6 ± 0.6
Lemon (Galego)	33.4 ± 0.8
Tangerine	23.6 ± 0.4
Passion flower	20.2 ± 0.6

We then compared preserved juice with fresh juice (Table V) prepared as a housewife would do from fruit available at the São Paulo market at the time. The fresh orange juice compares less favourably with the preserved juice because the latter is more concentrated, but was still found to have the highest vitamin C content of the fresh juices studied. In general, the fresh whole juices were found to contain more vitamin C than preserved whole juices. At the same time, we estimated the cost of supplying the daily requirement of 45 mg vitamin C with each of these fruit juices: the analysis showed again that orange whether fresh or preserved, is the cheapest and most convenient.

Clinical Signs and Symptoms of Vitamin C Deficiency

We surveyed the inhabitants of 11 towns for clinical manifestations of vitamin C deficiency. As shown by Table VI, families with a diet that was 100 % adequate were the minority: in only three towns did they represent over 50 %, and at least one-third of all families had a diet that was less than 80 % adequate. Where such a situation is chronic, clinical deficiency disease can become a widespread problem. On the basis of the available evidence, we can expect not only that this situation will continue but also that it will worsen with inflation.

Tab. VI: Dietary vitamin C intake in 11 towns of São Paulo state

Daily intake of vitamin C in % of dietary requirement	Proportion of families per town, %[1]										
	1	2	3	4	5	6	7	8	9	10	11
100.0 and more	31.8	30.5	14.3	54.2	35.8	17.9	27.4	33.3	58.4	34.4	56.0
80.0–99.9	4.7	7.1	4.8	5.1	–	10.7	14.3	7.1	8.3	4.5	4.8
60.0–79.9	9.5	10.7	20.0	12.2	21.4	7.1	11.9	10.7	7.1	14.3	7.1
40.0–59.9	11.9	32.1	26.6	11.2	10.7	14.3	13.1	17.9	10.7	9.8	4.8
20.0–39.9	15.4	12.5	24.8	6.1	10.7	28.6	10.7	19.9	9.4	17.0	8.3
0.0–19.9	28.7	7.1	9.5	11.2	21.4	21.4	22.6	13.1	6.0	16.0	19.0

[1] Totals all add up to 100 %.

Although, surprisingly, we found no cases of scurvy, some clinical signs not necessarily specific to vitamin C deficiency were recorded (Table VII.) The most prominent of these was atrophy of lingual papillae which was found in between 19.6 and 58.3 % of the population studied. Abnormalities of the gums, i. e. bleeding, erythema and oedema were also found. Perifolliculosis, perhaps the most specific sign encountered, was present in a fairly large proportion of the population surveyed. Epiphyseal enlargement, petechiae and purpurae, none of which is pathognomic of vitamin C deficiency, were reported in a small number of cases.

Tab. VII: Clinical signs attributable to vitamin C deficiency in 11 towns of São Paulo state

Clinical signs	Proportion of population per town, %											
	1	2	3	4	5	6	7	8	9	10	11	mean
Gums												
Marginal erythema	3.9	5.6	12.5	35.6	28.9	22.4	15.5	22.4	27.7	13.0	13.2	18.2
Marginal edema	2.0	7.8	25.0	10.2	22.2	19.4	13.2	28.0	31.9	51.0	11.8	21.4
Bleeding gums	–	–	–	13.6	17.8	13.4	11.5	29.9	18.1	27.0	6.6	16.8
Atrophy of												
lingual papillae	19.6	20.0	58.3	5.1	44.4	34.3	38.5	46.1	41.5	4.0	26.5	31.9
Perifolliculosis	2.0	–	–	30.5	8.9	11.9	1.1	8.1	16.0	5.0	–	6.9
Epiphysial enlargement	–	–	–	1.7	–	1.5	–	–	–	–	–	0.2
Petechiae	–	–	–	1.7	–	–	–	0.3	–	–	–	0.2
Purpurae	3.9	–	–	1.7	–	–	–	0.3	–	1.0	–	0.3

Conclusion

The results of our clinical survey do not indicate that vitamin C deficiency poses a health problem in São Paulo state. However, the findings of our nutrition survey indicate that it is only a matter of time before such a problem develops.

Prof. D. Wilson, Universidade de São Paulo, Faculdade de Saúde Pública, Caixa postal 8099, 01255 São Paulo, S.P., Brazil

Author Index

Amar, M. 167

Baker, H. 47
Barbosa, M.C. 117
Basu, T.K. 247
Bauernfeind, J.C. 307
Biesalski, K. 225
Buzina, R. 157

Cayazzo, M. 167
Chadud, P. 167
Chavez, A. 85

Daza, C.H. 9

Fatima Nunes Marucci, M. de 117
Frank, O. 47

Glatthaar, B.E. 139
Gunn, A.D.G. 213

Hallberg, L. 177
Hanck, A. 189
Hauser, G.A. 207
Hertrampf, E. 167
Hornig, D.H. 139

Kläui, H. 335

Layrisse, M. 105
Llaguno, S. 167

Mata, A. 85
Mejía, L.A. 75
Milatovič, L. 345
Mora, J.O. 19
Moser, U. 363

Netto, O.B. 117

Olivares, M. 167

Pietrzik, K. 61
Pizarro, F. 167

Sandoval, J. 85
Schaefer, A.E. 33
Schmidt, K. 363
Seib, P.A. 259
Simao da Costa, A. 117
Steiner, A. 117
Stekel, A. 167
Subotičanec, K. 157

Tolbert, B.M. 121

Vega, V. 167

Weisburger, J.H. 381
Weiser, H. 189
Wilson, D. 117, 403

Key Word Index

Acetylsalicylate 189
Adolescents 157
Adults 47
Analgesic properties 189
Anemia 75
Anthropometry 19
Anti-inflammatory 189
Anticonvulsants 247
Antioxidant 307
Ascorbate 247
Ascorbic acid 121, 139, 167, 335, 363
Ascorbic acid requirement 157
Ascorbyl palmitate 307
Aspirin 247
Assessment of nutritional status 9

Borderline deficiency 61
Brazil 117, 403
Bread gluten structure 335

Carbonated foods 307
Carotenoids and colour 345
Carrageenan, kaolin 189
Cell formation 61
Children 47
Colombian population 19
Colon cancer 381
Content in phagocytes 363
Cooking properties of pasta 345
Cured foods 307
Cyanocobalamin 189

Daily vitamin C requirement 139
Deficiency 403
Dehydroascorbic acid 121, 345
Derivatives 259
Dietary pattern 403
Diketogulonic acid 121
Drugs 247

Eating habits 403
Effect of smoking 139
Elderly 47
Esophageal cancer 381

Fats 307
Fermented or cultured foods 307
Fetal 47
Flour improvement 335
Folacin 247

Folate 61
Food consumption 403
Food enrichment 85
Food fortification 9, 167
Frozen foods 307
Functional parameters 61

Gastric cancer 381
Gluten 345

HPLC 225
Heat processed foods 307
Hematopoiesis 75
High temperature drying 345
Hyaluronidase 189
Hypovitaminosis A 75

Immunomodulation by ascorbic acid 363
Impaired vitamin C status 139
Incidence-treatment survey 213
Increased by smoking 139
Inhibition of transport 363
Inner ear 225
Iron 85, 157
Iron absorption 105, 167, 177, 335
Iron balance 177
Iron deficiency 75
Iron deficiency anemia 19
Iron interaction 75
Iron requirements 177
Iron-multivitamin-mineral preparations 207

5-Ketoascorbitol 121

L-Ascorbic acid 259, 307, 345
Latin American diets 105
Lipoxigenase 345
Lutein 345

Maternal 47
Metabolism: distribution, function 121
Micronutrients 85
Milk, infant foods 167
Monoesters 259
Monoethers 259

Nitrate 381
Nitrite 381
Nitrosamines 381
Nutrition education 9

Nutrition survey applications 33
Nutritional status 19

Oils 307
Olfactory bulbus 225
Oxidation 259
Oxygen scavenger 307

Pasta processing 345
Phenylbutazone 189
Photosensitivity 225
Phylloquinone, analogs 189
Physical working capacity 157
Pineal gland 225
Population groups 9
Pregnancy 207
Premenstrual syndrome 213
Prevention and control 9
Prophylactic, therapeutic use 189
Prophylaxis 207
Public health significance 9
Pyridoxine 157, 213

Rat paw test 189
Redox reaction 345
Riboflavin 157
Risk factors 207
Risk group 247

School children 117
Semolina 345
Sodium ascorbate 307
Soft wheat flour 345
Spaghetti 345
Stimulation of transport 363
Sugar 85
Survey 403
Symptoms 403
Synergist 307
Synthesis 259

Tocopherol 307
Transport into phagocytes 363

Visual accuracy 117
Vitamin A 75, 117
Vitamin A derivatives 225
Vitamin A fortification 75
Vitamin B_6 213
Vitamin C 139, 157, 177, 189, 363, 381, 403
Vitamin deficiencies 9, 19
Vitamin deficiency stages 61
Vitamin requirements 207
Vitamin supplementation 47
Vitamins 47, 85, 189, 247

Women 177